THE AGORA BONE WELL

Hesperia Supplements

The *Hesperia* Supplement series (ISSN 1064-1173) presents book-length studies in the fields of Greek archaeology, art, language, and history. Founded in 1937, the series was originally designed to accommodate extended essays too long for inclusion in the journal *Hesperia*. Since that date the Supplements have established a strong identity of their own, featuring single-author monographs, excavation reports, and edited collections on topics of interest to researchers in classics, archaeology, art history, and Hellenic studies.

Hesperia Supplements are electronically archived in JSTOR (www.jstor.org), where all but the most recent titles may be found. For order information and a complete list of titles, see the ASCSA website (www.ascsa.edu.gr).

Hesperia Supplement 50

THE AGORA BONE WELL

Maria A. Liston, Susan I. Rotroff, and
Lynn M. Snyder

with a contribution by
Andrew Stewart

American School of Classical Studies at Athens
2018

Library of Congress Cataloging-in-Publication Data

Names: Liston, Maria A., author. | Rotroff, Susan I., author. | Snyder, Lynn M., author.
Title: The Agora Bone Well / by Maria A. Liston, Susan I. Rotroff, and Lynn M. Snyder, with a contribution by Andrew Stewart.
Description: Princeton, New Jersey : American School of Classical Studies at Athens, 2018. | Series: Hesperia supplements, ISSN 1064-1173 ; v. 50 | Includes bibliographical references and indexes.
Identifiers: LCCN 2018023617 | ISBN 978-0-87661-550-8 (alk. paper)
Subjects: LCSH: Agora (Athens, Greece) | Athens (Greece)—Antiquities. | Infants—Mortality—Greece—History—To 1500. | Human remains (Archaeology)—Greece—Athens. | Animal remains (Archaeology)—Greece—Athens. | Burial—Greece—Athens. | Wells—Greece—Athens.
Classification: LCC DF287.A23 L57 2018 | DDC 938/.508—dc23
LC record available at https://lccn.loc.gov/2018023617

PREFACE

This project began 80 years ago with Dorothy Burr Thompson's excavation of what promised to be an ordinary Athenian water source. Thompson was the mother of a young family when she completed the excavation of the Agora Bone Well in 1938, with twin toddlers and a three-month-old daughter. The clearing of the lower depths of the well and its attached cistern, a task left over from the previous year, was her only assignment that summer, carried out at the tail end of the excavation season. Family obligations presumably left her time for little more. In the diary that she kept for most of her life (now in the Bryn Mawr College Special Collections; we thank archivist Marianne Hansen for sending us scans of the relevant sections), June 1938 is dominated by her children's ailments: ear infections, stomach upsets, and a mild case of dengue—if nothing else, a reminder of the normality of frequent illness in small children. The diary records some distaste for the excavation ("more vile bones of dogs etc."), adding only that J. Lawrence ("Larry") Angel looked at the bones on June 22 and found "many of them human—infants chiefly." Thompson's comments in her excavation notebook are brief and businesslike, and she makes no mention of infant bones.

However muted her reaction at the time, the well—which ultimately disgorged the bones of hundreds of infants and dogs—made a lasting impression on Thompson. She brought it to Susan Rotroff's attention in the 1970s, urging her to try to solve the mystery. Her own pet theory was that both infants and dogs had succumbed to some mysterious ailment that particularly targets these two populations, and she had from time to time asked medical professionals if they could suggest a likely disease. In 1989, Maria Liston briefly explored the possibility of the collection as a dissertation topic, when it looked like the necessary permits to study bones from Kavousi would not be granted. At that time, however, the science of skeletal study was not sufficiently advanced. It was not until 1996, and by chance rather than by design, that the right combination of scholars for this project appeared on the Agora's horizon. Lynn Snyder was attracted to the deposit by its dogs, a subject of special interest to her, and approached T. Leslie Shear Jr., then director of the excavations, with a proposal to study them. Susan Rotroff was examining pottery from the well for the publication of the Hellenistic plain wares from the Agora. Lisa Little, a graduate student in physical anthropology at Indiana University, was working on Agora material for her dissertation. Sitting around the Agora tea table, they devised a project to publish the well and its contents, and they reported on the early stages of their work at the 100th Annual Meeting of the Archaeological Institute of America in 1998 (Little 1999; Rotroff 1999; Snyder 1999). All had other commitments, however, and the work went slowly. Maria Liston joined the project in 2005, replacing Little as physical anthropologist and undertaking a complete restudy of the human skeletal material. In 2014, Andrew Stewart added a discussion of the herm from the well, which he was studying in the context of his research on Hellenistic sculpture at the Agora. The full team was at last in place.

In the course of our work we have incurred debts to a long list of people. First, we would like to thank John McK. Camp II, director of the Agora Excavations, for permission to study and publish this material and for his careful reading of and comments on the manuscript. The Agora staff has been unfailingly supportive, often going beyond the call of duty to facilitate our work. Jan Jordan, Sylvie Dumont, and Pia Kvarnström were tireless in their efforts to provide access to the material and check details for us when we were absent. Craig Mauzy took many new photographs, often at a moment's notice. Amandina Anastassiades contributed expertise from the conservation laboratory, and her father, rheumatologist Tassos Anastassiades, consulted with Liston on the diagnosis of the ailment that afflicted the adult in the well. We would also like to single out IT guru Constantinos Tzortzinis for his assistance in the School's computer lab at Athens.

Many scholars have been kind enough to take an interest in our project and offer advice and assistance on such diverse subjects as ancient bronze, Roman pottery, elephant ivory, similar concentrations of infants, and much more, and we offer them in return our heartfelt thanks: Chryssi Bourbou, Kevin Clinton, Edgard Espinoza, Sherry Fox, David Gill, Carolyn Koehler, Mark Lawall, Neda Leipen, Kathleen Lynch, John Milakson, John Morgan, James Muhly, Clare Pickersgill, James Russell, James Santangelo, Debby Sneed, Dimitris Sourlas, and Michael Vickers. We are also grateful to Stephan Schmid and Karl Reber, who, just as this project was reaching completion, generously invited Liston to study the human bone from two wells at Eretria that constitute striking comparanda for the Agora Bone Well. We thank Robert Lamberton for his translations of the passages from Poseidippos and the letter of Hilarion.

The Mütter Museum of the College of Physicians of Philadelphia provided comparanda for Liston's work, and we are all grateful to the American School of Classical Studies at Athens for the work space and laboratory and library facilities that it provides to its members. For funding, we are indebted to the Malcolm H. Wiener Laboratory for Archaeological Science, the Loeb Classical Library Foundation, and Washington University in Saint Louis.

As this scholarly project nears the end of its trajectory, we want to express our gratitude to our editor, Colin Whiting, who has shepherded this manuscript through the publication process with tact, intelligence, and efficiency, and to the staff of the School's Publications Office for the care and meticulous attention they have devoted to the production of our monograph.

CONTENTS

ILLUSTRATIONS

TABLES

CHAPTER 1

The Well and Its Neighborhood

The first days of life were perilous in the ancient world. Birth accidents, infections, neglect, or worse resulted in significant neonatal mortality, documented by the high numbers of infants in ancient cemeteries as well as by concentrations of infant bones in contexts beyond the graveyard. Just such a concentration came to light in 1938 in a Hellenistic well on the fringes of the Agora of ancient Athens (Fig. 1): the bones of over 450 infants and a few older individuals, along with a remarkable collection of animal bone, including the remains of over 150 dogs—an unparalleled collection of skeletal material that quickly earned the feature its excavation nickname, "The Bone Well."[1] J. Lawrence Angel examined the bones shortly after excavation and included the human remains in his catalogue of skeletal material from Attica published in 1945.[2] But, despite—or perhaps because of—its spectacular character, the deposit has never received full publication. It has, however, raised speculation, the large number of infant dead evoking a series of dramatic explanations: symbolic sacrifice, famine, plague, or infanticide.[3]

Our aim in the present study is not to exhaust all of the possibilities of the deposit, but rather to present the data in full, place it within its social and historical context, and offer a plausible suggestion about how, when, and why this remarkable assemblage of humans, animals, and artifacts came to be deposited in the well. To anticipate, we conclude that the well was filled in the second quarter of the 2nd century B.C.,[4] that the majority of the individuals died of natural causes, and that the well served as a burial place for individuals who, either because of their young age or their low social status, did not receive conventional funerary rites.

1. It is more formally known in the excavation records as well G 5:3 or the well at 97/Γ in Section ΛΛ.

2. Angel 1945, pp. 311–312, nos. 114–116, fig. 12.

3. Shear 1939, p. 239 (symbolic sacrifice); Angel 1945, p. 311 (starvation or plague); G. R. Edwards, quoted in *Agora* XI, p. 168 (plague or epidemic); Osanna 1988–1989, p. 92 (epidemic or undefined ritual); Dasen 2013, pp. 33–34 (infanticide).

4. All dates are before Christ unless otherwise indicated. For earlier summaries of our conclusions, see Liston and Papadopoulos 2004, pp. 23–25; Liston and Rotroff 2013a, 2013b.

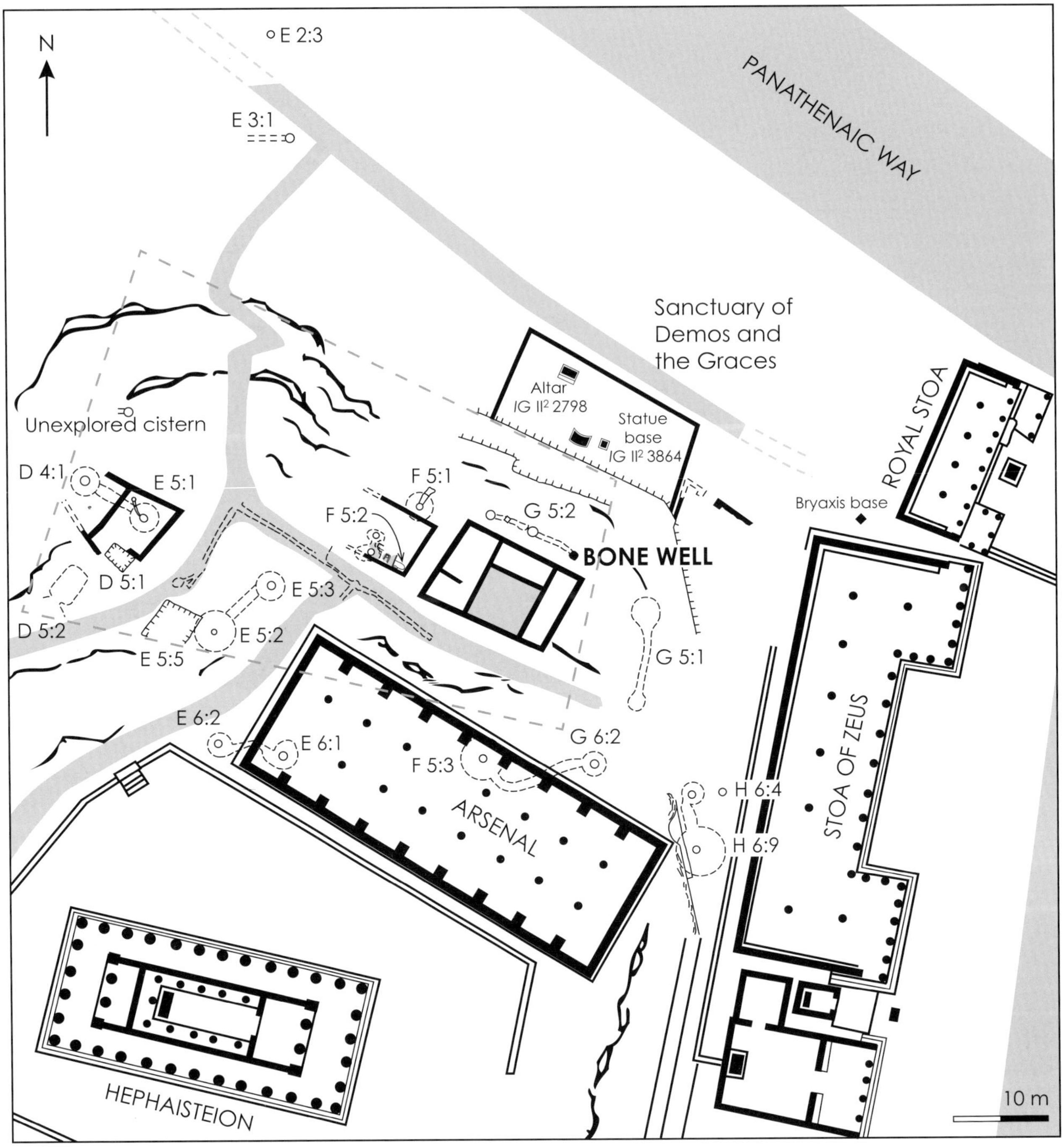

Figure 1. Reconstructed plan of the northern slopes of the Kolonos Agoraios and the area outside the northwest corner of the Agora square in the 2nd century B.C., with Hellenistic water sources indicated. The dashed line indicates the approximate extent of excavation Section ΛΛ. S. I. Rotroff

THE EXCAVATION, CONSTRUCTION, AND STRATIGRAPHY OF THE WELL

The exploration of the Agora Bone Well was part of a much larger project: the excavation of the Athenian Agora, the public space of the ancient city, by the American School of Classical Studies at Athens under the direction of the elder T. Leslie Shear.[5] The goal of that project, as conceived at its inception in 1931, was to uncover the complete extent of the political center (agora) of the ancient city. Work was interrupted by World War II but revived thereafter, and excavation continues today, as the northern border of the public space has still not been completely explored.[6]

The locale once occupied by the Agora was a densely inhabited urban space in the 1930s, and excavations proceeded plot by plot, as property became available. The Agora Bone Well lay in an area (christened Section ΛΛ)[7] that had remained free of modern construction, just outside the northwest corner of the ancient public space and north of the Hephaisteion.[8] Excavation here was supervised by Dorothy Burr Thompson, an experienced field archaeologist and specialist in Hellenistic terracotta figurines who had joined the excavation in 1932 as an Agora Fellow.[9] She devoted four and a half months in 1937 to the exploration of the largely Roman and Byzantine structures that survived there. The clearing of the well had to wait until the last week of the field season (June 14–19), and Thompson's men had reached a depth of only 11.05 m by the season's end. She resumed the unfinished project the following year (June 6–17), digging to a depth of 21.45 m and discovering the remarkable contents that give the well its name.[10]

Measuring about 1.00 m in diameter, the well descends through bedrock and is lined with terracotta tiles beginning at a depth of 18.20 m. At a depth of ca. 1.00 m an irregular passage leads to the northwest, descending into a large, bottle-shaped cistern (G 5:2; Fig. 2). This arrangement was probably intended as an aid to transferring water drawn from the well to the cistern, but it seemed to the excavator clearly to postdate the construction of the cistern. The cistern in turn is part of a larger water system that extends further to the west. A gallery leads from its neck, with a rectangular access shaft at a distance of 3.50 m and a shallow circular drawshaft at a distance of ca. 6.00 m. The entire length of the water system, from the Agora Bone Well to the westernmost shaft, is about 12.50 m.

The final fills of this system are of various dates: Late Roman in the cistern, Byzantine in the passage connecting the cistern to the well,

5. For the origins of the project, see Capps 1933.

6. For a brief sketch of the history of the excavations, see Mauzy 2009.

7. From the earliest American excavations in the Agora, the term "section," rather than the more familiar "sector," has been used to denote areas of the excavation.

8. See below, p. 8, for more information about this excavation section.

9. For Thompson's career, see Uhlenbrock 2004.

10. Published briefly in the director's annual report (Shear 1939, p. 239).

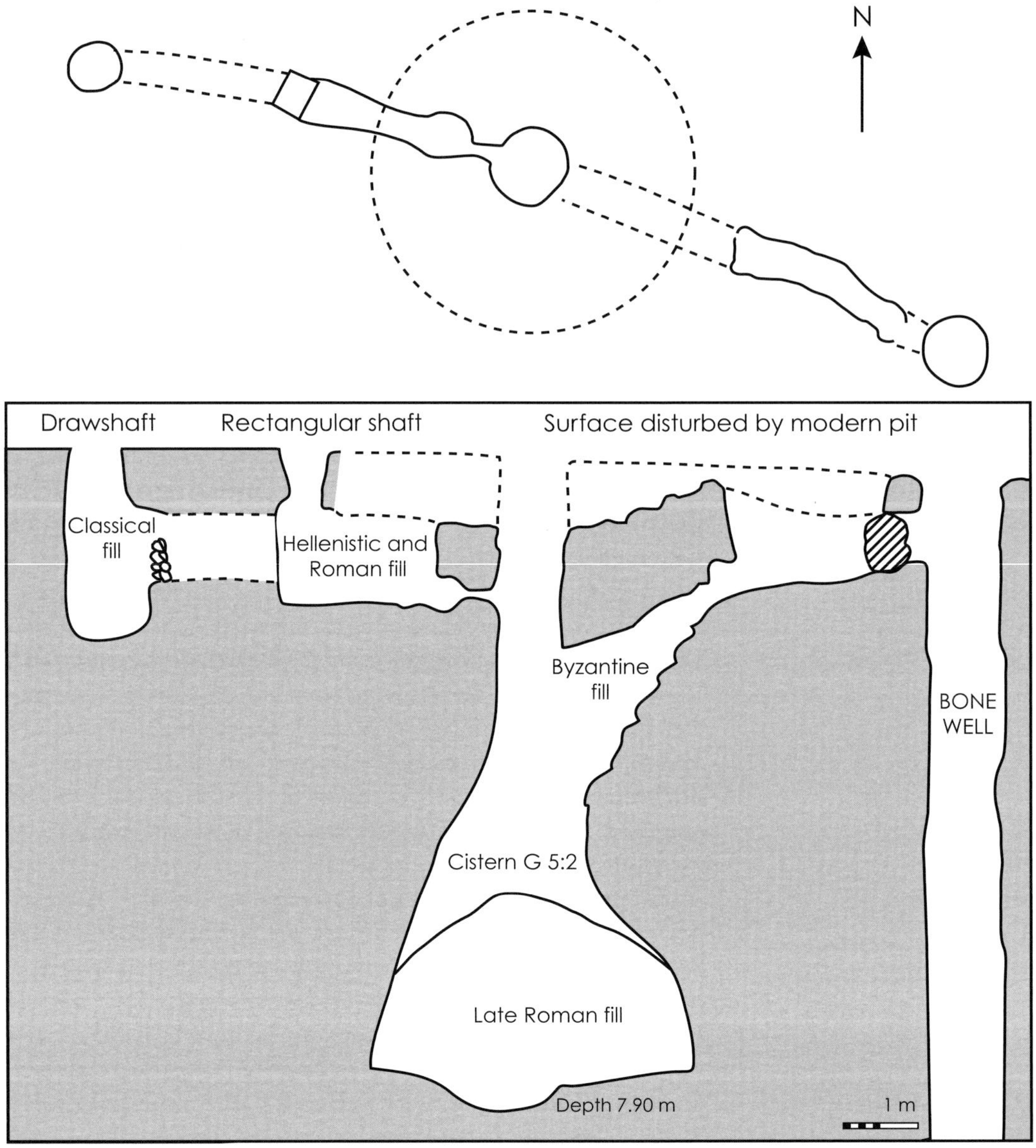

Figure 2. Plan and section through the water system to which the Agora Bone Well belongs, looking north. S. I. Rotroff, based on measured sketches by D. B. Thompson, notebook ΛΛ 8, pp. 1404, 1419

and a mixture of Hellenistic and Roman in the rectangular shaft.[11] The westernmost shaft and the passage leading to it, however, contained material dating largely between the mid-5th and the mid-4th centuries, together with masses of marble working chips,[12] suggesting that the system was in

11. Lots ΛΛ 265, ΛΛ 266.

12. The lowest 0.20 m of the drawshaft consisted of a silty water deposit documenting the shaft's use; it is reported to have contained only a few sherds, "looking mostly V[th] c[entury]" (Agora field notebook [hereafter "notebook"] ΛΛ 7, p. 1370). This layer was sealed in by 1.50 m of fill (lots ΛΛ 304, ΛΛ 305), which extended a short way into the passage (lot ΛΛ 306) and contained small amounts of pottery of the 5th and 4th centuries. The uppermost 0.90 m of the shaft contained Roman pottery (ΛΛ 303). Of course, the lower fills could have entered the system any time between the Classical and Roman period, but the Classical pottery in the silt accumulated while the drawshaft was active and the absence of later material there and in the fill above it argue for the use of the system in the Classical period.

use at least that early. It appears, then, that the water system was constructed in the Classical period to supply water for the activities of artisans working in the area (see pp. 8–19).

A concentration of Byzantine material was found in the mouth of the well,[13] but Thompson described the fill in the uppermost 2.15 m of the well as "mostly L[ate] H[ellenistic] but now and again a Byz[antine]-painted."[14] Pottery recovered on the two subsequent days of digging (down to 6.90 m) was "as before." Fill below 6.90 m was "pure Greek," but pottery remained scanty to a depth of 13.02 m. Water was reached at a depth of about 11 m, and stones began to appear in the fill at 12.00–13.02 m. From 13.02 to 14.70 m the fill was red, but still mixed with stones, and, for the first time, Thompson noted the presence of bones, some of them, she thought, human. Figure 3 summarizes the notebook account and filling from this point to the bottom. There was still little pottery, but two unguentaria (**36**, **37**) and two stamped amphora handles (**73**, **75**) were recorded at about 13.00 m. Another change in the fill was noted at 14.70 m; the earth now contained masses of coarse pottery along with abundant bones, and a heavy concentration of bronze appeared at 16.00–18.45 m (**82**–**87**). From 18.45 to 20.05 m the pottery was less but bones continued to be abundant, and pieces of wood were encountered. Below this level the fill was red and nearly sterile ("clean like clay"); digging ceased at 21.45 m without the bottom of the well having been reached. It is unlikely, however, to have been far away, for few Hellenistic Athenian wells are over 22 m deep.[15] Figure 4 presents a schematic representation of the relative position of bones, pottery, and bronze in the fill.

Only rarely did Thompson record the depths at which individual objects were found. Among the faunal material, she exclaimed over the discovery of "7 dog skulls!" at 14.70–15.28 m, and thereafter skulls were noted daily. Skulls of dog, horse, and boar were specified at 16.00–16.85 m, and a ram's skull at 18.45–19.75 m, but this is the extent to which we can place the animal bones within the well. While some of the more complete artifacts were inventoried and their depths recorded as excavation was going on, most of the pottery was not entered into the records until after the excavation was complete. There is evidence of haste. Objects were entered in the finds notebook under the heading, in Homer Thompson's hand, "The following objects have come from the filling *from the surface to 20 m.* No chronological difference could be detected in the material from this depth and it has all been placed together" (emphasis ours).[16] He entered a running number and a title for each inventory entry; measurements were added later in a different hand (perhaps that of Lucy Talcott,

13. Separately stored in lot ΛΛ 351.

14. The day-to-day account of the excavation may be found in notebook ΛΛ 8, pp. 1460, 1471, 1472, 1475, 1574–1576, 1582.

15. See Camp 1977, pp. 208–226, for the depths of Classical and Athenian wells around the Agora. The greatest depth recorded is 23.50 m (well G 14:2).

16. Notebook ΛΛ 9, p. 1763. Homer Thompson was Dorothy's husband and, after World War II, succeeded T. Leslie Shear Sr. as director of the Agora Excavations (1947–1967).

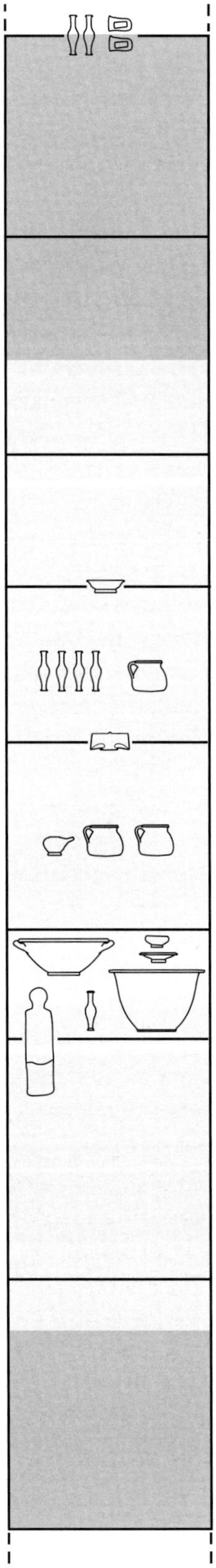

		ARTIFACTS	EARTH, BONES
	13.02	@ 13.00, unguentaria [**36**, **37**], stamped amphora handles [**73**, **75**]	"At 13 m red earth appears, but stones and pottery remain the same. Many bones, some worked, some human?"
June 9			
	14.10		
June 10		"masses of coarse Hell."	"At 14.70 earth changes. 7 dog skulls! Many animal bones."
	15.28		
June 11		"A dish [**2**] and Megarian bowl frags, much coarse."	"More skulls."
	16.00	@16.00, bowl with outturned rim [**2**]	
June 13		"Bronze tools, lead sheet, and a fine bone sword sheath handle [**81**]. Much coarse pottery [**60**], unguentaria [**32–35**]."	"Numerous skulls of dogs, horse, boar."
	16.85	@16.85 chape [**81**]	
June 14		"Pots [**26**, **61**, **62**]." [feeder, chytrai]	"Same. "
	17.85	"Much bronze broken bits. Pots [**8**, **12, 31**, **40**, **46**]." [echinus bowl, rilled-rim plate, unguentarium, lekane, deep bowl]	
June 15			"Few skulls. At 18.20 the tiled curbing of the well appears in situ. "
	18.45	@ 18.45, herm (**80**)	
June 16		"pottery less; . . . large bits of wood."	"Skulls still, including a ram's . . . mud begins."
	19.75		
	20.05		
June 17			"Bones practically cease. At 20.05 red earth which is practically sterile, clean like clay."
	21.45		

Figure 3 *(opposite)*. Graphic representation of the notebook account of the excavation of the Agora Bone Well (ΛΛ 8, pp. 1576–1577, 1582). Descriptions in quotation marks come directly from the notebook entries for each day (and thus in the range of depth excavated that day), with descriptions of artifacts to the right of the well shaft and earth and bones on the far right. Items preceded by @ are those for which a specific depth was recorded. Divisions within the well indicate the sections as they were dug day by day, with depths given to the left of the well shaft and the dates on which excavation took place at the far left. Shading within the shaft indicates recorded changes in the earth fill. S. I. Rotroff

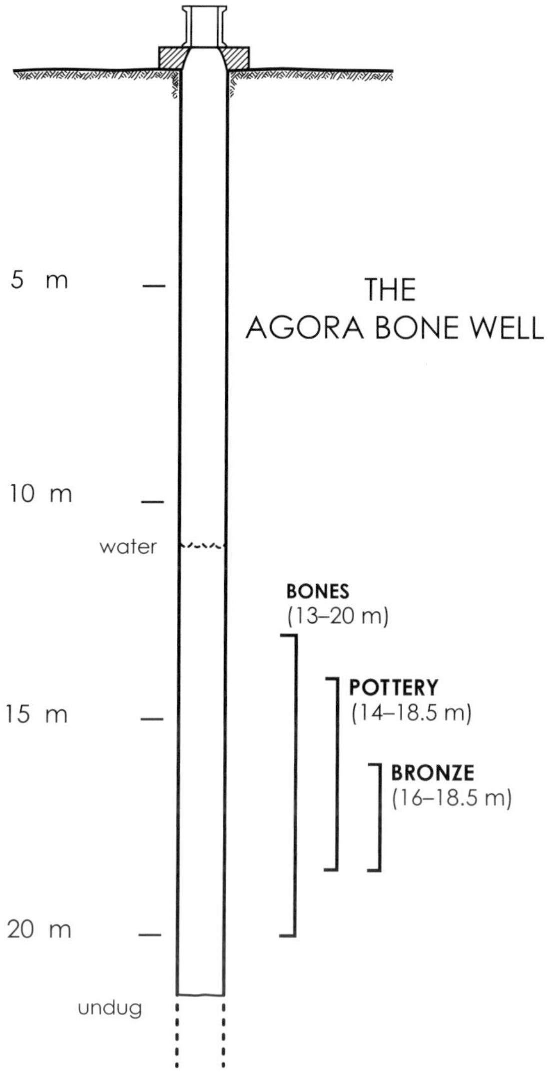

Figure 4 *(right)*. Distribution of the greatest concentration of bones, pottery, and bronze in the shaft of the Agora Bone Well. S. I. Rotroff, based on inked drawing by M. Djordjevitch

longtime secretary of the excavations).[17] The descriptions on the inventory cards were apparently supplied by the excavation staff; they do not exist in the notebook. This abbreviated procedure makes it impossible to reconstruct the fill in detail. Furthermore, since uninventoried material from all levels (including the upper 13 m, where the fill was clearly of a different character) was stored together, some of the objects that we now have at our disposal must not have been found in association with the bones. The notebook is explicit, however, about the scantiness of the pottery in the upper reaches of the well, and it is probably safe to assume that the whole or nearly whole objects were found with the bones, and mostly at a depth of 14.70 to 20.05 m.

17. Talcott was secretary (the equivalent of registrar) of the excavations from their inception until 1958. In that capacity she devised the inventory procedure and its elaborate system of cross-references, which has served as a model for many other Mediterranean excavations. She was in addition an expert on Athenian pottery and coauthor of *Agora* XII.

THE DATE OF THE WELL DEPOSIT

Although early accounts associated the well with the siege of Sulla in 86 B.C.,[18] we can now confirm that it was filled much earlier. The latest closely datable objects in its fill are two Knidian stamped amphora handles (**74**, **75**) naming the eponyms Aristarchos and Asklepiodoros, who date within Virginia Grace's Period IV A.[19] Grace's dates for the period are 188–167, but some downward adjustment is almost certainly in order, and these two handles may date within the 160s (see below, pp. 87–88). An approximate *terminus ante quem* comes from the absence of long-petal bowls among the moldmade bowls extracted from the well. The date of the introduction of the type at Athens is uncertain, but it was rare before the third quarter of the 2nd century.[20] The closing date of the deposit, then, probably falls within the second quarter of the 2nd century. Close examination of the pottery, and particularly the moldmade bowls, suggests that it is to be dated within a fairly narrow range. Most of the bowls (both those that are nearly complete and fragments) belong to classes that probably began to be made in the decade 170–160 (**15–18**), and, perhaps more telling, bowl types characteristic of the period ca. 225–175 are present in only a few small fragments (see below, pp. 73–74). This suggests that the fill began to enter the well considerably later than ca. 175, and hence that the deposit accumulated over a period of no more than 15 years, from ca. 165 to 150.

THE NEIGHBORHOOD OF THE WELL

Excavation Section ΛΛ, which includes the Agora Bone Well and its surrounding neighborhood, was defined by the Athens–Piraeus Railroad on the north, the modern boundary wall of the Hephaisteion terrace on the south (now demolished), and the steep slope of the Kolonos Agoraios and the Annex of the Stoa of Zeus on the east (Figs. 1, 5, 10). Theseion Street formed its western boundary, over an area that remains unexplored. Excavation of Section ΛΛ, from its modern surface to ancient levels, continued from February 1 to June 19, 1937, with two weeks of supplementary work in 1938 (June 6–17) devoted to the continued excavation of the Agora Bone Well and cistern G 5:2, which had been left unfinished at the end of the 1937 season.[21]

This northern half of the Kolonos Agoraios suffered minimal disturbance in the Ottoman and modern periods. An east–west road crossed its

18. Shear 1939, p. 238; Angel 1945, p. 311, under no. 116; Grace 1949, p. 186, under no. 8.

19. For Grace's periodization of Knidian amphora stamps, see Grace 1985, pp. 31–35. For Rhodian handles we use Grace's periods, with the chronology as revised by Finkielsztejn (2001).

20. The long-petal bowl was well established at Corinth before the city's destruction in 146 and occurs as well in the fill of the Great Altar at Pergamon, probably no later than the 160s. Only a few fragments, however, have been found in deposits dating earlier than the mid-2nd century at Athens, suggesting that the form was rare until the third quarter of the century there. Conversely, deposits datable after the middle of the century regularly include a high proportion of long-petal bowls. See *Agora* XXII, pp. 35–37; Rotroff 1988, 2001, 2011b.

21. For a plan showing the location of Section ΛΛ, see *Agora* XXVI, pl. 35. The excavation is recorded in notebooks ΛΛ 1–9 and was published in a laconic two pages by the then director, T. Leslie Shear Sr. (Shear 1938, pp. 339–340).

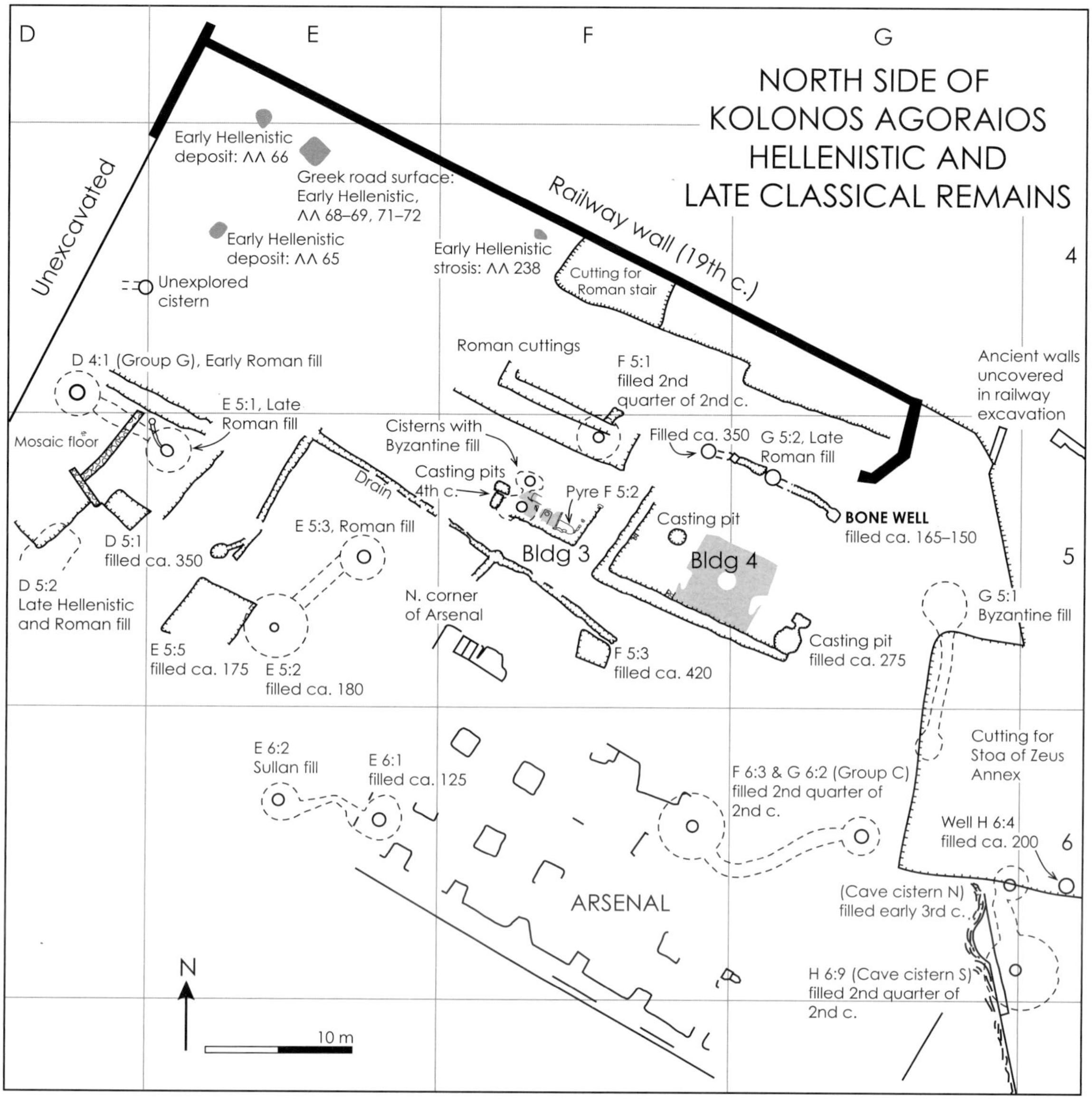

Figure 5. Extant Hellenistic and Late Classical remains on the north side of the Kolonos Agoraios. For the approximate location of Section ΛΛ, see Fig. 1. S. I. Rotroff, based on plan of Section ΛΛ drawn by D. B. Thompson at the time of excavation

northernmost sector in Ottoman times, while the southern part was perhaps given over to agricultural use thereafter.[22] The area was intensively occupied, however, in the Late Roman and Byzantine eras. At least seven Byzantine buildings, many with numerous large pithoi set into their floors, were built here. Their foundations had been cut into the northern slopes of the hill, obliterating most earlier remains there, except for the underpinnings of a massive stairway of the Early Roman period. Ancient remains were better preserved to the southeast, but even there only scraps of walls, cuttings, and disturbed stroseis survive. These may be combined to present a picture, albeit a sketchy and incomplete one, of the neighborhood and its history in the Hellenistic period.

22. Attested by the "Turkish Garden," a series of holes for plantings, with roots in situ, found in the southwest part of the section and in Section KK, to the south (lots ΛΛ 65, KK 1049–KK 1051).

The most important fact that emerges from study of the topography of this area is its isolation, despite its elevated location on the Kolonos Agoraios and close to the public buildings of the Agora (Fig. 1). This is particularly true of the area just around the Agora Bone Well. It lay uphill from and behind the Stoa of Zeus, which effectively cut it off from the Agora. To the south, the long, featureless wall of the Arsenal,[23] built in the Early Hellenistic period, formed an impenetrable barrier, cutting the area off from the sacred precinct of the Hephaisteion. At the foot of the Kolonos Agoraios to the north lay a road that ran from the Sacred Gate at the Kerameikos to the northwest corner of the Agora, ending behind the Royal Stoa.[24] In its Roman phase this road was as much as 6.00 m wide, but it was more modest in the Hellenistic period, probably no more than a narrow alleyway.[25] The rock of the hill had been cut back in a long, straight scarp just below (north of) the Agora Bone Well; between this scarp and the road lay the sanctuary of Demos and the Graces, established in the last quarter of the 3rd century.[26] A fine marble altar dedicated to Aphrodite and the Graces (*IG* II^2 2798), dating to 194/3,[27] was found here in situ during excavation of the railroad bed in 1892, along with several inscriptions honoring foreign benefactors of Athens that were to be set up in the sanctuary (*IG* II^2 844, 908, 909, 987). They are approximately contemporary with the Agora Bone Well deposit, ranging in date from 181–170 to after 150, but before the construction of the monumental stair later on, there was no easy access from the hill to the road below. The area in which the Agora Bone Well was situated, then, was accessible only from the west. A narrow road, marked by the course of a rock-cut drain (Fig. 5 [E–F 5]) running south of Buildings 3 and 4 (see below), may have approached from that direction, providing the only easy access to this isolated spot.

Building 4

Excavation revealed traces of Hellenistic buildings on the north side of the hill. Most interesting for our purposes is Building 4, the best preserved, which lay just to the southwest of the Agora Bone Well (Figs. 5 [F–G 5], 6, 7). The lines of its western and southern walls are documented by cuttings in bedrock: vertical scarps and low wall beddings measuring 0.80–1.10 m in width. Only traces of the walls themselves were found, built of stones set in clay and faced with stucco. The south cutting, both ends of which are preserved, measures 14.50 m in length. The cutting for the west wall survives for a distance of ca. 7.50 m; a corner indicates the position of the east wall, of which no trace remains. Two or perhaps three rooms can be

23. Pounder 1983.

24. A monumental propylon connected this road to the Panathenaic Way in Roman times (Shear 1973b, pp. 370, 374–375, fig. 3). Its construction destroyed all Hellenistic remains here, so there is no evidence for the layout of this area contemporary with the Agora Bone Well.

25. Traces of the polygonal retaining walls that flanked the earlier road indicate a width of 1.85 m. In the first half of the 3rd century a cistern (E 3:1; see Fig. 1) was located in what was later the middle of the Roman street further west (see *Agora* XXIX, pp. 444–445). Its fill (from a potter's workshop) and a nearby pit full of iron slag (deposit E 2:3, *Agora* XXIX, p. 444) attest to the industrial character of the area in the Late Classical and Early Hellenistic periods.

26. Travlos 1971, p. 79; Mikalson 1998, pp. 172–179; Monaco 2001.

27. For the significance of the dedication and the role of Aphrodite Hegemone in the cult, see Mikalson 1998, p. 176.

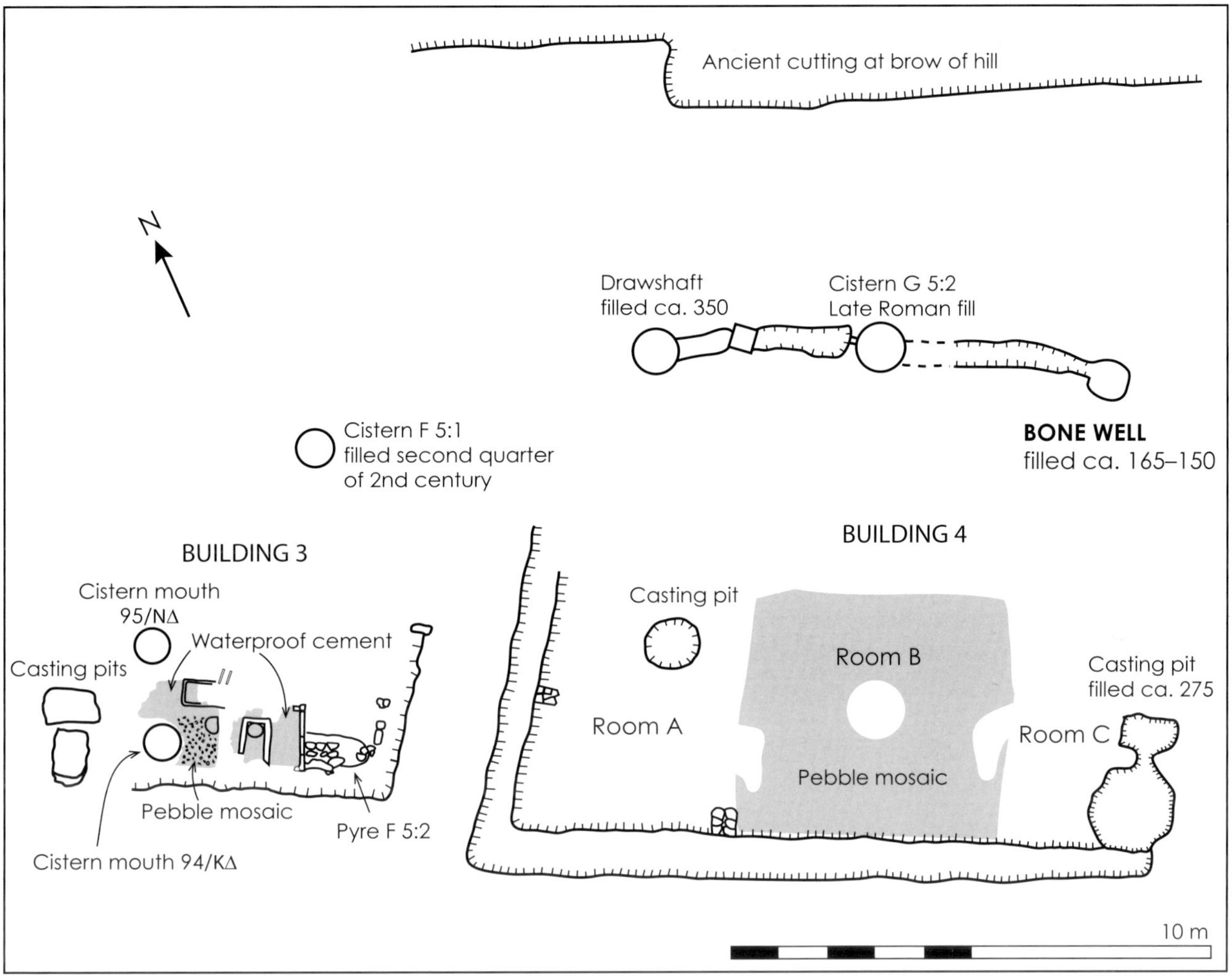

Figure 6. Extant remains of Buildings 3 and 4 and the water system to which the Agora Bone Well belongs. S. I. Rotroff, based on notebook sketches of D. B. Thompson (ΛΛ 4, p. 624) and her plan of Section ΛΛ

distinguished. A meter or so of internal rubble wall defines a westernmost room ca. 4.00 m in width (room A). At some point this space was divided into a southern and northern area by another rubble wall, creating a southern room measuring less than 3.00 m north to south. To the east, room B was paved with a pebble mosaic, the dimensions of which suggest a room measuring about 5.50 m on a side. The surface of the mosaic was coated with waterproof cement, suggesting that this was a courtyard. Room B may have extended to the eastern limit of the building, but the absence of mosaic flooring there suggests that area may have been occupied by a third room (C), though a very narrow one, no more than 2.00 m in width. The northern part of the building is gone, but the water system to which the Agora Bone Well belongs lies only 4.00 m to the north of the surviving remains, providing a hint to the northern limit of the building and giving it a north–south measurement of about 10.50 m. It is possible, of course, that these water sources were located within the building rather than outside it, but the steep slope of the hill just beyond them indicates that the building cannot have extended much further in that direction. Although abundant metal waste and other industrial material found in the building attest to

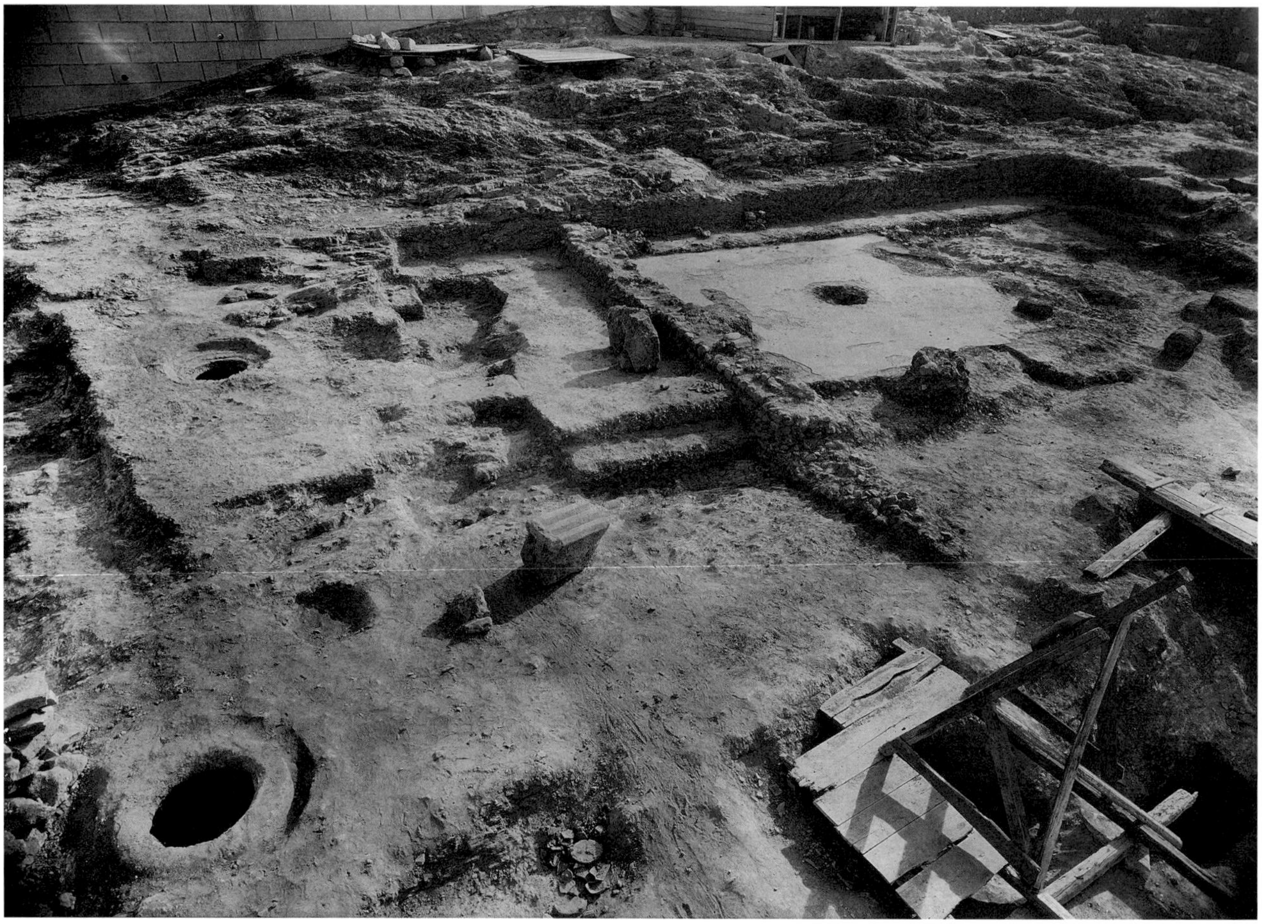

Figure 7. Building 4 shortly after excavation, looking southwest. The Agora Bone Well is at the lower right. Photo Agora Excavations

its use as a workshop, the abandonment debris also included pieces of fine red, white, and blue stucco, some with edges imitating drafted masonry. Some of the rooms, then, were nicely decorated and were presumably living quarters; perhaps they were located on an upper floor, to which a stairway in the narrow room C could have provided access. We might then identify the structure as a house, but one that also included workshop space, a common arrangement in houses around the Hellenistic Agora.[28]

The fact that the limits of the water system of which the Agora Bone Well is part fall just inside the lines of the east and west walls of the house can hardly be coincidental. Those who lived and worked here must have used that system when it was an active water source, and consequently the history of the house is of considerable interest in the context of the present study. The layers above and within the house are difficult to read, and joins between many of the lots bespeak mixing between them—whether in antiquity or in the course of excavation, it is impossible to say. In some cases, the excavation account does not make it clear what lay over a given deposit, but an effort has been made to reconstruct the relationship of these strata to the history of the house even when specific information is lacking. The stratigraphy is subject to differing interpretations, but the following outline of the history of the house seems probable.

28. Tsakirgis 2005, 2009.

The fill of a casting pit under the floor of room C provides a *terminus post quem* of ca. 275 for the construction of the house (see Fig. 8 for a schematic representation of the stratigraphy of Building 4).[29] Floor surfaces contemporary with the building proved difficult to recognize, but a patch in the southwest corner of room B and a strip at the north of room C, just south of the Agora Bone Well, produced pottery ranging in date from the 5th century to at least as late as the end of the first quarter of the 2nd century.[30] No distinction was made, in excavation, between floor surfaces and floor makeup, and the latest sherds are probably those that were trodden into the floor in the course of the building's use. More prominent were deposits of red earth that seemed to the excavators to represent the debris of the house. These occurred in two areas in room A, in a patch in room B, and in the southwest corner of room C. There is evidence of intrusion, in

29. *Keyhole-shaped casting pit.* Widened at one end, under the southeast corner of room C. Lot ΛΛ 59 (half a tin): six pieces of identifiable fine ware, including four pieces of a large rolled-rim plate (ca. 300); fragments of one form 3 lopas indicating date of 285 or later. Lot ΛΛ 58, characterized as a "loose intrusion" in the pit's fill, contained an unguentarium fragment dating after ca. 200.

Floor over pit. Lot ΛΛ 57 (half a tin): largely coarse, with fragments of three identifiable fine-ware shapes, the latest a Classical kantharos or cup-kantharos of ca. 275.

A circular pit and a pile of small pieces of slag over bedrock in room A suggest the presence of another casting pit here, but there is no evidence for its date. Also beneath the level of the floor were the following: (1) Deposit of "green earth" in Room A. Its relationship to the floor of the room is uncertain, since it was dug as the bottom of a modern disturbance. Pottery as late as last quarter of 3rd century (lot ΛΛ 48, half a bag): fragments of seven identifiable pieces of fine ware, including a West Slope kantharos (275–225) and a moldmade bowl (probably 225–200). One rim fragment may come from a Late Hellenistic chytra. Perhaps part of the abandonment debris of the house, shifted to this low level by later digging in the area. (2) Small deposit in southeast corner of room A, eight fragments of pottery, not closely datable, but possibly late 4th century (lot ΛΛ 49). (3) Single Classical sherd from under mosaic (lot ΛΛ 53). (4) Knidian amphora handle from under floor of north side of room C, early period V (146–108; SS 7754, eponym Kallidamas [KT 902]); probably intrusive.

30. Pottery from floors:

Room B. Lot ΛΛ 52 (less than one bag): fragments of ca. 10 identifiable fine-ware pieces, the latest being two fragments of a white-ground lagynos (a shape first attested in Athens in the first quarter of the 2nd century; see *Agora* XXIX, p. 227). Unguentarium foot of category 5 (2nd century). Rim of local imitation of *orlo bifido* pan is much later (1st century), probably intrusive. A terracotta figurine may also come from this level (T 1506).

Room C. Lot ΛΛ 56 (half a tin): fragments of ca. 20 identifiable fine-ware pieces, including two fragments of moldmade bowls (ca. 200 or later), lagynos-ware pyxis (first quarter of 2nd century or later), and Cypriot(?) plate with incurved rim (2nd century). Second-century material among coarse wares: fragments of two or three large funnels (ca. 175 or later); unguentarium of category 5; lopas of form 4 or 5 (ca. 180 or later). Small fragment of Early Roman sigillata chalice is intrusive and joins fragment from lot ΛΛ 45, which lay higher up. Further evidence of mixing between this material and the upper stratigraphy is provided by joins with fragments of a gray-ware vessel in lot ΛΛ 54. Coin ΛΛ-556 (*Agora* XXVI, p. 41, variety 43, 330s–322/317). Parian stamped amphora handle (SS 7756).

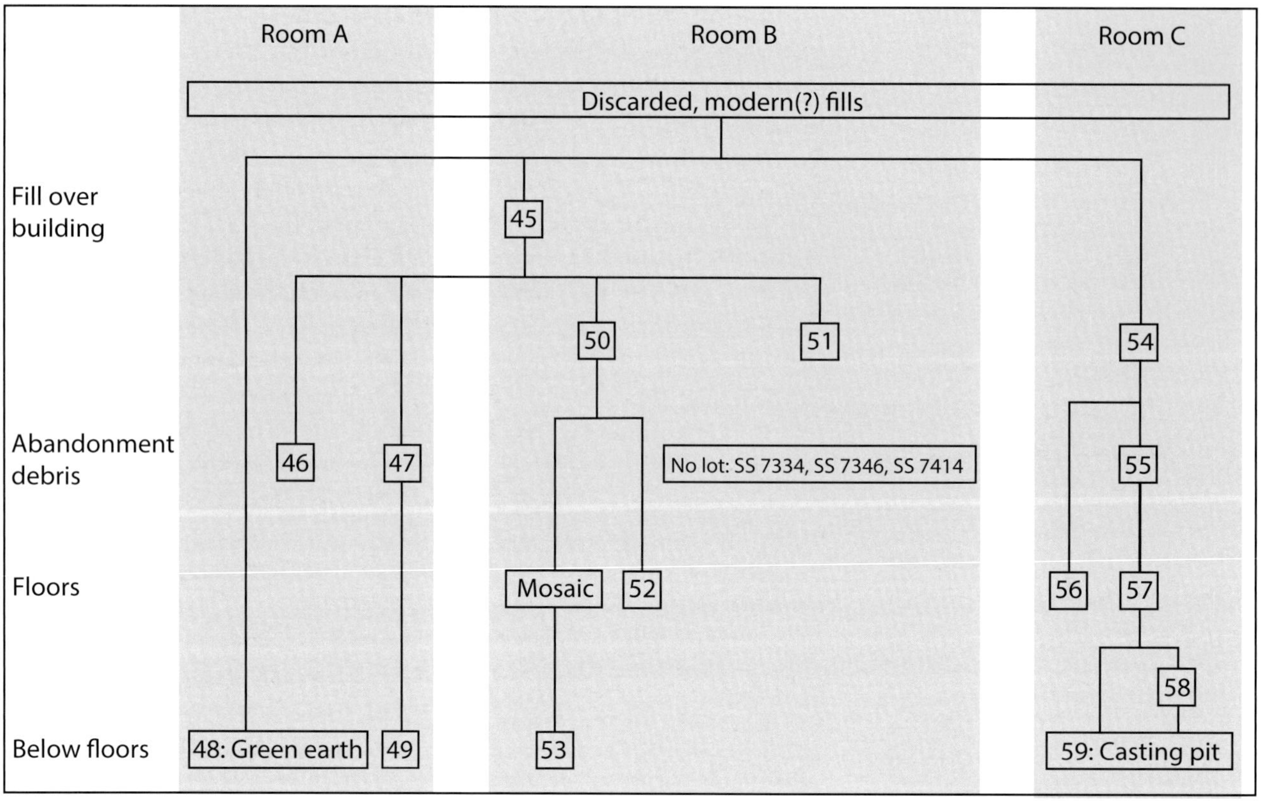

Figure 8. Schematic diagram of the stratigraphy of Building 4. Numbers refer to pottery lots in Section ΛΛ (in the excavation records, they bear the prefix ΛΛ). S. I. Rotroff

the form of occasional Roman pieces and joins with material from superposed strata, but the latest Hellenistic material is contemporary with that in the floor levels.[31] Taken together, the evidence suggests that the house was occupied for something under a hundred years, falling into disuse early in the 2nd century. This confirms what would almost certainly have to be the case, that the house had been abandoned by the time the Agora Bone Well began to be used as a burial place. A thorough search was conducted for joins between material from all levels of the house and that from the well without result, which further suggests that the house was not in use when the well was active as a dump.

31. Pottery from abandonment debris:

Room A. Lot ΛΛ 47 (from west side of room, perhaps remnants of mud-brick wall; one bag): largely fine ware, from Classical to at least late 3rd century; latest pieces are two fragments of moldmade bowls (ca. 225–175), with five intrusive Roman fragments of 2nd century A.D. or later. Join with fragment from uppermost deposit in room (lot ΛΛ 45) suggests some mixing with that material. Lot ΛΛ 46 (half a bag): fragments of about 15 identifiable fine-ware pieces, mostly before ca. 250, but with fragments of moldmade bowl (ca. 200 or later). Two intrusive Roman fragments of 2nd–4th century A.D. Two terracotta figurines (T 1436, T 1437). Join with fragment in lot ΛΛ 55 (abandonment debris in room C).

Room B. No lot. Two Rhodian stamped amphora handles (SS 7334, SS 7346), the latter of period IIa (shortly after ca. 234), and a Knidian amphora handle (SS 7414, eponym Nikasimachos [KT 1660], early period IV [180s or later]), the latter found on floor in southeast corner of room. Figurine mold (T 1442); handle of coarse jug (P 9698).

Room C. Lot ΛΛ 55 (half a bag): fragments of about 10 identifiable fine-ware pieces, moldmade bowl. Two unguentarium fragments probably date at least as late as late 3rd century. Fragments of lopas of form 4 or 5 date after 180, but possibly intrude from lot ΛΛ 54 above, where a fragment of the same vessel was found. Join with fragment in lot ΛΛ 46 (abandonment debris in room A). West Slope cup (P 10173, *Agora* XXIX, pp. 411–412, no. 1673, fig. 100, pl. 133).

The whole area of the house and that to the north was covered by a loose, dark, gravelly fill, full of tiles, marble chips, metal waste, and large amounts of pottery. Although its contents are largely Hellenistic, the top of the fill lay at about the level of the bottom of a Byzantine wall that ran across the house, and it may have been put in place, or at least leveled, at a much later date. To the south, over the preserved remains of the house, the material dates largely before the end of the 2nd century; none of the stamped amphora handles found in undisturbed areas there is later than Knidian period V (146–108).[32] The part of the fill that lay further north—red earth in the northeast corner of room B and dark fill to the north of room B—is later, reaching to the Sullan sack and beyond, with amphora handles of period VI (108–88) and one of period VII (after 88).[33] If this fill was brought in from elsewhere, the difference in date might reflect two different sources. But, in any event, it does not seem to be related to the occupation or destruction of the house. Its source may have been the debris of the Arsenal, which was destroyed in the Sullan sack.[34]

The industrial activities that preceded the construction of the house probably continued throughout its occupation, for chunks of iron and iron

32. Fifty-seven stamped amphora handles were found in this fill (strosis 1, lot ΛΛ 45 and perhaps also ΛΛ 50), three from disturbed areas (marked by an asterisk): SS 7342, SS 7347, SS 7348, SS 7399–SS 7404, SS 7408, SS 7409, *SS 7410, *SS 7412, *SS 7418, SS 7490–SS 7494, SS 7497–SS 7508, SS 7533, SS 7723–SS 7735, SS 7739–SS 7743, SS 7747–SS 7751, SS 7757, SS 7758. Twenty-six of these come from the southern part of the area, the latest naming Knidian eponyms Dionysios II (SS 7490 [KT 1131]) and Philombrotidas (SS 7491 [KT 1241]), of period V (146–108).

Upper part of fill over rooms A and B. Lot ΛΛ 45 (one tin): much Classical and Early Hellenistic, with latest Hellenistic material dating late 2nd to early 1st century; two fragments of long-petal bowls; West Slope reversible lid with trefoil garland; small funnel; brazier with plain lug; fragment of Eastern Sigillata A; five fragments of 2nd-century plates. Around 28 fragments dated 1st to mid-5th century A.D., two Byzantine sherds, one Turkish sherd. Joins with lots ΛΛ 47 (abandonment debris in room A) and ΛΛ 56 (floor in room C) suggest that those who spread this material dug down into lower levels. Coin ΛΛ-426 (no identification); a Turkish coin is also recorded (notebook ΛΛ 6, p. 1069, V/7/37, no. 3). Inventoried: fragments of Pergamene West Slope amphora (P 33955), Hellenistic cup (P 33956), head vase (P 33958, 1st–2nd century A.D.).

Fill over room B. Lot ΛΛ 50 (half a tin): largely Hellenistic, before middle of 2nd century, except for a fragment of Eastern Sigillata A (after 150) and an Ionian platter (1st century). Nineteen Roman fragments, largely 2nd century A.D., with two 4th–5th century, one Turkish fragment. Inventoried: Late Hellenistic–Early Roman redware dish (P 33959).

Fill over room C. Lot ΛΛ 54 (one tin). Largely Hellenistic before mid-2nd century, except for fragments of two long-petal bowls (probably after ca. 150), pyxis lid of Large Leaf Groups (125–86), thin-necked West Slope oinochoe (ca. 125 or later?). Later objects include local imitation of *orlo bifido* pan (1st century), Ionian platter (second half of 1st century), and 15 Roman fragments, mostly Early Roman (cf. lamp L 3010 below), but one 3rd–4th century A.D. Joins with fragments in lot ΛΛ 55 (abandonment debris in room C) and ΛΛ 56 (floor in room C). Inventoried: Campana B plate (P 33957).

Other objects inventoried from strosis 1 but not associated with specific lots. Stamped plate (P 10847, *Agora* XXIX, p. 418, no. 1726, fig. 102, pl. 148), type 52C lamp (L 3010, *Agora* IV, p. 185, no. 724, pls. 28, 51), glass base (G 107), stone button (ST 190), lead token (IL 590, *Agora* X, p. 113, no. L 268c, pl. 29), iron chisel (IL 616), stamped loomweight (MC 384), terracotta molds (T 1427, T 1428, T 1441) and figurines (T 1429, T 1546 [Thompson 1954, pp. 99–102, pl. 23, with joining fragments from much further northwest], T 1547 [Thompson 1954, pp. 99, 102, pl. 22, with joining fragments in cistern F 5:1]).

33. Lot ΛΛ 51 (red earth in northeast corner of room B; half a tin) contains some pottery typical of Sullan destruction debris: fragments of one long-petal bowl, two semiglazed bowls, and an Eastern Sigillata A plate. Three amphora handles: SS 7744–SS 7746, one of which dates to period VI B, shortly before 88 B.C. (SS 7744, eponym Hermon [KT 485]). Four or five Roman fragments of late 1st–early 2nd century A.D. The latest of the 31 stamped handles from the northern dark earth of strosis 1 dates to period VII, after 88 (SS 7735, late Knidian [KT 2481]), and three more, also Knidian, date to period VI B, ca. 98–88 (SS 7731, eponym Hermon [KT 1531]; SS 7750, eponym Aristokrates [KT 877]; SS 7742, *duoviri* of term of Aristodamos [KT 1515]).

34. Pounder 1983, pp. 254–255.

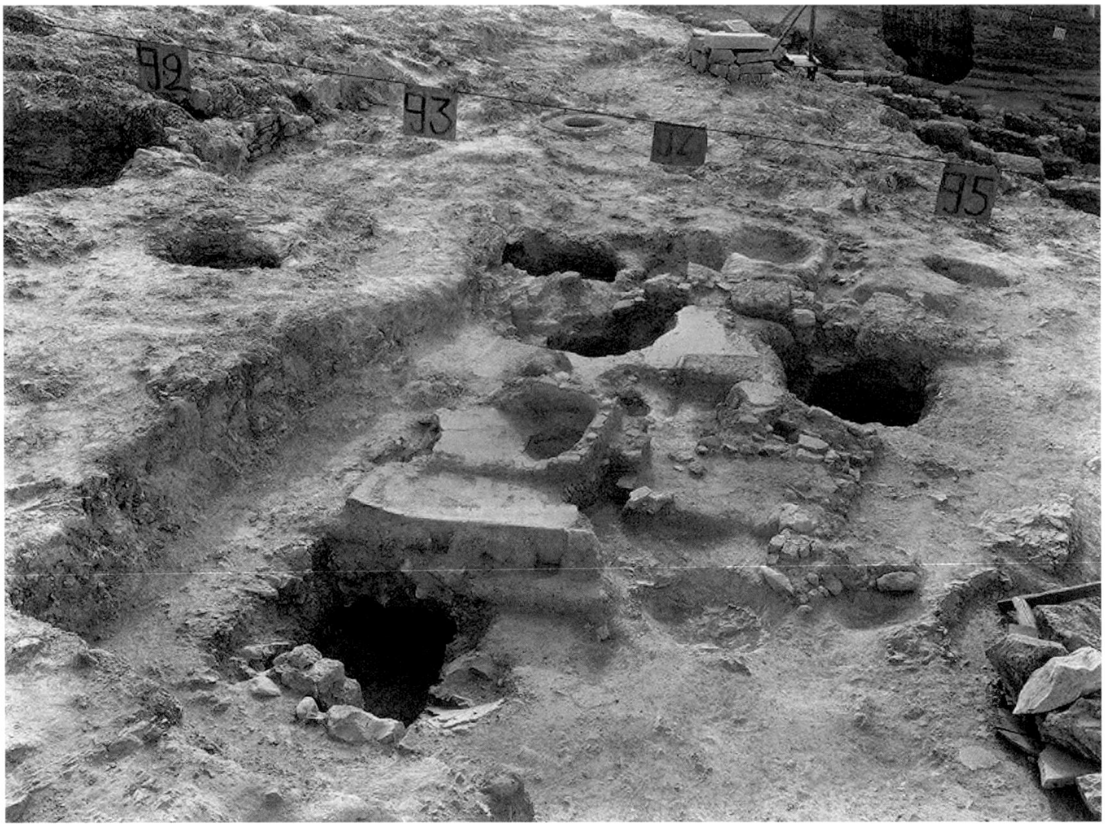

Figure 9. Building 3, looking east.
Photo Agora Excavations

objects (including an identifiable chisel, IL 616), slag, lumps of pigment, chips of different kinds of marble (some with worked surfaces), and a grinding stone were found in the vicinity. Unfortunately, these were stored together, regardless of the layer in which they were found,[35] so it is impossible to determine how much might be from the upper fills and thus postdate the life of the structure. Industrial activity is more abundantly attested in the nearby Building 3, which was probably constructed somewhat earlier, but was refurbished at about the time that Building 4 was built and may be part of the same industrial complex.

Building 3

Building 3 lay to the west, separated from Building 4 by an alley two meters in width (Figs. 6, 9).[36] Two cuttings in the rising bedrock form the southeast corner of the building and preserve measurements of ca. 5.00 m east–west by 3.00 m north–south. Bedrock drops off to the north, and any substantial expansion of the structure in that direction, if it existed, has been destroyed by the massive cutting for the Roman stair. Thus we have traces of a single room, the dedicated industrial purpose of which is attested by its internal arrangements: a plastered tub with a settling basin, set at right angles against the south wall of the room, and plastered areas of floor with tile borders. In the western part of the room is one mouth of a double cistern (94/ΚΔ), the floor around it plastered with waterproof cement; the other mouth is two meters farther north (95/ΝΔ). Although this cistern

35. In lots ΛΛ 61–ΛΛ 64.
36. For the notebook sketch on which the drawing of Building 3 in Fig. 6 is based, see Rotroff 2013, p. 123, fig. 50.

system was filled in Byzantine times, it is certainly part of the Hellenistic establishment. Yet another cistern, larger but with a single chamber, lies a few meters to the north (F 5:1). A saucer pyre (deposit F 5:2) had been buried in the southeast corner of the room in a ritual of the first quarter of the 3rd century.[37] Two floors were excavated in the room, the lower one, through which the pyre was cut, perhaps dating within the 4th century,[38] the upper one including material that dates as late as ca. 200.[39] The building, then, was probably built in the Classical period, then refurbished in the early 3rd century. Two small casting pits just to the west, filled with debris of the 4th century, may be contemporary with its occupation;[40] another, located under the room and disturbed by the diggers of the pyre, must be earlier.[41] The fill that overlaid the floors and the basins, clearly deposited after the abandonment of the structure, contained material largely of the 3rd century (with Roman intrusions) and was deposited no earlier than the first quarter of the 2nd century;[42] this building, then, probably went out of use at about the same time as Building 4 next door. The northerly cistern (F 5:1), however, remained empty until the second quarter of the 2nd century, when it was filled with material closely contemporary with that in the Agora Bone Well.

Development of the Complex

If we consider these two structures as a single complex, its possible history may be summarized as follows. Metalworking began in the area in the Classical period, possibly as early as the 5th century, as evidenced by the casting pit under Building 3. Stonecutting also seems to have been practiced here, judging from the abundant working chips in the westernmost shaft of the cistern system, which contained material dating chiefly before

37. Shear (1938, p. 355, fig. 42) illustrates a lamp from the pyre, which he describes as "a child's grave." For recent discussion of the deposit, see Rotroff 2013, pp. 123–124, no. 21, figs. 50, 51. The relationship of the pyre to the floors is unclear. The cross-section in the notebook shows it covered by the upper floor of the room, while the lower floor is described as "broken away round protruding tops of stones" of the uppermost level of the pyre (notebook ΛΛ 4, p. 703). Probably the pyre was dug into the lower floor and covered over by the upper floor.

38. Strosis 4. Lot ΛΛ 34: six fragments of pottery, not closely datable.

39. Strosis 3 (0.07 m thick). Lot ΛΛ 33 (one-third tin): largely 3rd century with one moldmade bowl fragment of ca. 200 or later. Includes fragments of pyre material, probably from pyre F 5:2.

40. *Pit A.* Lots ΛΛ 39 (one-fourth bag), ΛΛ 40 (one bag): includes skyphos base of late 4th or early 3rd century, coin of 322/317–307 (ΛΛ-266; see *Agora* XXVI, p. 43, variety 46).

Pit B. Lot ΛΛ 42 (one-third tin): first half of 4th century.

41. Lot ΛΛ 38: nothing necessarily later than 5th century, with fragment of pot support (P 9695; see Morris 1985, p. 404, pl. 101:c).

42. Lot ΛΛ 32 (half a tin): latest datable Hellenistic consists of five fragments of moldmade bowls (225–200 or later), unguentarium fragment (probably second half of 3rd century). Rhodian stamped amphora handle apparently from this layer brings date down to end of first quarter of 2nd century (SS 7257, eponym Kallikratidas II, ca. 175/173). Thasian amphora handle (SS 7258; see *EtThas* IV, p. 212, no. 721) is earlier. Thirty-three Roman fragments date at least as late as 4th century A.D.

ca. 350. Building 3, built in the 4th century, served as the work space of the founders who used the casting pits that lie to the west of Building 3 and under Building 4. Around 275, Building 3 was refurbished, an event perhaps commemorated in ritual by the burial of the saucer pyre in its southeast corner,[43] and at the same time, the larger and nicely decorated Building 4 was constructed immediately to the east, perhaps to serve as a dwelling for the craftsmen who worked here. The workers used water from the Agora Bone Well system, as well as from the cisterns under and to the north of Building 3, and their business flourished for most of a century. The worked bones noted by Dorothy Thompson and described below (pp. 56–57) may be tools associated with the metal workshop and casting pits here, left behind when the neighborhood was abandoned and later thrown into the well. When the last of these craftsmen died or moved away, his house and workshop at the end of a dead-end street remained unoccupied. The buildings slowly crumbled; possibly scavengers rooted in their floors, which would account for some of the later material found close over bedrock here. A more general abandonment of the wider area was to follow soon, in the course of the second quarter of the 2nd century. In addition to the Agora Bone Well and cistern F 5:1, which served this complex of buildings, two other former water sources on the northern Kolonos Agoraios were filled with debris at that time: the Cave Cistern (H 6:9), located on the eastern slopes of the hill and some distance to the south, at the northeast corner of the Arsenal;[44] and the two-chamber system that contained Homer Thompson's Group C (G 6:2), on the north side of the Arsenal.[45] The area seems to have become a dumping ground at this time.

The Agora Bone Well, which had been kept clear of accumulation while the house was occupied, began to collect silt, forming the sterile layer that was found at its bottom. Soon it began to be used as a dumping place for infant bodies and animal bones. Perhaps it had ceased to provide sufficient water for regular use, since such dumping would be unlikely in a viable water source; it is even possible that the impending failure of the well contributed to the abandonment of the nearby house. With one exception (**40**), the artifacts that survived their fall into the well intact or only chipped are small, sturdy items (**2, 8, 12, 29, 31–38, 60–62, 78, 81**). Most of the larger and more fragile vessels are broken, suggesting that water did not break their fall, though they might, of course, have been broken by objects thrown in after them, or by striking the wall of the well during their fall. On the other hand, the extraordinarily good preservation of the bones of both humans and animals indicates that the bones continuously remained in a stable, presumably wet, environment until they were excavated. But even if the well was not dry, its water was clearly useless for human consumption after dumping began. After a little while, other material joined the human and animal debris, mostly pottery, but a large piece of bronze furniture and other items as well. The dumping of corpses and animal waste continued, even after other garbage stopped entering the well. Then, rather suddenly, all dumping ceased and the well was filled up with a nearly clean fill of earth and rocks, with only an occasional Classical or Hellenistic sherd. The fill in the 2 m above the bone deposit is remarkable for the heavy concentration of stones it contained. For the two days of excavation prior to reaching

43. For the association of pyres with remodeling and reflooring, see Rotroff 2013, pp. 61–64.

44. Rotroff 1983, pp. 273–275.

45. Thompson 1934, pp. 345–369; for the date, see Rotroff 1983, pp. 276–278.

the bone levels, the complete descriptions of the excavated contents of the well read: "Dig to 12 m. Stones and scanty 4th c[entury] pottery" and then "Still stones. Dig to 13.02 m." Bones were first encountered on the following day, in a fill still rich with stones.[46] This thick layer of stones, earth, and little else seems to indicate an emphatic and purposeful closing of the burial deposit. Settling of this fill by the Byzantine era prompted a small subsequent deposit in the well's mouth; it then sat unnoticed until its discovery in 1937.

Other Hellenistic Remains

A few words will suffice to describe further Hellenistic remains on the hill. A series of walls, cuttings in bedrock, a paved court, and a fragment of pebble mosaic in the southwest corner of the area bear witness to Hellenistic activity there (Fig. 1; Fig. 5 [D–E 5]). Not all of these features are at the same alignment, so they may represent more than one phase or more than one building—the reconstruction in Fig. 1 is highly conjectural. Two different cistern systems here probably also go back to Hellenistic times, although they were filled later (D 4:1 + E 5:1, D 5:2),[47] and probably functioned with the building(s). The structure overlay a stuccoed pit that had been filled by a massive pottery dump around the middle of the 4th century (D 5:1),[48] but no trace of the stratigraphy associated with the building above it survives. A little to the southeast, a pit cut into bedrock measuring about 4.50 m square was filled in the Hellenistic period, probably around 175 (E 5:5).[49] Its purpose is, to quote the excavator, "obscure,"[50] but close by is yet another cistern system, the southernmost chamber of which (E 5:2) was abandoned at about the same time,[51] attesting to another establishment of some sort here. Material in the fill of the pit includes charcoal, lumps of iron, iron nails and tacks, lead clamps, small pieces of sheet lead, a lump of red pigment, a worked bone, and many fragments of figurines, and again emphasizes the industrial character of this quarter of the city. In sum, the vestiges of Hellenistic activity are slight, and it all seems to have come to an end within the first half of the 2nd century.

46. Notebook ΛΛ 8, pp. 1488, 1574–1576.

47. Cistern D 4:1 (Robinson's Group G: *Agora* V, pp. 22–45), with a fill dating from the late 1st century B.C. to the early 2nd century A.D., is joined by a tunnel to Cistern E 5:1, which was filled in Late Roman times (*Agora* V, pp. 124–125). Cistern D 5:2 contained a fill of ca. 150 to the early 1st century B.C. mixed with Late Roman material (*Agora* XXXIII, p. 348).

48. *Agora* XII, p. 387.

49. Lots ΛΛ 23–ΛΛ 27. Latest Hellenistic material in lowest, largely undisturbed part of fill (lot ΛΛ 26): unguentaria with solid feet (categories 4 and 5, 2nd century), five fragments of moldmade bowls (probably first quarter of 2nd century). Two later pieces: grayware lamp (late 2nd–1st century?), handle of Roman jug. Nine coins (ΛΛ-120, ΛΛ-121, ΛΛ-183, ΛΛ-216–ΛΛ-218, ΛΛ-222, ΛΛ-223, ΛΛ-236); the latest two are Euboian bronzes of 253–245 (ΛΛ-222, ΛΛ-236; *Agora* XXVI, p. 209, variety 613). Inventoried: cooking-ware lid (P 33954, *Agora* XXXIII, p. 320, no. 722, fig. 90).

50. Notebook ΛΛ 2, p. 316.

51. *Agora* XXXIII, p. 351. The northern chamber (E 5:3) was filled in Byzantine times.

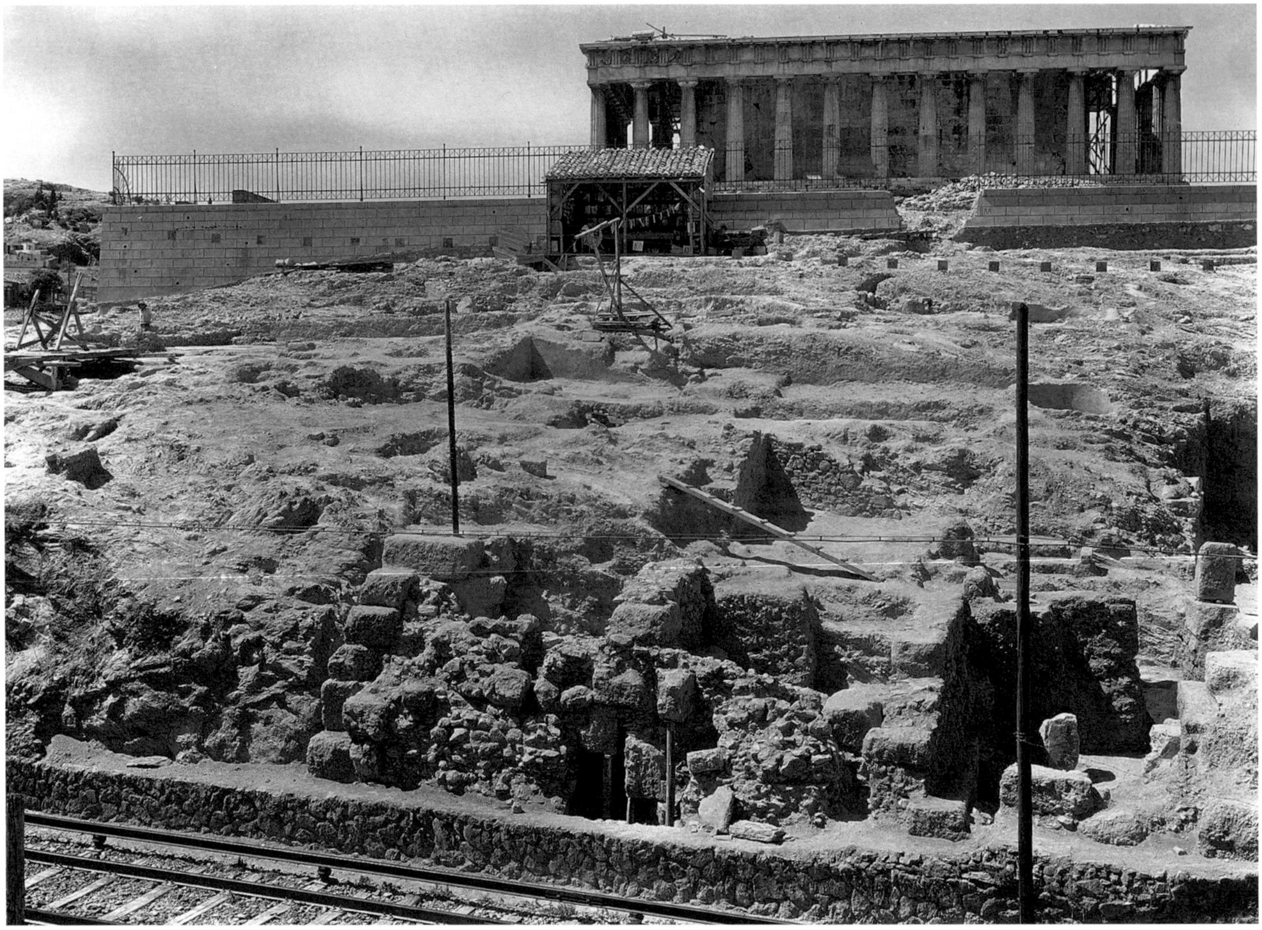

Figure 10. The central part of Section ΛΛ during excavation, looking south, with the railroad in the foreground and the Hephaisteion and its modern terrace wall (now demolished) in the background. The foundations for the Roman stair are in the center of the photograph, just beyond the railway. The Agora Bone Well is at the far left. Photo Agora Excavations

The Sanctuary of Aphrodite Ourania

It remains to consider the question of the location of the sanctuary of Aphrodite Ourania and its relevance, if any, to the well. Pausanias (1.14.7) is our only witness. He places the shrine near (πλησίον) the Hephaisteion and describes it immediately after the Hephaisteion and before the Stoa Poikile. For this reason, earlier scholarship located it on the northern side of the Kolonos Agoraios. The only ancient structure of monumental scale that has been found there is the Roman stair mentioned above: a large cutting, occupied by an imposing foundation about 8 m wide, consisting of a grid of conglomerate blocks with a heavy stone packing. It sits on the northern brow of the hill and is preserved to a maximum length of about 3.20 m in a north–south direction (Figs. 5, 10); the northern part was cut away by the builders of the modern railway. Nonetheless, the foundations reach a height of 3.20 m where they descend the steep slope of the hill at their northern end. At the time of excavation, these were recognized as the foundations of a stairway that connected the hill with the road at its base; further traces were subsequently found at the foot of the hill, north of the railway.[52] Evidence for the date of the stairway is limited. Thompson associated it with a large fill to the south, which she described as chiefly Late Hellenistic but with some fragments of Early Roman pottery (e.g., western sigillata); she concluded that the stair was probably built in the

52. For the upper foundations, see Shear 1938, p. 339. The lower foundations appear on a plan published by T. Leslie Shear Jr. showing the area at the base of the hill in the Roman period (Shear 1973b, p. 371, fig. 3, between South Building I and the "Altar of Demos and the Graces").

1st century A.D. Although the relevant pottery can no longer be identified, other associated lots support a Roman date. Nine fragments extracted from the earth between and under the stair blocks, probably about the middle of the southern foundation wall, include a possible fragment of a micaceous water jar, pushing the date to at least the 1st century A.D.[53] Pottery from a layer that ran under the stair on its western side is largely Classical and Early Hellenistic, but with some Roman fragments.[54] On the basis of Pausanias's topographical hint, John Travlos suggested in 1949 that these foundations belonged to a Roman temple of Aphrodite Ourania: he reconstructed a prostyle Doric building with its porch resting on the preserved foundations, and approached by a monumental stairway.[55]

In a plan drawn by William Dinsmoor Jr. and dated 1978, the temple was replaced by a stairway plain and simple;[56] clearly its identification as the Aphrodite sanctuary—about which doubts had already been expressed[57]—had been rejected, but without published comment. Subsequently, however, Massimo Osanna revived Travlos's idea, arguing not only that the sanctuary was located on the northern slope of the Kolonos Agoraios, but also that the Agora Bone Well lay within its temenos.[58] The clearly domestic and industrial character of the structures immediately to the south of the well rule this out; furthermore, there is insufficient space between Buildings 3 and 4 and the brow of the hill for even a very modest temenos. It is not impossible that the shrine was located elsewhere on the hill, but it cannot have been in the immediate area of the Agora Bone Well.

53. Lot ΛΛ 75, "from cleaning under and between stones in good spots" (notebook ΛΛ 7, p. 1332) and "under cross-wall" (notebook ΛΛ 9, p. 1616); the other fragments include two pieces of Classical black glaze, two possible lekane fragments, and four nondescript household-ware wall fragments.

54. Lot ΛΛ 238, from strosis 14: "The wall of stone packing for the Stair along its west side rests upon this strosis which therefore antedates the stairway" (notebook ΛΛ 7, p. 1274). About half a tin of pottery retained. All fine ware is Greek, the latest fragments Early Hellenistic: kantharos with molded rim (cf. *Agora* XXIX, p. 246, no. 40, pl. 4, 310–300 B.C.[?]), fragment of early West Slope plate or cup (for decoration, cf. *Agora* XXIX, p. 275, no. 315, pl. 32, 275–265 B.C.). Roman material: eight wall fragments with wheel-ridging, sliced handle, and coarse base, not closely datable. Apparently an Early Hellenistic level disturbed at the time of the building of the stairway in the Roman period.

55. Travlos 1949, pp. 391–392, fig. 2; 1971, pp. 79–80, fig. 102. He found evidence for the south wall of the cella in a shallow cutting in bedrock (0.60 m wide and 0.10 m deep) with a few stones in situ, some 7 m south of and parallel to the east–west foundation of the stair, and turning a corner at its west end, apparently in alignment with the western edge of the stair foundation (see Fig. 5 [F 4–5]). At its east end, however, this cutting continues eastward beyond the line of the eastern edge of the stair foundation. This trench was filled with Late Roman and Byzantine pottery (lot ΛΛ 93); the relatively careful workmanship of the cutting suggests that it is ancient, but there is no further evidence for its date. Of the large and impressive cutting that Travlos shows surrounding the walls of the cella, only the southeast corner and the south side is preserved; it extends well beyond the line of the west side of the stair, at which point any further extension has been destroyed by subsequent cutting of the bedrock there. This cutting does not seem to be centered on the stair foundation, as Travlos drew it. Dorothy Thompson associated it with a Roman house, itself too poorly preserved for reconstruction. Pottery at the bottom of the cutting (lot ΛΛ 92), over bedrock, is largely Roman (much of it 1st century A.D., with several examples of *Consp.* form 34 [cf. *Consp.*, p. 112] but with pieces possibly as late as ca. 100–150 A.D. [including a local copy of Eastern Sigillata B form 60; cf. Hayes 1985, p. 64, pl. XIV:5–8]), with a substantial proportion of residual Hellenistic, but it is not possible to tell how long after the cutting was made that this earth and pottery came to rest there. We are grateful to Clare Pickersgill for assistance in dating the Roman pottery.

56. First published, as far as we are aware, in 1982 (*Agora* XXII, pl. 99). The revision of the plan was undertaken in the context of Robert Pounder's study of the Arsenal (Pounder 1983), during which Dinsmoor reviewed evidence for the structures on the north side of the Kolonos Agoraios. The stairway appears in all subsequent Agora plans.

57. See *Agora* XIV, p. 142, n. 127, where Homer Thompson suggests the foundation may instead have supported a propylon.

58. Osanna 1988–1989.

In 1981, another candidate for the sanctuary of Aphrodite came to light: the remains of an Archaic altar and a Roman temple on the northern side of the Agora, just west of the Stoa Poikile.[59] The altar was built around 500, damaged sometime thereafter (perhaps by the Persians in 480), and rebuilt in the decade 430–420. In the early 1st century A.D. the area was restructured: the altar was carefully buried and covered by a paved platform, and a south-facing temple was constructed immediately to the north. The shrine apparently continued to function in this new form until the 4th century A.D. While the case is not ironclad, objects found in the area suggest that this may have been the shrine of Aphrodite Ourania.[60] Items with feminine associations were found in the vicinity of the altar and within the ash inside it,[61] and a few figurines of doves, found immediately to the west of the altar, are suggestive of Aphrodite.[62] A fragmentary Classical relief depicting a woman descending a ladder, probably to be identified as Aphrodite Ourania, was found in Byzantine levels some 10 m to the east.[63] Preliminary reports that dove bones figured within the sacrificial ash have proven incorrect; the offerings were chiefly young ovicaprids, a common choice for sacrifice in many cults.[64] The Roman rebuilding almost certainly served the same cult as the Archaic altar, whose integrity it respected, and if this is indeed the sanctuary of Aphrodite Ourania, any direct connection of the goddess with the Agora Bone Well can be dismissed.

One might object that a position just west of the Stoa Poikile does not accord perfectly with Pausanias's account (1.14.6–15.1). In this section of his text, having completed his circuit of the Agora and returned to its northwest corner, where he had entered, he writes:

> ὑπὲρ δὲ τὸν Κεραμεικὸν καὶ στοὰν τὴν καλουμένην Βασίλειον ναός ἐστιν Ἡφαίστου. καὶ ὅτι μὲν ἄγαλμά οἱ παρέστηκεν Ἀθηνᾶς, οὐδὲν θαῦμα ἐποιούμην τὸν ἐπὶ Ἐριχθονίῳ ἐπιστάμενος λόγον: τὸ δὲ ἄγαλμα ὁρῶν τῆς Ἀθηνᾶς γλαυκοὺς ἔχον τοὺς ὀφθαλμοὺς. . . . πλησίον δὲ ἱερόν ἐστιν Ἀφροδίτης Οὐρανίας. . . . ἰοῦσι δὲ πρὸς τὴν στοάν, ἣν Ποικίλην ὀνομάζουσιν ἀπὸ τῶν γραφῶν, ἔστιν Ἑρμῆς χαλκοῦς.

> Above the Kerameikos and the Royal Stoa is a temple of Hephaistos. That a statue of Athena stands by him caused me no surprise since I know the story about Erichthonios. I observed that the statue of Athena had blue-gray eyes. . . . Nearby is a shrine of Aphrodite Ourania. . . . As you go to the stoa which is called Poikile because of the pictures, there is a bronze Hermes.[65]

He locates the Hephaisteion with reference to the Kerameikos (his term for the Agora) and the Royal Stoa. Then, after a short digression on the statue of Athena in the Hephaisteion, he goes on to describe the sanctuary of Aphrodite nearby (πλησίον). The altar and the Roman temple, however, lie about 100 m from the Hephaisteion to the northeast; is this too far away to meet the demands of Pausanias's description?

Pausanias uses the word πλησίον with some flexibility; while it frequently means "right next door," it can also encompass a considerable distance. For instance, the Enneakrounos (probably to be identified in his

59. Shear 1984, pp. 24–40, figs. 1, 3.

60. Shear 1984, pp. 37–40. Osanna (1988–1989, p. 86), Weber (2006, pp. 182–183), and Lippolis (2009, p. 263) reject the identification.

61. Inscribed and otherwise altered knucklebones and an iron ring in the ash of the altar, and a miniature pyxis and a spindle whorl in stratified layers nearby (Shear 1984, p. 38, nn. 61–63, pl. 8:d, i, j; G. V. Foster 1984, p. 79, pl. 20:e, f).

62. Shear 1984, p. 38, n. 64, pl. 8:f, as well as a few unpublished examples found subsequently in layers immediately predating the construction of the altar (T 4208, T 4215, T 4223). These layers also produced some small, plain votive plaques (only traces of paint remain) and tiny fragments of what may be votive shields. They document worship on the site in the later 6th century but provide no assistance in identifying its object.

63. Edwards 1984.

64. See G. V. Foster 1984 for the original analysis and Reese 1989 for the correction.

65. Trans. R. E. Wycherley, Princeton 1957, adapted.

account with the Southeast Fountain House) is described as near (πλησίον) the Odeion (1.16.1), while it is in fact about as far away from the Odeion as the Archaic altar is from the Hephaisteion. The sense in which Pausanias uses it here becomes apparent when we consider his standpoint as narrator. It is clear that at some point he climbed the Kolonos Agoraios and inspected the Hephaisteion at close quarters, for he comments on the eye color of Athena's statue. His πλησίον, however, was written from the perspective of a viewer standing on the Agora floor, near the Royal Stoa—the location from which he initially describes the Hephaisteion—just across the Panathenaic Way from the Roman temple that replaced the Archaic altar. Having completed his account of the statue, he turns to that area, about 30 m to his right, well within the limits of πλησίον.

CHAPTER 2

Human Skeletal Material

Having examined the structures and established the character of the immediate surroundings of the Agora Bone Well, we may now turn to its most disturbing contents: the human remains. We are accustomed to imagine the end of life marked by formal ceremony, acknowledging the humanity of the deceased; the well, with its masses of haphazardly discarded bone, confounds these expectations.

The human bones from the well were recovered as commingled remains, together with many animal bones, and with no documentation of individual bodies or articulation of the remains. On June 9, 1938, Dorothy Thompson notes, "at 13 m . . . many bones, some worked, some human?"[1] This suggests that one of the older individuals, both of whom had intact skulls (see below), was near the top of the deposit, as it is unlikely that the infant bones would have been immediately recognized as human in the field. On following days, the quantity of bones is again noted. After excavation, the bones from the well were stored in a number of boxes and bags, and some of the material retains designations by box number and subunit (a, b, and so on). There is no evidence that these numbers have any contextual significance, and there is no record of the numbers other than on the bags themselves. They appear to simply represent an earlier inventory designation of the massive quantity of bones.

The human bone was initially examined by Angel; on the basis of the 155 pairs of left and right scapulae that he identified, he estimated that there were about 175 infants and late-term fetuses in the well.[2] Angel offered no explanation of how he arrived at this number, and he left no notes on his calculations.[3] Most likely the estimate was based on the volume of bone and Angel's count of the easily identified scapulae, perhaps also making allowances for bone that was not recovered or went unrecognized in his initial sorting of the material. He further speculated that the infants had died simultaneously, perhaps due to starvation or plague associated with Sulla's siege. Angel also observed that most of the skeletons were of full-term infants or late-term fetuses, with several older infants as well. It is clear that Angel never sorted all of the commingled remains of humans and animals and did not intend to produce a complete report. He noted

1. Notebook ΛΛ 8, p. 1576.
2. Angel 1945, pp. 311–312, fig. 12.
3. Angel's field and laboratory notes are archived at the National Museum of Natural History in Washington, D.C., and were examined by Liston.

the material mainly as a curiosity in his catalogue of skeletal material from various sites in Attica, in which he was concerned primarily with morphological typology in adult remains.[4] The presence in the animal-bone bags of large numbers of readily identifiable human bones from the infants and two older individuals suggests that no serious attempt to sort all of the bone was ever made prior to the present study.

When this project began, the human and animal bone had been partially cleaned and sorted, and was stored in nine wooden drawers. Many of the previously identified major long bones of the human infants and fetuses had been sorted by anatomical element, and the left and right bones for each element were stored in separate sections of the drawers. Some of the infant cranial bones likewise had been partially grouped by bone, but many of the cranial and postcranial bones remained mixed with the animal bone.

Because almost all of the infant bones fall within a very limited size range of infants, only four relatively complete skeletons of older individuals—an adult, an older child, and partial skeletons of two post-neonatal infants—can be identified from the mass of human bones. Two other slightly post-term infants may be represented by a few isolated bones. The remaining skeletons must be considered as a single commingled sample, not as individuals; for any given skeletal element, there are multiple bones of each incremental size. The adult and older child were identified separately in Angel's study of skeletal material from Attica and given the AA (Athens Agora) designation he used for bones from this site. He assigned number AA 24 to the adult and AA 25 to the child. All of the infant bones received a single number for the collection, AA 26.[5] In order to distinguish them from the mass of younger infants, the partial skeletons that have been identified as belonging to the two older infants are now designated AA 26a and AA 26b.

While the large number of infants is the distinguishing feature of this well, the two older individuals' burials, AA 24 and AA 25, deserve some consideration as well. It is unclear where they were located in the mass of bones, although, as noted earlier (p. 25), at least one probably rested near the top of the bone deposit, since the presence of human remains is mentioned early in the excavation of the well. It is not known what their relationship is, if any, to the infant burials. However, their presence in this unique assemblage must be addressed.

THE ADULT MALE (AA 24)

AA 24 is a nearly complete skeleton of an adult male. The bones are in an excellent state of preservation, although there has been some postmortem breakage. The bones are heavily stained with copper, and most of them are bright green in color. The antimicrobial properties of copper compounds may have contributed to the outstanding preservation of the bones, as did the constantly wet environmental conditions of the well. The individual is male, with clearly masculine features of the skull and pelvis.[6] The age at death is estimated at 45–55 years, based on the morphology of the preserved pubic symphysis and auricular surfaces of the pelvis.[7] The stature is

4. Angel 1945.
5. Angel 1945, p. 311.
6. Buikstra and Ubelaker 1994, pp. 16–21; Bass 1995, pp. 211–213.
7. Todd 1920, pp. 301–314; Lovejoy et al. 1985, pp. 22–26; Meindl et al. 1985, pp. 36–44.

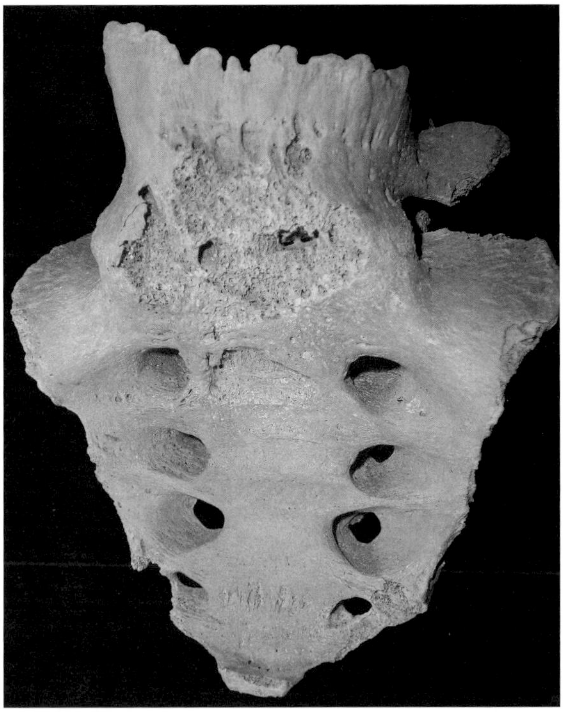

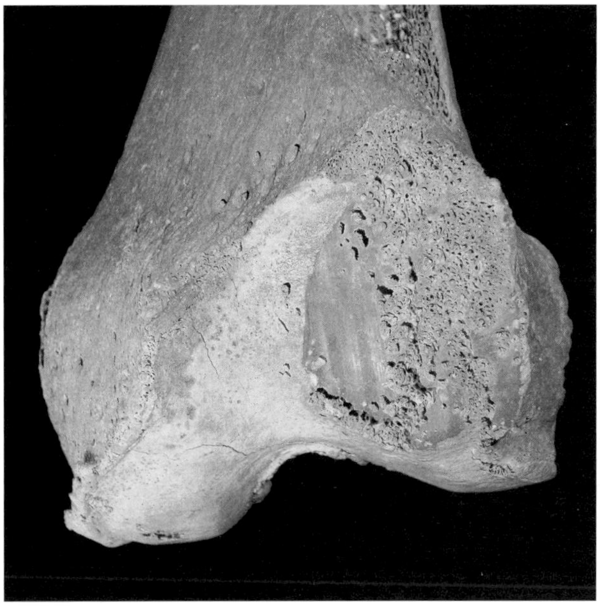

Figure 11 ***(left).*** **Sacrum of adult AA 24, showing fusion with fifth lumbar vertebra.** Scale 1:2. Photo M. A. Liston

Figure 12 ***(right).*** **Eburnation and pitting of joint surface of left femur of adult AA 24.** Not to scale. Photo M. A. Liston

estimated at 158 ± 3.27 cm, based on measurement of the complete right femur.[8] While many of his teeth were lost postmortem, those that remain are heavily worn, with complete loss of the enamel of the tooth crown, also supporting the evaluation of age as that of a mature adult. As also noted by Angel,[9] a small, circular, depressed fracture on the right frontal bone and fractured nasal bones, both healed, suggest an earlier episode (or episodes) of trauma, probably interpersonal conflict. The bones show well-developed muscle insertions, particularly in the arms and hands, indicating active use of major muscle groups despite the presence of debilitating arthritic lesions of the joints.

There are extensive pathological lesions on the joints found on both the axial and appendicular skeleton. The vertebrae, knees, elbows, and shoulders are particularly involved. Multiple vertebrae are affected. Extensive marginal syndesmophytes (bone spurs) have resulted in ankylosis (fusion) of the eighth and ninth thoracic vertebrae, and the fifth lumbar vertebra is fused to the sacrum (Fig. 11). In addition to bone proliferation around the joint capsules, there was also complete destruction of the joint cartilage, resulting in eburnation of the bone surfaces in the knees, elbows, and neck (Fig. 12). In the hands, the joints between the second and third metacarpals and their associated proximal phalanges have marginal osteophytes and eburnation, indicating bone-on-bone wear with complete loss of cartilage. The left thumb has osteophytes but no eburnation on the metacarpal. The right thumb was not recovered. It is unusual, given the severity of the lesions on the affected joints, that the hips and the other joints of the hands and feet, often sites of severe osteoarthritis, are relatively normal, with only slight to moderate changes typical of age-related degeneration. The pattern of joint involvement is important for a differential diagnosis of the pathologies.

8. Trotter and Gleser 1952, p. 483.
9. Angel 1945, p. 311.

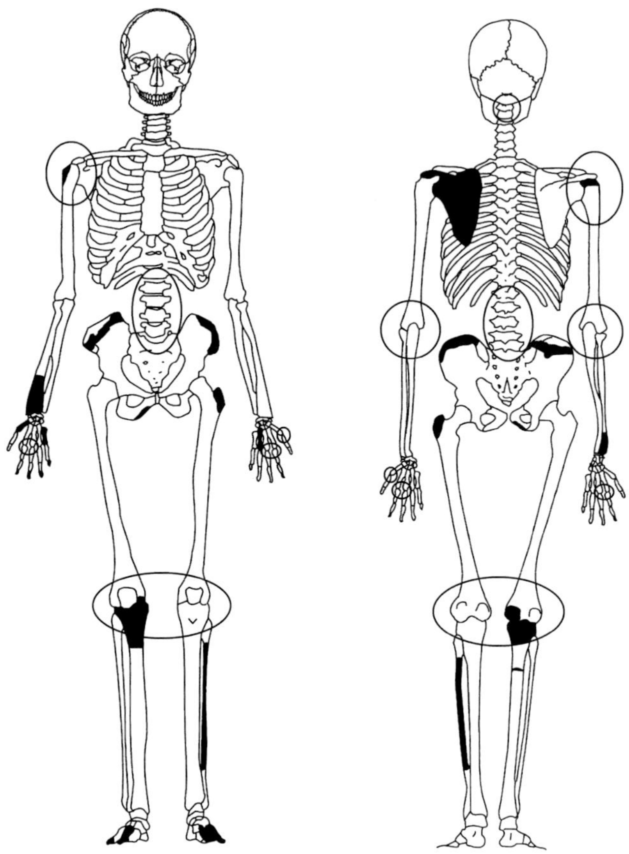

Figure 13. Joints affected by hemochromatosis in adult AA 24 (circled). Shaded areas are missing. Drawing M. A. Liston

In addition to the joint disease, this individual also appears to have suffered from some degree of osteopenia, or loss of bone mass. The bones of the arms in particular are quite light, and the humeri exhibit cortical thinning and unexpectedly diffuse trabecular bone visible at the broken surfaces. Radiographs confirm that the cortical bone in the humeri is quite thin, and the trabecular bone in the proximal humeri, femora, vertebral bodies, and innominates is markedly reduced from the normal pattern. While osteopenia is not unknown in males, it is unusual in an individual this young, as osteopenia and osteoporosis are generally confined to females over 50 years and much older ages among males.[10] The extensive bone loss and pattern of joint destruction suggests a precipitating pathology rather than age-related bone loss.

The differential diagnosis for this individual's skeletal pathologies is hereditary hemochromatosis. This is a genetic disease involving increased intestinal absorption of iron, resulting in a buildup of toxic levels of iron in the body. Hemochromatosis causes a variety of visceral and metabolic complications in adults, including diabetes, cirrhosis of the liver, skin pigmentation, cardiac failure, and multiple arthropathies. The skeletal effects of hemochromatosis are quite severe and widespread. They include arthritic changes of multiple joints, including spine, shoulders, knees, hands, and feet.[11]

The pattern of joints affected is often diagnostic of hemochromatosis and is quite obvious in skeletonized remains (Fig. 13). The most commonly involved joints are the first and second metacarpophalangeal joints, with

10. Parfitt 1998, pp. 360–361; Ortner 2003, pp. 410–411.

11. Jäger et al. 1997; Rihl and Kellner 2004, pp. 26–28.

the vertebrae, shoulders, knees, and feet also frequently affected. Normally other major weight-bearing joints, particularly the hips, are spared.[12] This is in sharp contrast to the pattern seen in common osteoarthritis, where the hips are frequently involved and the distal interphalangeal joints are more affected than the metacarpophalangeal joints.[13] In addition, osteopenia has been noted in modern clinical cases of hereditary hemochromatosis.[14] In individuals with hemochromatosis, the accumulation of toxic levels of iron begins in early adulthood and clinically significant symptoms usually begin in the fourth decade of life, increasing in severity over time. While both men and women may be affected, severe symptoms in women often are delayed until menopause, because of blood loss through menstruation and pregnancy.

AA 24, an adult male in his late 40s or early 50s with severe but unusually patterned joint disease and osteoporosis, fits the profile of an individual suffering from untreated hereditary hemochromatosis. The severe lesions on the second and third metacarpophalangeal joints, and the absence of lesions from most of the rest of the joints of the hands, are particularly diagnostic. Isolated arthropathy of these joints in the hands has been described as pathognomonic for hemochromatosis.[15] Osteoarthritis, diffuse ideopathic skeletal hyperostosis (DISH), pseudo-gout, gout, and other calcium pyrophosphate depositional diseases all may potentially have affected an adult male in this population.[16] The pattern of lesions, however, most closely resembles that seen in hemochromatosis, particularly considering the absence of involvement of the hip joint, the severe involvement of the second and third metacarpophalangeal joints, and the exclusion of most other joints of the hands.

Hereditary hemochromatosis is an autosomal recessive disease, and today is the most commonly identified genetic disease among Caucasians, affecting between 0.25% and 0.50% of individuals. In the past, it may have conveyed a selective advantage, with increased resistance to certain infections associated with excessive iron levels and possibly protection against coronary artery disease.[17] This would account for the high frequency of the disease, even though, when untreated, it results in severe disability and death, normally in older adults. Death normally results from liver cancer or heart failure.[18] Ironically, the modern clinical treatment for hemochromatosis is the traditional staple of ancient medicine, bleeding the patient.[19] Had this individual been bled regularly throughout his adult life, he would have avoided most or all of the symptoms exhibited on his skeletal remains.

12. Hirsch, Killien, and Troupin 1976; Lacombe 2004, p. 487; Franchini and Veneri 2005, pp. 348–349.

13. Ortner 2003, pp. 546–549.

14. Jäger et al. 1997, p. 1205.

15. Tassos Anastassiades, pers. comm. Our sincere thanks for his assistance and direction in identifying the specific disease process in this skeleton, and in particular for pointing out the significance of the pattern of joint involvement in the hands.

16. Rogers and Waldron 1995, pp. 32–54, 78–86; Ortner 2003, pp. 546–550.

17. Jäger et al. 1997, p. 1199; Franchini and Veneri 2005, pp. 347–349; Moalem, Weinberg, and Percy 2004, pp. 135–136, 138; Rihl and Kellner 2004, pp. 22–23.

18. Jäger et al. 1997, pp. 1200, 1205.

19. Franchini and Veneri 2005, pp. 350–351.

THE CHILD (AA 25)

AA 25 is the partial skeleton of a child. The bone is very heavily stained with copper and is very well preserved. While not all of the bones are present, there is no systematic exclusion of any portion of the body, suggesting that the missing bones are the result of incomplete recovery at excavation, not the secondary deposition of a partial skeleton into the well.

This child was about 8–10 years old at the time of death, based on the development of the dentition.[20] The skeletal age of the child is somewhat younger, 6.5–8.5 years, indicating that there were probably disruptions in growth and that the child was small for his/her age. There are multiple growth arrest lines (Harris lines) visible in radiographs of the long bones, confirming an interruption of growth during life.[21] The presence of extensive skeletal pathology suggests a chronic or long-term disease process. Evaluation of the preserved ilia suggests that this individual is probably male. Although determination of sex in children is particularly problematic,[22] the very narrow sciatic notch, lack of ventral arc, and depressed auricular joint surface of the ilium all would tentatively suggest a male child.

There is moderate *cribra orbitalia* in both eye orbits, also noted by Angel,[23] indicating an anemic condition; this was probably ongoing at the time of death, although there is evidence for remodeling in these lesions. The child also has evidence of marked bone pathology involving the vertebrae, scapulae, and cranium. The lesions on the vertebrae are lytic rounded foci in the vertebral bodies, with some active bony reaction on the margins visible grossly as thickened trabeculae as well as smooth margins around the openings into the anterior face of the vertebral bodies (Fig. 14). The lesions exhibit a range of size and involvement, progressing on subsequent vertebrae from enlargement of the normal foramina found in juvenile vertebrae to tunnels, and then to coalescing lesions that consume nearly the entire centrum. In two cases, the lesions perforate the superior and inferior surfaces of the centra as well. On the interior surface of the vertebral arches, there is a layer of rough, apparently reactive, bone, and in some cases extensive deposits of a layer of subperiosteal bone, all of which appear to have been actively forming at the time of death.

The endocranial surfaces in the skull also have extensive areas of periosteal bone deposits with no evidence of remodeling (Fig. 15). These are clearly visible because the bronze staining has affected the disorganized bone quite differently from the normal bone surfaces. These deposits are found on all seven major bones of the cranial vault. The only other areas on the preserved skeleton that exhibit a pathological process are the scapular spines. Here there is bilateral evidence of a periosteal reaction extending from the dorsal surface of the acromial process laterally down the scapular spine. In places there is a clear sheet of remodeled periosteal bone now separating from the underlying surface. Here again, the process appears to have been active at the time of death, and there is little or no evidence of remodeling.

The differential diagnosis for this skeleton is difficult. Tuberculosis must be considered, but while tuberculosis was unquestionably present in the Mediterranean by the Bronze Age and Galen clearly describes the disease,

20. Angel 1945, p. 311; Ubelaker 1989, pp. 63–65.
21. Aufderheide and Rodríguez-Martín 1998, pp. 422–424.
22. Weaver 1980, p. 191.
23. Angel 1945, p. 311.

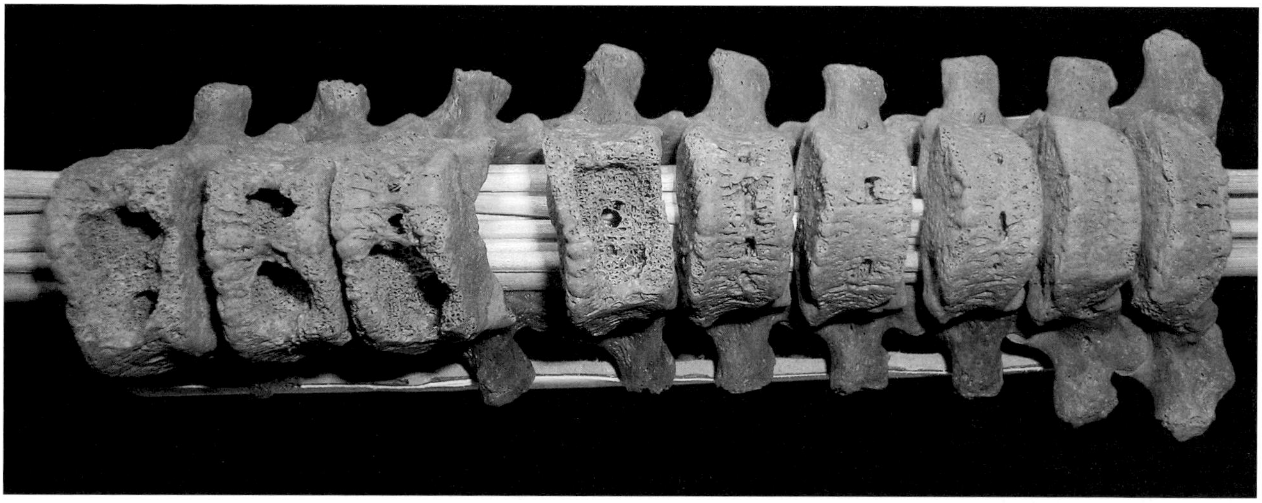

Figure 14. Vertebrae of child AA 25.
Scale 1:1. Photo M. A. Liston

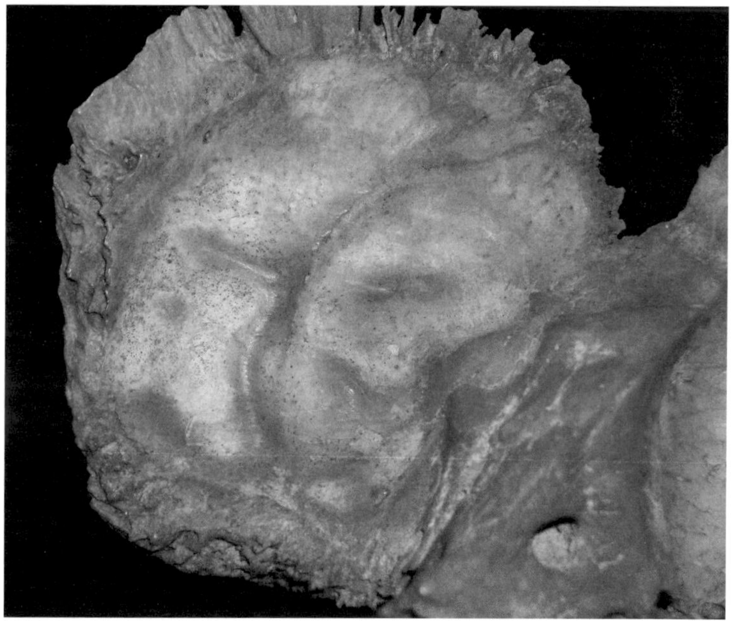

Figure 15. Endocranial surfaces of the skull of child AA 25, with extensive areas of periosteal bone deposits.
Not to scale. Photo M. A. Liston

there is limited skeletal evidence in Greece and no definitive cases have been identified.[24] Despite the extensive vertebral lesions, there is no evidence of vertebral collapse in this child, even in the most severely affected vertebrae, yet this is typical of tuberculosis. Together with the presence of inflammatory bone on the vertebral arches, which is not seen in tuberculosis, this largely eliminates tuberculosis as a possible causative factor. The absence of lytic foci on other bones is also a confounding factor. Fungal infections have been documented much more rarely in the Old World than the New World but can produce the extensive vertebral destruction without collapse seen here.[25] Finally, the hollowed lesions and coarsened vertical trabeculae of the vertebral bodies suggest one of the benign vascular tumors, including hemangioma or lymphangioma,[26] but this would not produce the new bone formation in the skull and scapulae.

24. Roberts and Buikstra 2003, pp. 170–171.
25. Ortner 2003, pp. 228–231, 326–327.
26. Resnick 1995, vol. 6, pp. 3821, 3823, 3830.

In the Greek environment, the most likely disease to have produced these lesions in the child is brucellosis. This disease is a zoonosis, carried normally by goats *(Brucella melitensis)* and cattle *(Brucella abortus)*. There are other species of *Brucella,* but these are the ones most commonly transmitted to humans, generally through the handling and consumption of raw meat and milk products. The disease causes systemic infection that can affect any organ system, and skeletal involvement is common, occurring in as many as 40% of cases. It affects the spine and sacroiliac joints, and complications include inflammation of the meninges, which could result in endocranial lesions. The lesions on the vertebrae of this child are remarkably similar to those found on a child's skeleton from Butrint, Albania; DNA from *Brucella abortus* was identified in these remains.[27] It is also possible, of course, that the child suffered from more than one infection, which produced the unusual distribution of lytic and reactive bone lesions.[28]

THE OLDER INFANTS

AA 26A

The oldest of the infant skeletons, AA 26a, consists of both a partial cranium and partial postcranial skeleton. Although association of the disarticulated skeletal elements is difficult, a mandible and partial skeleton appear to be associated with the partial cranium on the basis of the developmental stage and the degree of green staining from the bronze in the well. Both the skull and skeleton are distinctly larger than those of the other infants in the well, and there is no duplication of elements that would indicate more than one individual. Most of the major limb bones are represented on one side or the other, and there are some ribs, vertebrae, and other elements.

The preserved teeth in the mandible suggest that this infant died at around 16–18 months of age. The length of the long bone diaphyses, however, suggest that it died at 6–12 months.[29] Tooth development is less subject to environmental influence, and therefore the dental age is more likely to approximate actual chronological age.[30] The discrepancy between dental age and skeletal age suggests the child's growth was delayed, either by disease or by inadequate care or nutrition.[31]

Infant AA 26a has an array of traumatic injuries, some healed, some healing, and some perimortem fractures, which would be consistent with a case of Battered Child Syndrome. The most obvious injury is an antemortem fracture located on the posterior right parietal, adjacent to the lambdoidal suture (Figs. 16, 17). The injury consists of four stellate fracture lines ema-

27. Mutolo et al. 2012, pp. 258, 261, figs. 2, 5.

28. Young 1995, pp. 284–285; Ghosh, Gupta, and Prabhakar 1999, p. 59; Kochar et al. 2000, pp. 171–172; Mutolo et al. 2012, p. 256.

29. Scheuer and Black 2000, pp. 158–161.

30. Liston 2017, p. 522.

31. Lewis 2007, pp. 1017–1018.

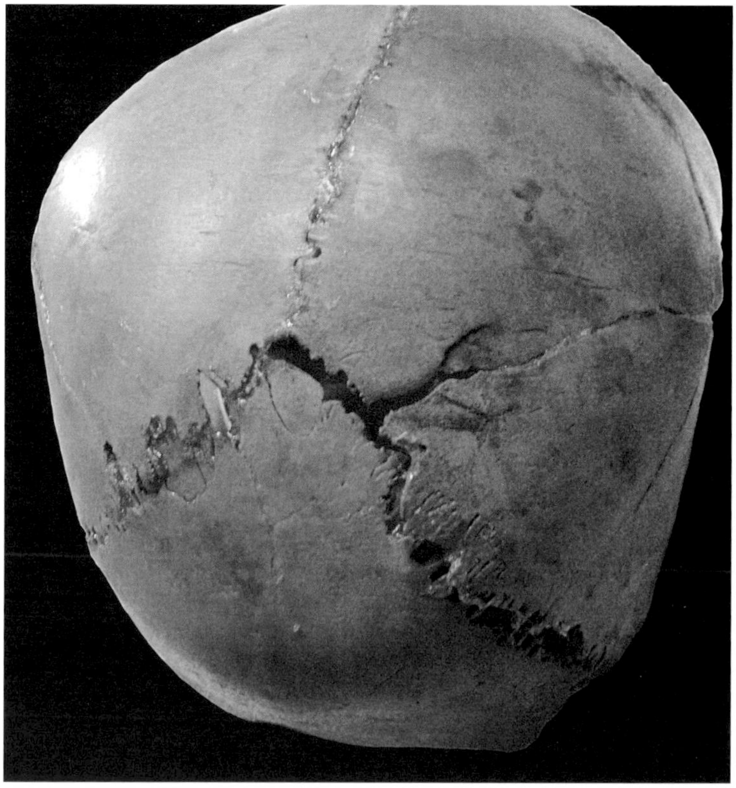

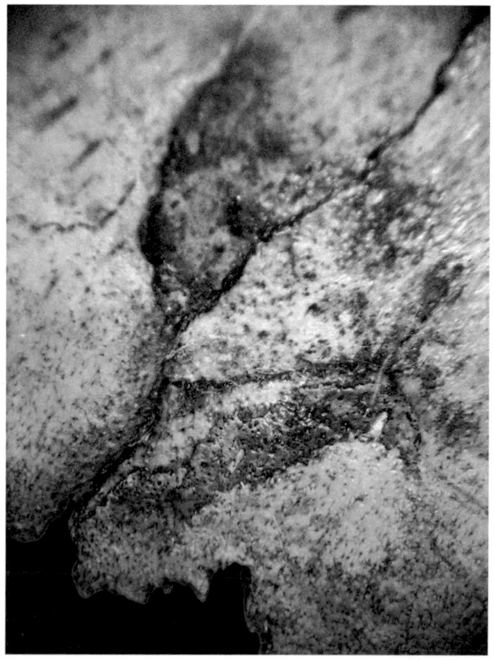

Figure 16 *(left)*. **Antemortem fracture on the posterior right parietal of infant AA 26a.** Not to scale. Photo M. A. Liston

Figure 17 *(right)*. **Detail of the fracture on the skull of infant AA 26a.** Not to scale. Photo M. A. Liston

nating from a focused central point of impact. Stellate fractures normally are the result of low-velocity impact with heavy objects, producing strong in-bending of the cranial bones and fracture lines radiating outward from a focused point of impact.[32] The presence of grossly visible periosteal bone indicates the child survived for at least 4–5 days, but the absence of evidence for callus formation at the fracture indicates death probably occurred within 12–21 days of the injury.[33] Fatalities from cranial injuries following a lengthy period of lucid consciousness have been documented in falls of as little as 0.60 m in infants and children, but the child also may have had an impaired level of consciousness for periods following the injury.[34] Despite the lengthy post-injury period, the fracture may have contributed to the death of the infant.

The exact cause of this injury cannot be identified with certainty. The infant was old enough to have begun to walk, which increases the risk of head injury. It also could have rolled or fallen off of a surface, striking its head. The injury also could have resulted from the child accidentally striking an object when dropped, or from a deliberate impact. The location of this injury, on the back quarter of the skull, does not rule out any of these possibilities, although stellate fractures such as those seen on this infant's skull are most likely to occur from deliberate blows to the head.[35]

Further examination of the postcranial bones suggested a more ominous pattern of injury beyond this fracture. There are three healed rib fractures near the sternal (anterior) end of the ribs on the anterio-lateral area of the

32. Walker, Cook, and Lambert 1997, pp. 196–197; Galloway 1999, pp. 68–69.
33. Prosser et al. 2012, p. 1014.
34. Plunkett 2001, pp. 1–2.
35. Hobbs 1989.

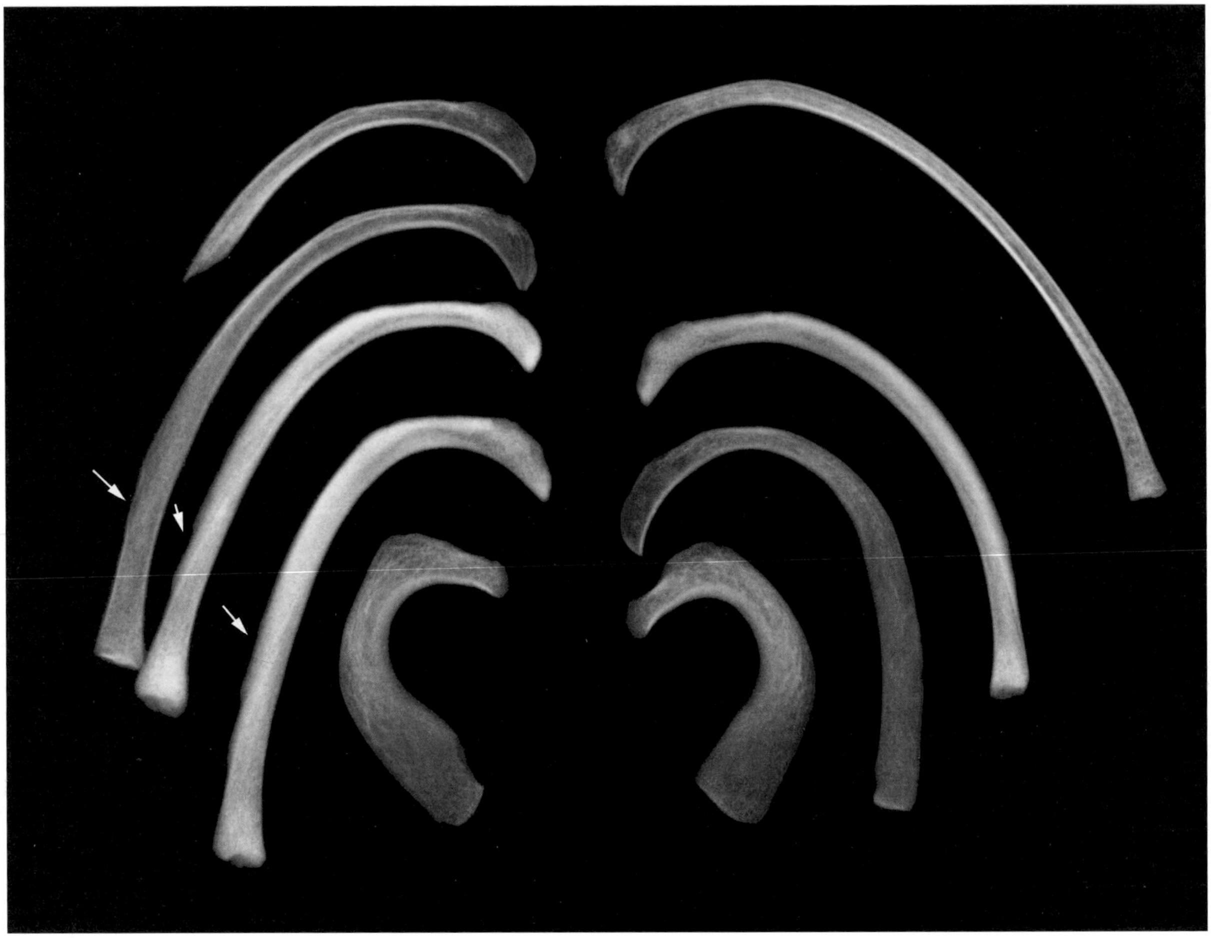

Figure 18. Radiograph of the ribs of infant AA 26a, with sites of fractures indicated. Not to scale. Radiograph S. Fox

rib cage. Two are grossly visible on the ribs, and the third was revealed in a radiograph. The fractures are in the same location on three adjacent ribs, probably on ribs 5, 6, and 7 or 8. These fractures are well healed and remodeled, with minimal distortion of the rib morphology. The degree of healing and remodeling indicated in radiographs of the bone (Fig. 18) would probably have required at least 12 months, indicating that the injuries took place early in the child's life.[36] Rib fractures can occasionally occur accidentally in infants under one year old, but a review of multiple clinical studies found that multiple fractures are more common after abuse than other trauma and that rib fractures were strongly associated with abuse,[37] suggesting that the cranial fracture was not the first non-accidental trauma this infant had endured.

More subtle signs of abuse are found on the mandible, the humeri, and the single right femur. There are extensive areas of periosteal bone formation. This is new bone that forms when the periosteal membrane surrounding the bone is bruised or separated from the bone, usually by impacts, violent squeezing, or twisting of the limbs.[38] On the mandible, there is an area of new periosteal bone on the exterior right surface of the body and ramus, suggesting the child may have been hit on the side of the

36. Prosser et al. 2012, p. 1015.
37. Kemp et al. 2008, p. 5.
38. Greenguard 1964.

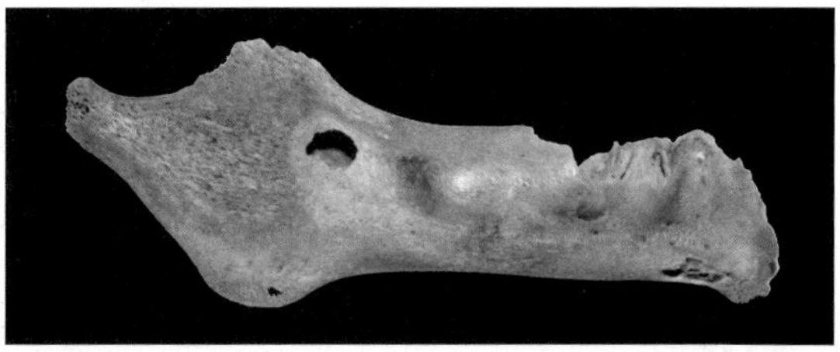

Figure 19. Right half of mandible of infant AA 26a, showing areas of new periosteal bone on the lateral surface. Scale 1:1. Photo M. A. Liston

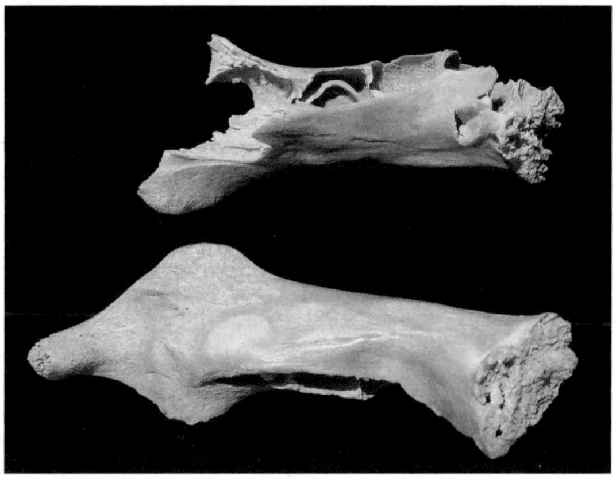

Figure 20. Left and right halves of mandible of infant AA 26a, showing the perimortem fracture at the midline. Scale 1:1. Photo M. A. Liston

face at some point not long before death (Fig. 19). While there are diseases that can cause periosteal reactions on the limb bones, the deposits of bone are normally symmetrical. On this infant, periosteal bone deposits formed on the left and right humeri; these are asymmetrical and irregular, which is consistent with abusive trauma.[39] In addition, the periosteal bone on the humeri and femur shows differing degrees of development and remodeling, indicating the injuries took place at different times, all of which suggests repeated trauma.

There are also fractures that probably occurred in the perimortem interval, no more than 4–5 days before death. The bone around the fractures has bent and splintered, but there is no evidence of healing, which can appear in as little as 4–5 days in infants and young children.[40] There is a perimortem complete fracture of the mandible (Fig. 20). The bone is separated into two parts, at the midline, and then continues through the posterior portion of the crypt for the developing central incisor. In a child of this age, the two halves of the mandible, which forms as two bones, would normally have been fused together. The fracture through the fused symphysis is unlikely to have occurred accidentally. On the left distal humerus there is also a possible corner fracture, an injury often caused by violent twisting of an infant's lower limbs that causes the cartilage of the epiphysis to tear away from the bone shaft, fracturing the immature bone forming at the metaphysis (Fig. 21).[41]

The analysis of this infant's skeleton suggests repeated trauma over much of the child's life. The pattern of multiple traumatic injuries with differing degrees of healing indicates that this infant is a victim of Battered

39. Walker, Cook, and Lambert 1997, p. 204.
40. Prosser et al. 2012, p. 1014.
41. Walker, Cook, and Lambert 1997, p. 203.

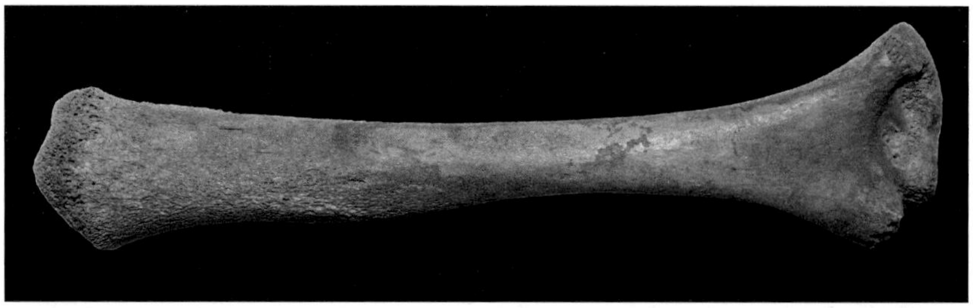

Figure 21. Possible corner fracture on the left distal humerus of infant AA 26a. Scale 1:1. Photo M. A. Liston

Child Syndrome.[42] Child abuse is recognized in the literature of Greek and broader Mediterranean antiquity. Although identified all too commonly in the modern world, and described in the literature of many cultures, the paucity of archaeological cases of abused children has led some scholars to speculate that physical abuse is a modern phenomenon.[43] Another case of a battered child has been identified in a toddler from the Romano-Christian Kellis 2 cemetery in Egypt.[44] However, the infant from the Agora Bone Well is the earliest case of child abuse reported thus far from the archaeological record worldwide.

AA 26b

AA 26b is the second of the two oldest infants in the collection. Unlike the abused infant, AA 26a, this individual's survival beyond birth indicates that considerable effort was put into supporting and caring for a child who would have become increasingly debilitated. The absence of any dental remains or clearly associated long bones prevents an exact estimate of age. However, the infant is well past the perinatal period, because the diploë, the spongy erythropoietic bone between the inner and outer tables of the skull, is well developed. There is little or no data on the timing of the appearance of the diploë, but it occurs well into the postnatal period.[45] The general level of maturity of the bone and the degree of suture formation between the bones suggests the child was perhaps six to eight months old at death.[46] Significant pathology in this cranium prevents the use of metric estimations of age.

The infant suffered from hydrocephalus, the accumulation of cerebrospinal fluid in the cranial space. This can be associated with a number of different diseases and developmental defects, and so is a symptom, not a diagnosis of a particular disease. A number of characteristics of the skull point to the identification of hydrocephalus. The sagittal fontanelle, which normally is obliterated at birth, is patent and clearly defined by the preserved right sagittal suture. The anterior and posterior fontanelles at the top of the forehead (at the bregma) and at the back of the skull (at the lambda) are also patent, with wide gaps of nearly 2 cm between the bones (Fig. 22). These gaps normally are completely closed by two years of age, and such large openings are typical only of infants less than six months of age; they should not be so wide in a child with otherwise well-developed closed cranial sutures.

In addition to the open fontanelles, the cranial bones are expanded and show signs of rapid abnormal growth. There are multiple vascular grooves on

42. Greenguard 1964.
43. Walker, Cook, and Lambert 1997. Waldron (2000, pp. 31–34) comments on other reasons why the syndrome is so rarely detected in archaeological specimens.
44. Wheeler et al. 2007, 2013.
45. Scheuer and Black 2004, p. 104.
46. Sim, Yoon, and Kim 2012, p. 33.

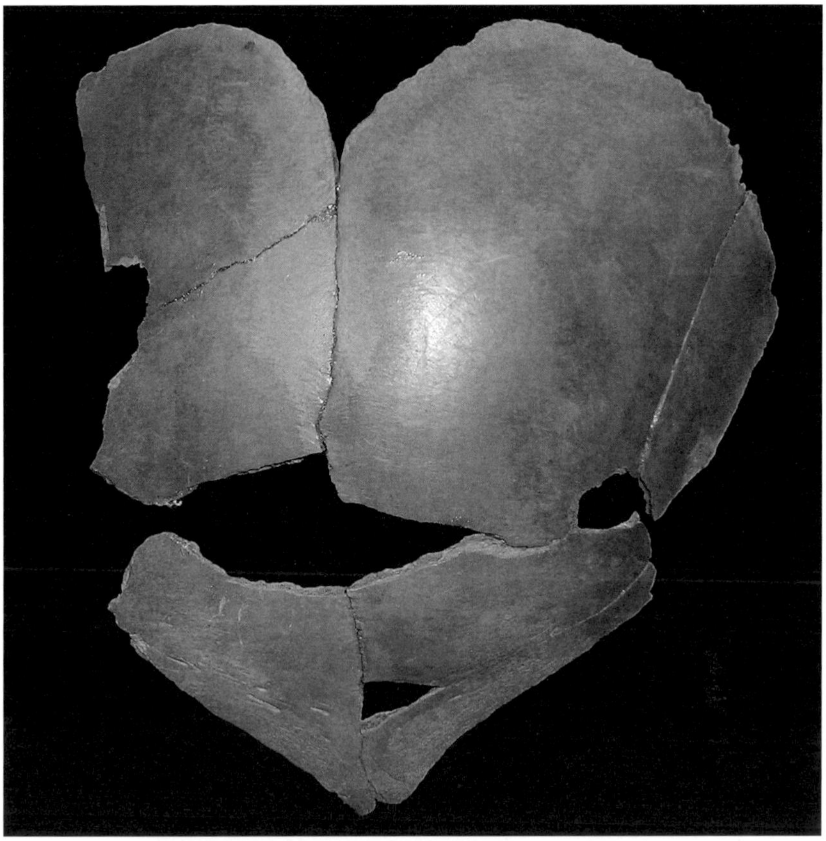

Figure 22. Anterior fontanelle of infant AA 26b. Note the V-shaped gap at the top of the bone. Scale 1:1. Photo M. A. Liston

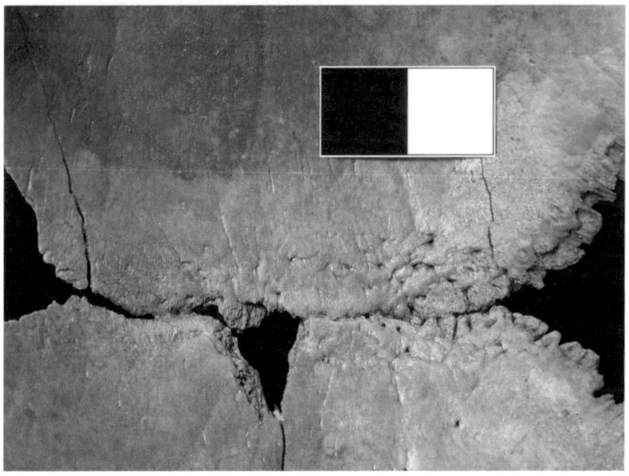

Figure 23. Endocranial surface of the skull of infant AA 26b. Scale 1:1. Photo M. A. Liston

the exterior surface of the frontal and parietal bones. There is disorganized woven bone, resembling periosteal bone deposits, on the posterior parietals and occipital fragments. On the endocranial surface, the bone adjacent to the cranial sutures is rough and irregular for a distance of about 1 cm from the coronal, sagittal, and lambdoidal sutures (Fig. 23). The bone appears to be rapidly formed and lacks the normal smooth inner surface. The normal overlap of the squamosal suture, between the parietal and temporal bones, is distorted on the right side, with the parietal bone extending outside of the temporal bone, instead of the normal pattern, with the temporal squama overlying the parietal. Although the vault is incomplete, the overall size of the reconstructed cranium is approximately that of a four-year-old child, which would be much older than the age that the other features suggest for this child. The upper surface of the preserved left eye orbit is also deflected downward approximately 30 degrees. This would force the globe of the eyeball downward in what is termed "setting-sun sign," where the iris and pupil are partially obscured by the lower eyelid, and a broad extent of the white sclera would be visible.

All of these features suggest an oversized and rapidly expanding cranial vault. This indicates an abnormally increased volume in the cranium, most often caused by an increase in the volume of cerebrospinal fluid, the condition known as hydrocephalus. The indication of "setting-sun sign" in the eye orbit is almost pathognomonic for hydrocephalus. Although not unknown in antiquity, the condition is rare.[47] Congenital hydrocephalus occurs in three to four infants per 1,000 live births. Most commonly, neonatal hydrocephalus is caused by defects in the structure of the brain and associated ventricles or intrauterine infections. It can also develop after birth due to perinatal infections or trauma. In older infants, it can develop following hemorrhage and viral or bacterial meningitis.[48] The skeletal results would be similar regardless of the underlying cause, making it impossible to determine why the infant developed the condition. What is clear is that the child was cared for during a period when it would have become progressively more debilitated and more disturbing in appearance. Infants with hydrocephalus, in addition to having a rapidly expanding braincase that is disproportionate when compared to the face and body, also exhibit increasingly severe developmental and motor delays and dysfunction. Infants may fail to develop mature reflexes, and spasticity of the limbs, particularly the legs, may arise. Lethargy, vomiting, seizures, difficulty with swallowing, and respiratory distress may also occur.[49] In order for this child to have survived the condition long enough for the changes to the cranium to have occurred, it would have required increasingly more attention from its caregivers, although after death, burial in the well was accomplished with little investment of effort or cost.

THE YOUNGER INFANTS (AA 26)

The bulk of the human bones that make this well so unusual consists of a mass of commingled remains of infants and fetuses. A total of 13,018 individual infant and fetal bones have been identified in the collection. These include not only the large cranial and long bones, but many smaller elements, including hand and foot phalanges less than 2 mm in length (Table 1). Although small elements are present in much smaller numbers, it is clear that the recovery process did not systematically exclude small bones and that the smaller skeletal elements were present in the well at the time of excavation. There is no evidence of environmental weathering, carnivore gnawing, extensive postmortem breakage, or other indications that the bones were previously buried elsewhere or exposed above ground before being deposited in the well.[50] These factors indicate that most, if not all, of the skeletons found in this deposit entered the well as intact bodies of infants and fetuses.

47. Richards and Anton 1991, pp. 185–187; Tillier et al. 2001, p. 166.
48. Bouterie 2004, pp. 577–578.
49. Bouterie 2004, p. 578.
50. Lyman 1994, pp. 363–365.

TABLE 1. SKELETAL ELEMENTS OF THE YOUNGER INFANTS

Skeletal Element	*Right*	*Left*	*Middle/ Unsided*	*Total*
Frontal squama	202	234	76	512
Parietal	–	–	3,196	3,196
Temporal squama	142	104	–	246
Temporal petrous	131	101	–	232
Occipital squama	–	–	313	313
Occipital lateral	69	60	–	129
Occipital basilar	–	–	5	5
Sphenoid wing	6	–	–	6
Sphenoid body	–	–	12	12
Palatine	–	–	14	14
Maxilla	89	75	–	164
Zygomatic	–	7	–	7
Mandible	–	–	192	192
Rib 1	79	71	–	150
Rib 2–12	–	–	1,869	1,869
Vertebra, centrum	–	–	22	22
Vertebra, hemi-arch	–	–	557	557
Scapula	211	208	–	419
Clavicle	180	145	–	325
Ilium	167	166	–	333
Ischium	12	12	–	24
Pubis	8	12	–	20
Humerus	416	413	–	829
Ulna	299	293	–	592
Radius	256	274	–	530
Femur	459	454	–	913
Tibia	412	409	–	821
Fibula	229	235	74	538
Metacarpal/tarsal	–	–	36	36
Phalanges	–	–	12	12
Total	*3,367*	*3,273*	*6,378*	*13,018*

The number of infants was initially estimated by Angel to be about 175, based on his count of 155 pairs of scapulae.[51] He later noted that he had measured 380 femora, but without any comment on the number of infants represented.[52] In his 1945 article, he published a photograph of the scapulae, although only 95 left and 94 right bones are depicted in it.[53] The number of complete scapulae found bagged together at the beginning of this project corresponds well with Angel's original count. However, after sorting all of the mixed animal and human bones, a complete count of all identifiable

51. Angel 1945, pp. 311–312. On p. 311, n. 73, Angel notes, "The human infant bones and fairly complete skulls of about 100 dogs are in good preservation, and a statistical study of each will be of interest to anthropologist, mammalogist, or dog-breeder."

52. Angel 1971, p. 92, table 9.

53. Angel 1945, p. 312, fig. 12.

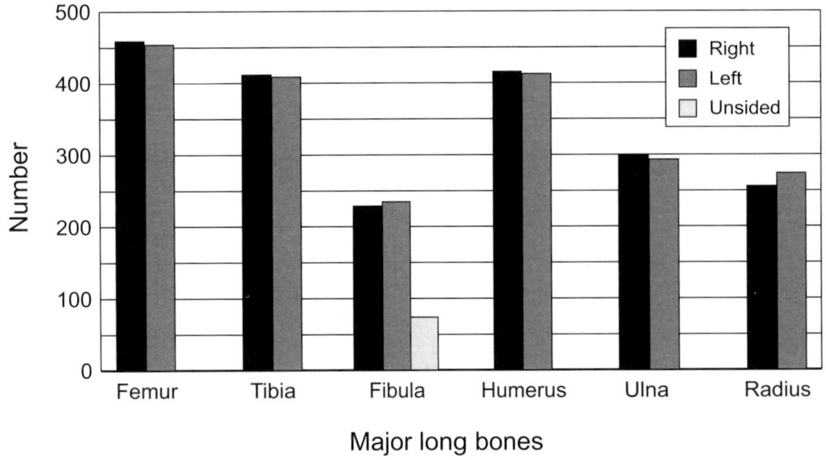

Figure 24. Counts for the major long bones of the infants

infant and fetal bones represented in the collection today yields a minimum number of individuals (MNI) of 459 based on the most common element, the complete and partial right femora. The actual number of individuals may be somewhat greater, but around 460 is a reasonable estimate of the approximate number of infants in the well. This number does not include the adult and older child, but does include three or four postnatal infants, two of whom are discussed above as AA 26a and AA 26b. The other older infants are represented by only a few cranial and long bones, and have no identifiable pathologies.

The right femur is the most frequently occurring bone in the collection, but the other long bones also are present in large quantities. The femur, tibia, and humerus, the largest of the fetal long bones, are represented in the greatest numbers. Smaller bones including the radius and ulna were recovered at a lower frequency. Counts for the major long bones are shown in Figure 24.

Cranial bones are also well represented, with over 5,000 identifiable pieces more than 1 cm in diameter (Fig. 25). Fragments small enough to pass through a 1 cm screen were not included in the count of cranial bones, nor were they included in the evaluation of pathologies.

The left and right frontal bones are the most common cranial elements, with 436 fragments that could be assigned to the right or left side. In addition, there are 3,196 fragments of the parietal squamae. Almost none of these could be assigned to the right or left side. The cranial bones as a whole make up approximately 50% of the infant bone assemblage by volume, but in no case did the count of uniquely identifiable cranial elements exceed the MNI count of 459 based on the right femora.

Age at Death

Age was estimated from measurements[54] of the diaphyseal length of the right femur and left humerus, the two most frequently occurring long bones (Fig. 26).[55] With the exception of the four older infants noted above, traditional regression estimates of age based on long-bone length indicate that most of the baby bones designated AA 26 correspond in

54. Measurements of the femora and humeri were also taken by L. M. Little in an early phase of this project, and we thank her for making her data available for the initial studies of the skeletons. All measurements presented in this volume were taken by Liston.

55. Fazekas and Kósa 1978, pp. 257–264; Scheuer and Black 2000, pp. 288–289, 297–299, 307–308, 394, 415–416, 425–426.

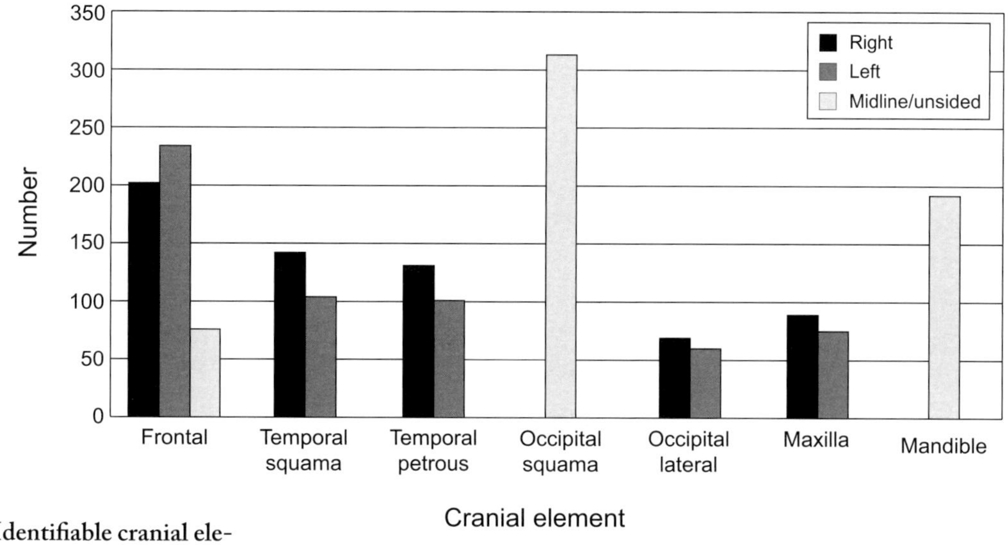

Figure 25. Identifiable cranial elements of the younger infants

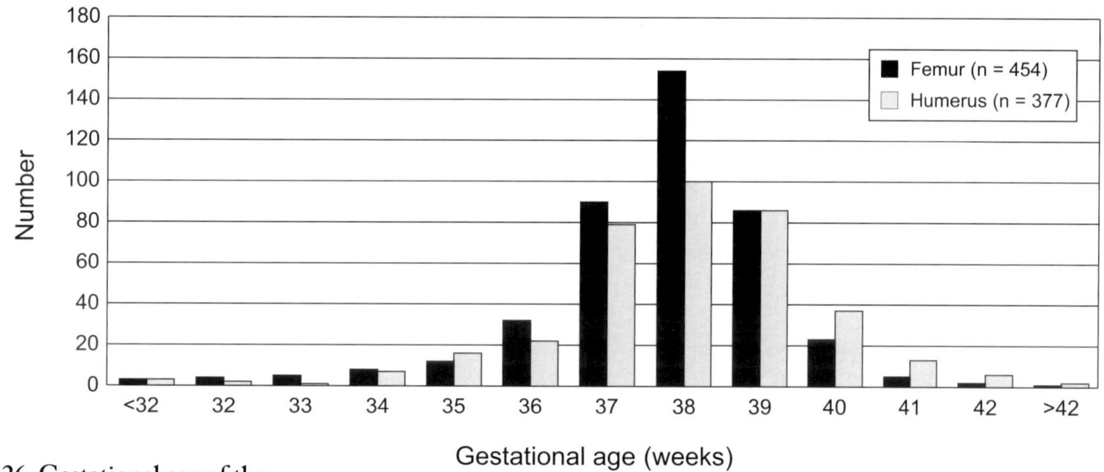

Figure 26. Gestational age of the younger infants at death, estimated from simple regression on the length of the right femur and left humerus

size to modern fetal and infant skeletons ranging in age from 30 weeks *in utero* to 42 weeks, or slightly more than full term (normally 40 weeks). There are a few outliers at each end of the age range. There are at least two very small fetuses, about 23–26 weeks *in utero*. There is also a larger infant whose skeletal age is about 47 weeks, or seven weeks after full-term birth.

There has been considerable debate in recent years concerning techniques for estimating fetal and infant age from long-bone lengths and the interpretation of mortality profiles. The use of simple regression to estimate age from long-bone lengths[56] has been challenged.[57] A more nuanced estimation of age at death in the perinatal infants can be accomplished using multifractional polynomial regression to regress femur length on age in weeks.[58] This can be compared to the age distributions of infants of the Native American Arikara tribe of the Great Plains area of the western United States. Since there is no evidence that the Arikara ever practiced infanticide in the historic or prehistoric periods, they can be used to model

56. Such as Scheuer, Musgrave, and Evans 1980, pp. 258–261; Scheuer and Black 2000, pp. 9–10, 28, 394; Sherwood et al. 2000.

57. Bocquet-Appel and Masset 1982; Konigsberg and Frankenberg 1992, pp. 238–239; Gowland and Chamberlain 2002, pp. 677–678; Lewis 2007, pp. 43–44.

58. Konigsberg and Liston 2013.

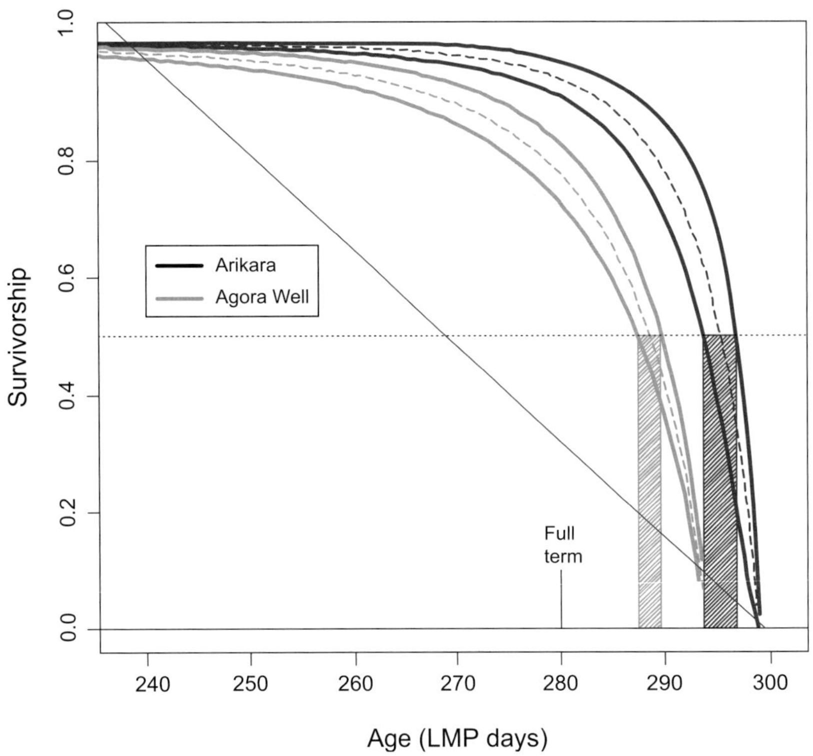

Figure 27. Age at death of Arikara infants and of the younger infants in the Agora Bone Well, in days from the last menstrual period, estimated by multifractional polynomial regression. L. Konigsberg

natural infant mortality distributions.[59] Using a skew-exponential power distribution, the model that best fits the Agora infant data indicates a median age at death at one week postpartum, and a 95% confidence interval of 8–10 days around the expected full-term birth at 280 days. These data closely mirror the Arikara patterns, although the median age at death was slightly higher among the Arikara (Fig. 27). These more precise data indicate that, except for the obviously older babies, nearly all of the Agora infants in this well died before the age of eight days.

It is clear that most of the infants in the well died at or near the end of a full-term pregnancy. Birth is a period of considerable stress, both from the actual process and because of the rapid adjustments required in the transition from the fetal environment to that of an independent organism.[60] As a result, birth is associated with elevated mortality in any population, and the presence in the Agora Bone Well of large numbers of infants who died at or shortly after birth does not require explanation by external mechanisms such as epidemic, famine, or infanticide.[61]

Identification of Sex

The determination of sex from the bones of non-adults has long been problematic. While there have been numerous attempts to develop morphological and metric methods of estimating sex, they have been hampered by the scarcity and small size of collections with known-sex children's skeletons. However, there is accumulating data indicating that there is a suite of sexually dimorphic features on the ilium, the largest of the three bones that make up the juvenile os coxa, and one that is markedly sexually

59. Owsley and Jantz 1985, pp. 321–323.
60. Lewis 2007, pp. 81–82.
61. Storey 1986, pp. 545–546.

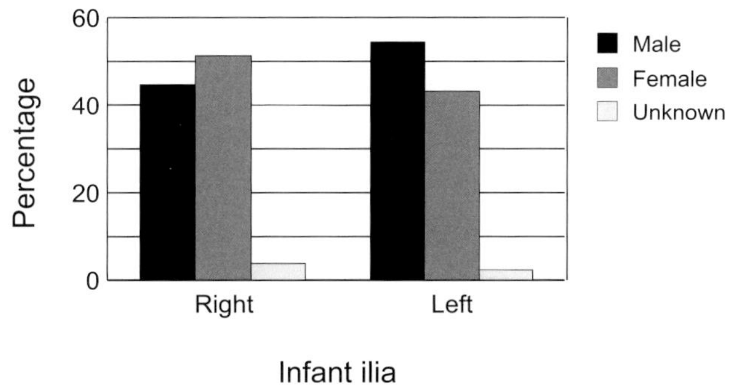

Figure 28. Distribution by sex of right and left infant ilia

dimorphic in adults. The features are most apparent on young infants but tend to be obscured by size increases in the ilia of older children.[62] Applied to individuals of known sex, these techniques have reliably identified sex in up to 100% of some forensic samples, including infants less than 0.1 years of age.[63] This suggests that morphological sex determination may be possible in samples of perinatal infants such as those found in the Agora well.

The infants in the Agora collection were evaluated using the morphology of the ilium, including the curvature of the iliac crest, the depth and angle of the sciatic notch, the "arch" criterion, which evaluates the relative positions of the sciatic notch and the auricular surface, and the elevation of the auricular surface.[64] The study was based on the 321 ilia sufficiently preserved for evaluation; a sample of the collection was also tested by two other researchers using a double-blind test.[65] The results (Fig. 28) suggest that the sex distribution is nearly equal, but with slightly more males, as would be expected in natural perinatal deaths; at all stages of development from conception through childhood, males suffer from slightly elevated mortality.[66]

The extraction and analysis of ancient DNA offer some hope for conclusively identifying sex in very young infant skeletons, but recent attempts to isolate DNA from the skeletons of Roman-period infants at Ashkelon and sites in Britain yielded results in less than 50% of the subset of bones sampled, although less than 20% of the individuals were tested.[67] The need to destroy bone in order to extract DNA is a further factor discouraging the widespread use of this technique. The chance of cross-contamination of the samples in the fetid mixture of organic material that was produced by placing over 450 bodies below the waterline[68] in the well leaves grave doubts as to the reliability of DNA testing in this sample even if it were attempted. For these reasons, we have chosen not to request permits for destructive sampling of the remains in this collection.

62. Lewis 2007, p. 51.

63. Weaver 1980, p. 195; Schutkowski 1987, pp. 350–351; 1993, pp. 203–204.

64. Weaver 1980, pp. 192–193; Mittler and Sheridan 1992; Schutkowski 1993, pp. 200–201; Wilson, MacLeod, and Humphrey 2008, pp. 270–272.

65. These were L. M. Snyder, the zooarchaeolgist on this project, and S. Fox, then director of the Wiener Laboratory. Their results corresponded closely to those of Liston on the same subsample.

66. World Health Organization 2006, p. 22.

67. Faerman et al. 1998, p. 863; Mays and Faerman 2001, p. 556.

68. Whatever the water level in the well at the time of the deposit, it was above the level of the bones at the time of excavation and probably had been so for many centuries. The remarkably good preservation of the organic remains indicates that they were in a constantly stable and probably oxygen-depleted environment.

Pathology and Cause of Death

Infant bone is notoriously difficult to study; the bones lack many of the characteristics that aid in the interpretation of more mature specimens. Much of what is ossified bone tissue in an adult or older child remains cartilage in infants and fetuses, and therefore does not survive in the archaeological specimens. In addition, normal rapidly growing bone in infants strongly resembles pathological rapidly growing bone to such a degree that many earlier studies have chosen not to evaluate pathologies on infant bone. In recent years, however, a number of scholars have begun to address the problems of pathology in infant and child bone, and have demonstrated the value of such work in evaluating morbidity and mortality in non-adult skeletons.

Premature Birth and Low Birth Weight

A normal pregnancy is calculated as 40 weeks (280 days) from the mother's last menstrual period. While the majority of the infants in the Agora Bone Well died at or near full-term size, approximately 34% were born preterm. Thirty-four percent of the femora and 34% of the humeri that could be measured correspond to the size of infants of 37 weeks gestation or less, a standard definition for preterm birth.[69] The presence of these skeletons in the well is probably the result of either fetal deaths or premature births, babies born too young to survive in antiquity. It is not possible to determine how many were stillborn, that is, born dead after 28 weeks *in utero*.[70]

Premature birth, both induced and unavoidable, is documented in the literature of ancient Greece. While numerous ancient authors argue that a child could safely be born in the seventh month,[71] this appears to have been a philosophical argument relying on the importance of cycles of seven days and months rather than a practical observation of fetal development.[72] In reality, birth at less than 37–38 postmenstrual gestational weeks would often have been incompatible with the survival of the infant. While many of these infants would survive today with medical support, in ancient Athens most if not all of them would have died from complications associated with their immature developmental state.[73]

Specific complications of preterm birth include an inability to nurse and swallow adequately due to central nervous system deficiency, intracranial hemorrhaging, and infection, which causes sepsis and meningitis four times more often in premature infants than full-term infants. A lack of body fat and ineffective thermoregulation would have further jeopardized a premature infant's chances of survival, particularly if born in either winter or the hottest portions of the summer.[74]

The frequency distribution of age at death, with its clear peak at 37–39 gestational weeks, also raises questions about the general health of the population that produced these babies. This peak falls slightly short of the normal 40-week gestation period; assuming that this peak represents the expected spike in births of newborns (that is, that these are full-term births),[75] a large proportion of the infants were small for their gestational age. Of course, our gestational-age estimates for the skeletal remains from the Agora Bone Well are based solely on the length of the femur and humerus, not an actual evaluation of development or time from conception, for

69. Beers and Berkow 1999, p. 2127.

70. Lewis 2007, p. 2.

71. Empedocles A75 [Diels-Kranz]; Hippocrates, *On Fleshes* 19 [Littré VIII.612–613]; Soranus, *Gyn.* 2.6.10; Censorinus, *DN* 11.2. References to Soranus follow the numbering in Temkin 1956.

72. Jouanna 1999, p. 122. See Parker 1999 for an exhaustive survey of this topic.

73. Little 1999 suggested that nearly all of the infants were viable, but this reflects modern forensic evaluations of viability, not the reality of 2nd-century postnatal care in Athens.

74. Beers and Berkow 1999, pp. 2128–2129.

75. Goodman and Armelagos 1989, pp. 226–227; Lewis 2007, pp. 81–82.

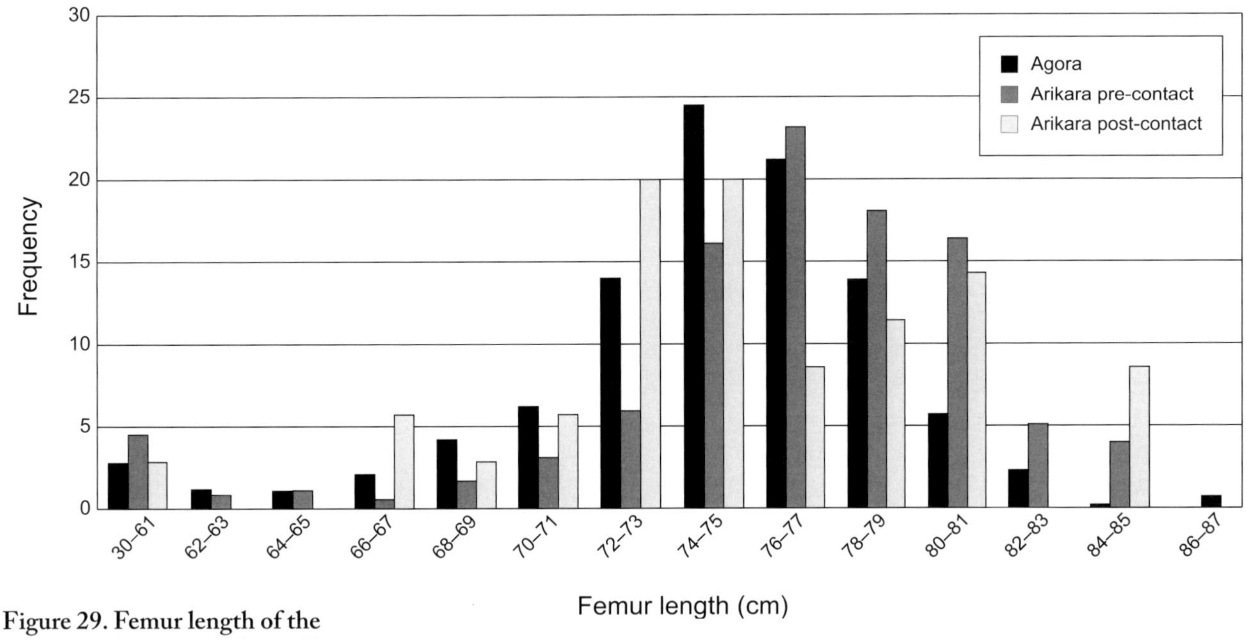

Figure 29. Femur length of the younger infants in the Agora Bone Well and of Arikara infants. A femur length of 74–77 mm indicates 37–40 gestational weeks.

which our material does not offer evidence. But a similar preponderance of small-for-gestational-age infants has been observed among individual Iron Age infant burials in the Agora, where skeletal size and dental development can provide independent estimates of age, since dental development is buffered from environmental stresses.[76] The frequency of preterm births is stable across various populations and cultures today,[77] and it is unlikely that 2nd-century Athens was experiencing an epidemic of preterm births. Rather, it appears that many of the babies were carried to full term, but were at the small end of the range for full-term pregnancies.

Infants with a low birth weight or that are small for their gestational age are at increased risk for perinatal mortality as well as long-term problems with growth, mental development, and immune response. In the United States, low-birth-weight births result in almost three-quarters of all neonatal deaths.[78] The high frequency of deaths among infants who were less than the optimal size for full-term infants suggests that low birth weight, rather than actual premature birth, may account for the deaths of a portion of these infants.

It is well documented that maternal health and socioeconomic status have a significant impact on birth weight and size. Increases in social and environmental stress have been demonstrated to result in reduced long-bone length of infant skeletons from Native American cemeteries of the post-contact Arikara (Fig. 29).[79] The predominance of small infants suggests that the population in Athens to whom these infants were born was stressed, probably by inadequate maternal nutrition and perhaps also by crowded and unsanitary conditions.[80]

76. Liston 2017, p. 522.

77. Haas, Balcazar, and Caulfield 1987, p. 470.

78. Martorell and González-Cossío 1987, pp. 195–196, 199.

79. Owsley and Jantz 1985, p. 321.

80. Storey 1986, pp. 545–546; Martorell and González-Cossío 1987, pp. 206–213.

Trauma

Traumatic injury from birth, accident, or abuse is the most readily identifiable skeletal pathology, particularly when there is evidence of healing on the bone indicating antemortem injury. While there are a great many broken long bones in this collection, most are clearly postmortem fractures. In addition, there are at least three incomplete or "greenstick" fractures that are common in young children's bone; these were found on the diaphyses of an ulna and two fibulae. There is no evidence of healing on these fractures, and it is entirely possible that these are perimortem fractures sustained shortly after death when the bodies were deposited in the well. Even if the water table was at approximately the same level as when the well was excavated, the infant bodies would have fallen 11 m before hitting the surface of the water, and could have struck the sides of the well on the way down with sufficient force to break some of the bones, resulting in these perimortem fractures. However, accident and abuse before death cannot be definitively excluded. As noted above, evidence of abusive treatment is clearly present on the oldest infant in the collection, AA 26a.

Infection and Hemorrhage

Infectious disease, particularly when the meninges of the brain are involved, is both a common cause of infant death in historic populations and in developing countries today, and one in which there is potentially rapid skeletal involvement on the endocranial surface of the skull.[81] The infant immune system is underdeveloped, and in the first few weeks of life, babies receive many of their antibodies from breast milk. Even with this source, however, the young infant may be unable to resist infection effectively and can develop serious complications. Congenital and neonatal infections are a common problem even in modern hospital births, and would have been a significant factor in infant morbidity and mortality in antiquity.[82] Infections, particularly tetanus, are a common cause of perinatal death in the third world today, and prior to the advent of antibiotics were responsible for 30% of neonatal deaths in London, with similar numbers found elsewhere in the western world.[83] In these studies pneumonia and septicemia were identified most commonly. Today *E. coli* and group B *Streptococcus* bacteria are among the most common causes of neonatal meningitis. Infections from the umbilical cord are quite common under conditions of poor sanitation; intrauterine infections probably are also a factor in these perinatal deaths. Therefore it is likely that infection played a significant role in the deaths of infants in ancient Athens.

The interior surface of the infant cranial bones preserves evidence of pathology involving the brain and its surrounding membranes. As a result of hemorrhage or infection, deposits of new bone may form on the endocranial surface of the bones of the cranial vault. Intracranial hemorrhage due to birth trauma is a common result of complicated or prolonged labor. Intracranial hemorrhage is also a common complication of premature birth.[84] Severe dehydration results in intracranial hemorrhage due to brain shrinkage and the tearing of membranes. Dehydration can develop due to excessive fluid loss associated with vomiting or diarrhea, or to limited fluid intake as a result of inadequate nursing.[85]

81. Naidu et al. 2001, pp. 445–446; Nasheit 2003, p. 66.
82. Kuo 2004, p. 108.
83. Bonar 1937, pp. 579–580; Bari et al. 2002, p. 217.
84. Beers and Berkow 1999, pp. 2132–2134.
85. Narchi 2013, pp. 213–214.

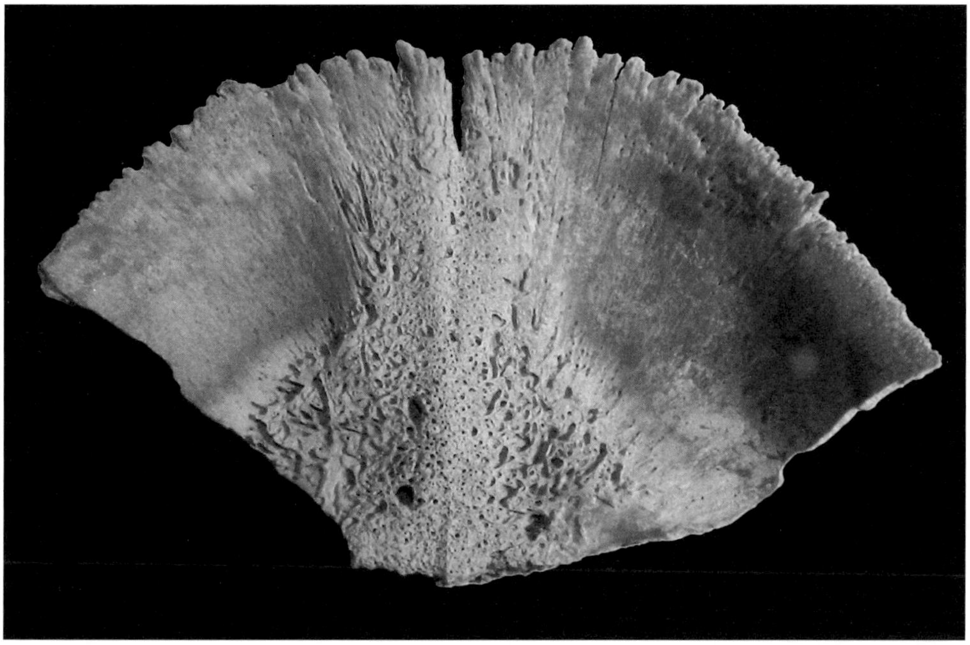

Figure 30. Lesions on the interior of the cranial vault of one of the infant occipital bones. Scale 2:1. Photo M. A. Liston

Infections causing meningitis or other endocranial infections may leave visible evidence on archaeological remains. Regardless of the cause, hemorrhage and infection may be manifested as endocranial lesions on the bones of the cranial vault.[86] In premodern skeletal populations, up to 80% of crania of infants and children, including neonates, have exhibited lesions associated with meningeal involvement in cranial hemorrhage or inflammation due to infectious process.[87]

In the Agora Bone Well collection, the endocranial surfaces of all cranial fragments more than 1 cm in diameter were examined using a hand lens. Cranial bones with suspected pathological lesions were then examined using the binocular microscope in the conservation laboratory of the Agora Excavations. Nearly 25% of the cranial vault bones had evidence of pathology, as indicated by areas of disorganized, rapidly growing bone deposits distinguishable from the stellate linear deposits of newly formed normal bone, or which clearly were deposited in additional layers above the normal bone surface. The cranial lesions in the Agora specimens resembled pathological bone described as porous or immature new-bone lesions in other studies.[88] These lesions have most often been documented on the occipital bone, but have been noted on the other bones of the cranial vault (Fig. 30).[89] Among the infant cranial bones in this collection, lesions were identified on the frontal, parietal, temporal, occipital, and sphenoid bones. Definite pathological activity was found on 18% of the frontal bones, 7% of the parietals, and 27% of the occipital bones. Lesser numbers of temporal and sphenoid fragments likewise had indications of pathological bone formation.

At any age, infection, dehydration, and hemorrhage, even when lethal, will result in visible bone involvement in only a small percentage of individuals. It is likely that many more of these infants died from common perinatal diseases, but did not survive long enough for skeletal involvement to occur.

86. Lewis 2004, pp. 82–83.
87. Jankauskas and Schultz 1995.
88. Lewis 2004, pp. 89–91.
89. Lewis 2004, p. 95.

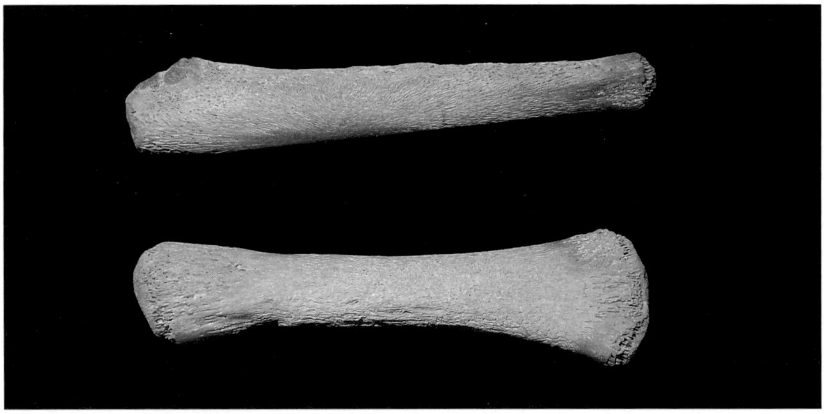

Figure 31. Malformed infant ulna (above) and humerus (below).
Scale 2:1. Photo M. A. Liston

Developmental Defects

Developmental defects are an inevitable part of human ontogeny. Both environmental teratogens and genetic variants contribute to disruptions in the normal development of a fetus, and some incidences of defects are of no known etiology. In ancient Athens, defects visible at birth or soon afterwards were considered appropriate reasons for not rearing a child (see pp. 120–121). A number of skeletal elements in this collection exhibit skeletal anomalies that would have been visible at birth and may have resulted in the exposure of these infants.

Although the skeletal elements were disassociated in the commingled remains, there are two bones, a right humerus and ulna, that appear to be malformed. The affected elements are misshapen and stunted, and it is probable that they are from the same individual. No affected right radius was found in the collection. The right ulna and humerus are markedly short and thick for their width. These arm bones are no longer than that of one of the smaller fetuses from the well assemblage, but the diaphyses are as thick as the bones of a near full-term infant (Fig. 31). There is also a right scapula with a dramatically reduced area of bone around the glenoid fossa, or shoulder joint. The dimensions of the bones suggest a severe growth anomaly resulting in stunted limbs. It appears that this anomaly affected only the right arm. As the limb-bone distortions are present in a perinatal infant, it is unlikely that they are the result of brachial plexus injury at birth, as the infant did not survive long enough for a loss of limb function to affect growth.[90] The combination of malformed radius and humerus, together with a small scapula, can be found in radial club hand or radial aplasia syndromes. These may be of genetic or teratogenic origin, but in most cases the etiology is unknown. The deformity probably would have included a marked abnormal appearance of the hand, possibly with a congenital absence of the thumb, and would have been immediately visible at birth.[91]

In modern Greece, limb reduction defect (LDR) of all causes has been identified in 1.97% of perinatal autopsies, of which 44.17% involved the upper limb.[92] While a stunted or malformed limb is normally not fatal,

90. Andersen et al. 2006, pp. 94–95.
91. Resnick 1995, vol. 6, pp. 4283–4284; Kozin 2007.
92. Goutas et al. 1993, p. 29.

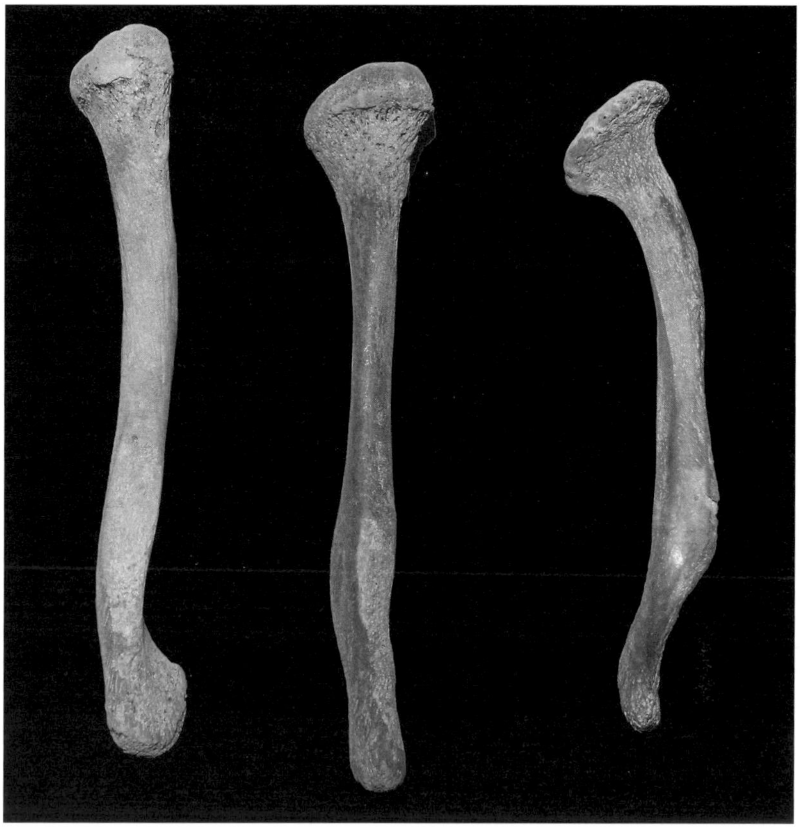

Figure 32. Infant clavicle with unusual morphology (right), with normal clavicles (left). Scale 2:1. Photo M. A. Liston

it certainly would have been visible at birth, and could have constituted a reason to choose not to rear a child.

Two other bones also exhibit anomalous structures. A left clavicle displays an unusual morphology, with a pronounced superior orientation of the medial end and an expanded medial articulation; at the lateral end there is a strong anterior curve, approximating 90 degrees (Fig. 32). If the associated structures were also positioned relative to the articular ends of the clavicle, the left shoulder would be positioned markedly lower and angled toward the front of the chest, rather than laterally. The defect would have been evident at birth, and like the stunted right arm, may also have resulted in the infant's rejection. It is also possible that the infant with the right arm deformity may have suffered from a bilateral condition, and the left clavicle is associated with the same deformity.

There is another skeletal birth defect present in the collection that may not have been visible, but is associated with increased risk of debilitating injury during birth. A left first rib from the collection has a complete cervical rib fused to the superior surface of the bone (Fig. 33). Cervical ribs result from a cranial shift in the cervicothoracic border, with ossification of the normal fibrous tissues originating on the transverse processes of the cervical vertebrae. This is a class IV cervical rib, the most extreme version of the anomaly, with a complete articular end and extending to the first thoracic rib. In this case, it is fused to the first sternal rib, not common for

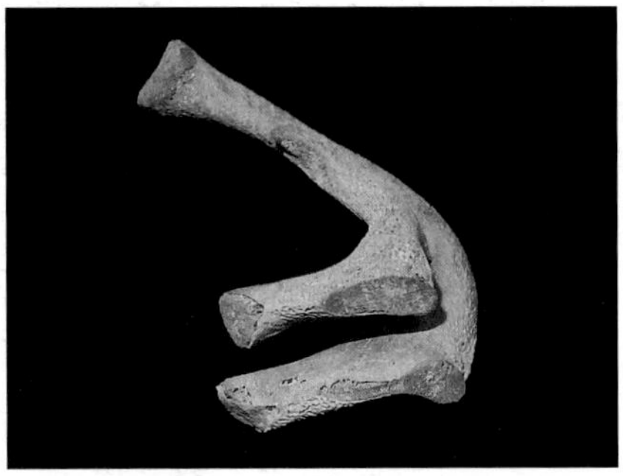

Figure 33. Infant cervical rib attached to right first rib. Scale 2:1. Photo M. A. Liston

these anomalous structures.[93] While cervical ribs do not cause debility in the majority of cases, class IV cervical ribs can cause compression on the brachial plexus and the subclavian artery, resulting in atrophy of the bones and impairing motor and sensory functions. Numerous cases of atrophy of the bones of the arm associated with cervical ribs are documented in adults from archaeological sites.[94] In clinical studies, cervical ribs have been found to be a contributing factor in brachial plexus injuries and paralysis in infants. They are associated with increased chance of injury from birth trauma, which can result in brachial palsy and paralysis. Even with modern medical intervention, the prognosis for full recovery is poor if the infant does not regain full limb function within a few weeks.[95] While the Agora infant with a class IV cervical rib may have died of natural causes, there was an increased chance of damage to the brachial nerves and impaired motion in the arms precipitated by the presence of the cervical rib. Such a deficiency could have marked the infant for rejection.

Cleft Palate

One of the most common developmental defects in the human skeleton involves the complete or partial failure of the structures of the face and mouth to unite at the midline during fetal development. The skeletal manifestation, cleft palate, is a different developmental process from cleft lip, although they may both be present.[96] Fetuses with cleft palate also experience more frequent and more severe soft tissue abnormalities than those without clefts.[97] A complete palate is essential for an infant because the hard surface is necessary for effective nursing. Without a complete palate, the infant has great difficulty feeding normally. When the oral cavity is open to the nasal cavity, as is the case in many infants with palate malformations, the infant is also at risk for aspirating breast milk and other fluids. Therefore a partial or complete cleft palate severely complicates feeding and decreases the likelihood of successfully raising the child. In addition, cleft palate is nearly always associated with bilateral otitis media, which untreated would have resulted in impaired hearing.[98]

93. Barnes 1994, pp. 100–101.
94. Barnes 1994, pp. 101–102.
95. Workum, Purvis, and Thomas 1971; Becker et al. 2002, pp. 741–742; Andersen et al. 2006, pp. 95–96.
96. Barnes 1994, pp. 174–175.
97. Kitamura and Kraus 1964, pp. 100–103.
98. Paradise, Bluestone, and Felder 1969, pp. 36–37.

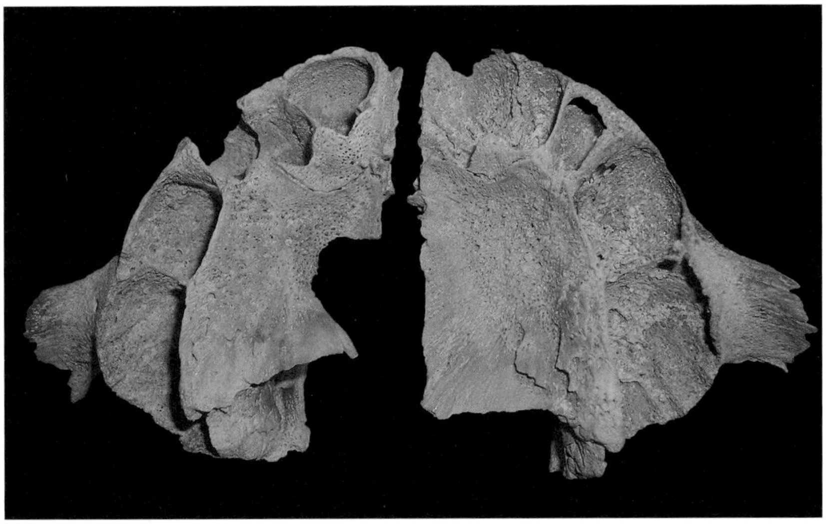

Figure 34. Normal palate (right) and cleft palate (left) of younger infants.
Scale 2:1. Photo M. A. Liston

At birth, the bony structures of the palate normally are completely formed, meeting at the midline to form a bony shelf across the top of the oral cavity and separating it from the nasal passages. The palate is formed from the left and right maxillae and the left and right palatine bones, which make up the posterior portion of the hard palate. Although they meet, the bones do not fuse together until later in childhood. After the soft tissue decayed, the maxillae and palatines from the Agora Bone Well skeletons separated, and were recovered as individual bones.

In the well, seven out of 164 maxilla halves exhibit definite cleft palate, as indicated by the absence of the palate shelf and the presence of rounded cortical bone surfaces, not broken edges on the margins of the defect (Fig. 34). Three additional maxilla halves also probably exhibit partial aplasia of the palate shelf, but postmortem damage to portions of the margin makes the identification less certain. Two of the definite cases involve clefting of not only the palate itself, but also the anterior margin of the maxilla, involving the alveolus, that is, the bone supporting the anterior teeth. This defect would have been immediately visible at birth, and the other cleft palates, even if not associated with cleft lip, would have been noted when the child was examined.

Cleft palate is known in all modern population groups; the incidence for Europeans ranges from 0.91 to 2.69 per 1,000 live births and late fetal deaths. Although there is some conflicting data, most studies document a higher incidence in males than in females.[99] Despite the frequency of the condition, there are very few cases known archaeologically, and these are of adult individuals.[100] The presence of well-preserved skeletons in the Agora Bone Well with aplasia of the bony palate provides confirmation of the presence of this condition in ancient Athens.

Many of the complications and associated deformities found with cleft palate potentially would have been fatal in antiquity. Thus the presence of these infants in the Agora Bone Well does not necessarily indicate that they were exposed, but parents may have hesitated to attempt to rear an infant with this debilitating deformity.

99. Vanderas 1987, pp. 217–218.
100. Barnes 1994, pp. 187–192; Ortner 2003, pp. 456–458.

SUMMARY

We have been able to determine the probable cause of death for many of the individuals in the Agora Bone Well. All of the older individuals suffered from conditions that would have severely compromised their quality of life and contributed to their deaths. The adult was crippled with hemochromatosis and the child suffered from an unknown ailment resulting in severe lesions of the spine and cranium; the older infants suffered from hydrocephalus and multiple trauma, possibly child abuse. These conditions help to explain their presence in the well (see below, p. 132).

There is abundant evidence of natural mortality among the young infants. Many were born preterm—some so early as to preclude survival—and many of those carried to term were small at birth. Both circumstances would have left them more than ordinarily susceptible to infection. Infections such as tetanus and gastrointestinal diseases, common causes of infant death today in urban conditions with poor sanitation and untreated water supplies,[101] would have left no trace on their bones, but many of the skull fragments of the infants in the Agora Bone Well exhibit pathological conditions, positive evidence of the ailments that killed them. The well contained a few infants with visible birth defects that may have made them candidates for infanticide, but the even distribution of male and female babies does not support gender-based infanticide as a major factor in the formation of the deposit.

101. Graham 1908, p. 1046; Simmons et al. 1982, p. 377.

CHAPTER 3

Faunal Skeletal Material

The remarkable quantity of animal bones, particularly skulls, was mentioned in Dorothy Thompson's notebook during the excavation of the Agora Bone Well, and they received more attention than the human bones in the early analysis of the material. A scant week after excavation was completed, Nils-Gustaf Gejvall produced a summary of the animal remains that was filed with the other excavation records.[1] He noted that the bones were in very good condition and stained with bronze. He then listed the species he found, beginning with 85 or more dog skulls, and then noting portions of two horses, four pigs, five goats, one cattle bone, two young cats, and one bird, as well as turtle-shell fragments. This is a considerably more detailed inventory than was conducted on the human remains in the years following the excavation.

While Thompson's description of the bone deposit during excavation indicates that it was concentrated in a portion of the well's fill, it is not possible from her notes to distinguish more specifically whether the dog skeletons in the well were intermingled with more common butchering and food debris and the human infant bones. All of the bones from the well were stored together without regard to stratigraphy, and therefore the entire bone assemblage from the well must be considered here as one undifferentiated deposit. It is not possible from the information available, therefore, to know if the more general food and butchering debris continued to be deposited during the interval in which the dog skeletons were placed in the well. Nonetheless, it is clear that the deposition of butchering and food debris would only have commenced after use of the well as a water source had ceased.

BUTCHERING AND FOOD DEBRIS

The animal-bone assemblage, with the exception of the concentration of dog skeletons discussed below, reflects common types of food refuse and a range of domestic animals. A total of 339 non-canid animal bones were recovered (Fig. 35; Table 2). The most commonly occurring bones were those of pigs, sheep, and goats, which collectively make up just over one-half of all non-canid bone debris. Cast-off primary butchering debris is represented by goat and sheep horn cores, which were roughly chopped from the skull. Possible food debris includes limb bones of pigs, sheep,

1. A typescript dated June 24, 1938, folded and tucked into a pocket of notebook ΛΛ 8. Gejvall was a Swedish osteologist and a pioneer in the study of both human and animal bone from archaeological contexts; for a brief sketch of his career, see Brothwell 1991.

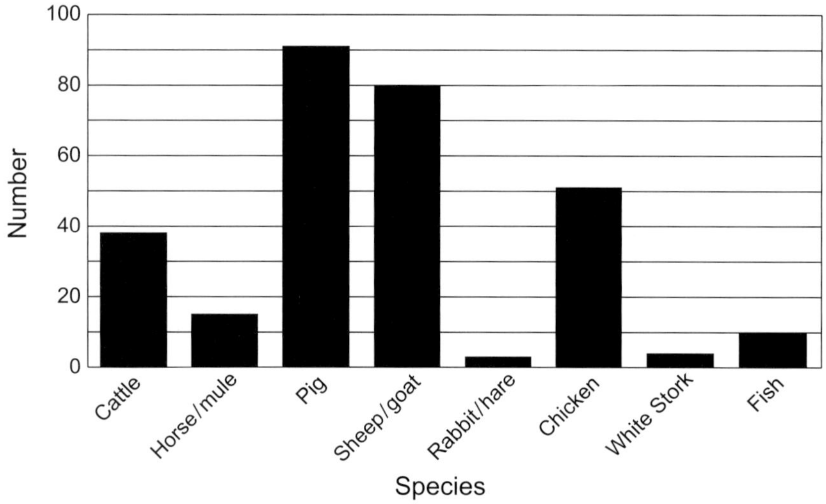

Figure 35. Number of bones of animals other than dog recovered from the well. Forty-seven turtle-shell fragments, also present, are not included.

TABLE 2. BONES OF ANIMALS OTHER THAN DOG

Species	*Number of Identified Specimens*
Cattle *(Bos taurus)*	38
Horse/mule (Equid)	15
Pig *(Sus scrofa)*	91
Sheep/goat (Caprine)	80
Rabbit/hare *(Leporidae)*	3
Chicken, domestic *(Gallus gallus)*	51
White Stork *(Ciconia ciconia)*	4
Fish	10
Turtle	47
Total	*339*

and goats. Cut marks on distal epiphyses indicate that limb segments were disarticulated, probably before cooking. Breakage of these bones through the diaphysis and the lack of burning on their surfaces suggest that these meat units may have been "pot sized"[2] for boiling or cooked on a small brazier rather than roasted on a spit. A hog jaw, first chopped from the skull, then split through the anterior symphysis by an additional blow, may also have been pot boiled as food.

In addition to adult food animals, a number of young animals are present in the deposit. At least seven piglets (Figs. 36, 37), one lamb, and one kid are represented by both cranial and postcranial elements, but are not represented by complete skeletons as are the dogs and human infants. None of the bones of these young animals show cut or chop marks, and the meaning of their presence in the well is unclear. They may have been utilized as food or in rituals related to the human deaths documented by

2. Oliver 1993, pp. 210–211.

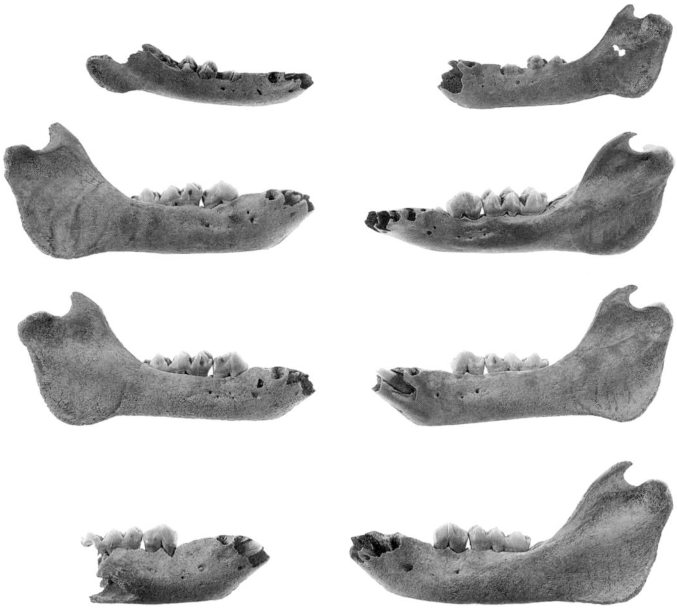

Figure 36. Left and right mandibles of piglets. Scale 1:2. Photo C. A. Mauzy

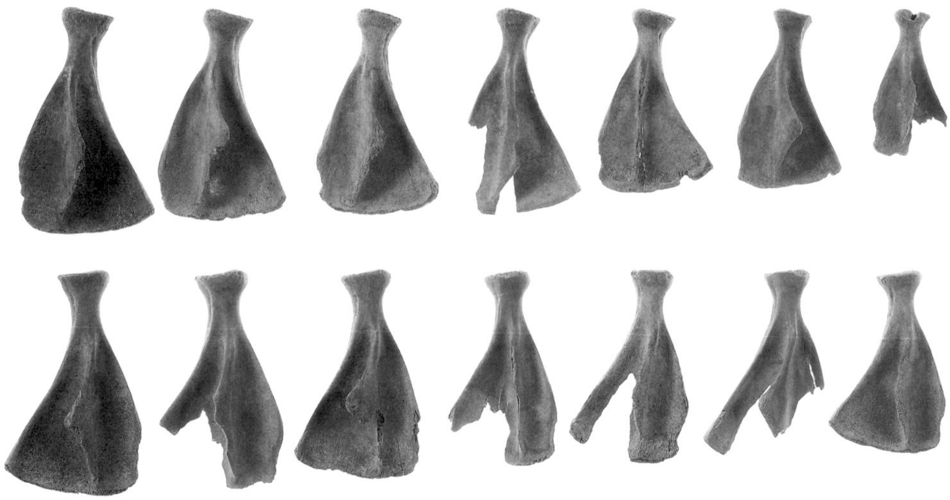

Figure 37. Left and right scapulae of piglets, representing a minimum of seven animals. Scale 1:2. Photo C. A. Mauzy

the well. Alternatively, these elements may simply represent animals that died at a young age and were disposed of in the abandoned well.

Smaller domestic and native animals are also at least minimally represented in the deposit. Three rabbit or hare bones, including a mandible, were recovered. Fifty-one domestic chicken bones represent at least three animals. Cut marks on a number of the bones indicate that these animals were used as food. The bones of one large bird, a White Stork *(Ciconia ciconia),* including the lower elements of a wing, a distal tarsometatarsus, and two phalanges, were found in the well. Cut marks on the articular condyles of the distal tarsometatarsus indicate that the bird had been deliberately butchered. Whether this animal was processed for food or harvested for its plumage is unclear. Fish are also minimally represented by several cranial fragments and one vertebra.

INDUSTRIAL AND MANUFACTURING DEBRIS

In addition to food and butchering debris, the industrial function of the area surrounding the well is reflected in bone debris from cattle, horses, and perhaps turtles. It is possible, of course, that some of these elements also represent food debris, but the heavy butchering marks on many of the elements suggest that the majority of these bones represent the remains of industrial and manufacturing processes.

Forty-seven turtle elements, primarily shell segments, may be debris from tortoise-shell production, or may simply represent one or more animals that died naturally in the area and were tossed in the well for disposal. None of the turtle elements show signs of deliberate modification.

Cattle are represented by one partial cranium, several vertebrae, and a number of postcranial elements. The basal part of a cattle skull is roughly chopped at the base of the occipital condyles; a set of articulating vertebrae (sixth cervical through third thoracic) may have come from the same animal and are also heavily chopped or trimmed on all margins. In contrast to the short, scattered cut marks on long-bone epiphyses and long, fine filleting marks on limb bones indicative of conventional butchering and meat removal,[3] most of the cattle long bones show heavy chop marks that, in some cases, appear to have been inflicted to trim the bone itself rather than remove meat from the bone. Both femora and humeri were treated in this manner. This rather heavy-handed trimming of cattle elements, seen on the crania, vertebrae, and limb elements recovered, suggests that if meat removal was the goal, it was done in a very rough, indelicate manner. It is possible that the heavy, thick-walled long bones, roughed out to form bone cylinders or blanks, represent manufacturing debris.

Horse elements from the well include two partial skulls, eight long bones, and three phalanges. As with the cattle elements, most of the horse long bones have been heavily chopped or trimmed, and they too may be remains of a manufacturing process.

The industrial and manufacturing nature of the northern slopes of the Kolonos Agoraios is also clearly reflected in a number of cattle ribs and scapulae, some of which were roughly shaped and then used as tools (Fig. 38). At least seven rib tools were made by chopping the head from the element, and in several instances by trimming the edges of the rib shaft itself. This may have been done to shape the rib shaft further or to remove all traces of flesh and connective tissue from the bone surfaces. These elements also show a high polish on one or more surfaces, and multiple fine striations generally parallel to the length of the element (Fig. 39). A minimum of seven additional bone tools were manufactured from cattle scapulae. These specimens appear to have served much the same function as the ribs. In several instances, the blunt, flattened glenoid or articular portion of the element has been removed or heavily reduced by chopping to produce a proximal or hafting element. In some cases, the thickened posterior margin of the broad scapular blade has also been trimmed. The remaining thin, plate-like blade of the scapula shows a high glossy polish over at least a portion of its surface, particularly toward the widened distal

3. Binford 1981, pp. 136–142.

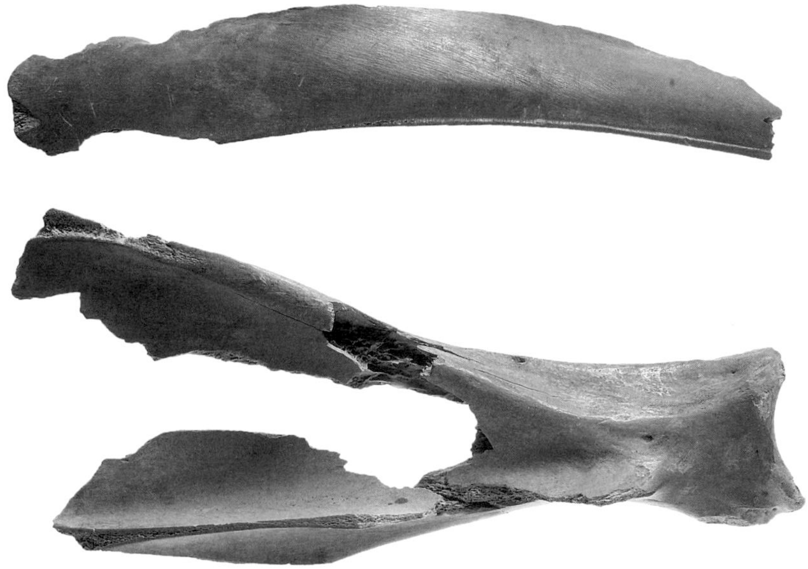

Figure 38. Cattle rib (above) and scapula (below) used as expedient tools in the casting process. Scale 1:3. Photo C. A. Mauzy

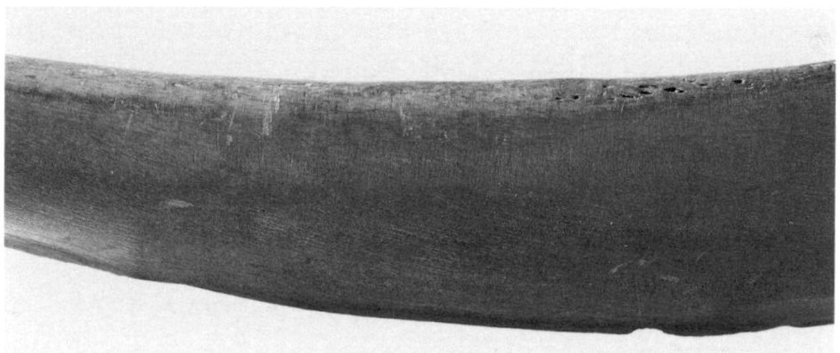

Figure 39. Detail of an expedient cattle-rib tool, showing fine parallel striations and general polish caused by abrasion during use. Scale 2:3. Photo C. A. Mauzy

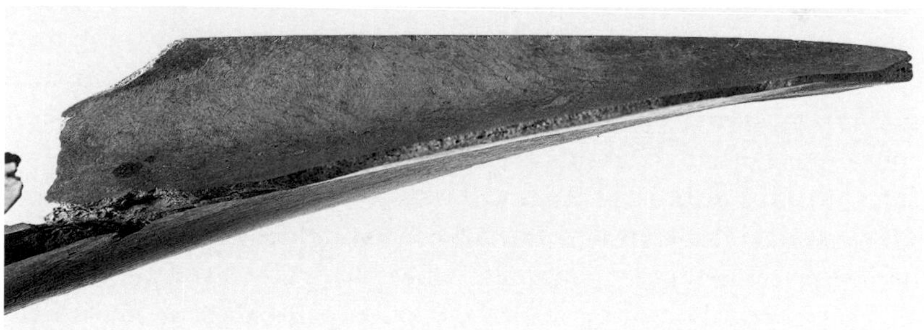

Figure 40. Detail of a fragment of a cattle scapula used as a tool, showing smoothing and polishing of the edges of the element and beveling of the distal (working) edge (to the left in the photo). Scale 2:3. Photo C. A. Mauzy

or working end of the tool (Fig. 40). On two fragments apparently broken from larger tools, the distal or working end of the fragment retains a high polish with fine striations, plus a distinct beveling of the working edge.

Given the location of the well, in an area of bronze-casting workshops, it seems likely that these cattle elements, both ribs and scapulae, were rather casually and quickly modified to produce digging or scraping tools. Such tools might then have been used to dig or maintain the contents of casting pits.[4]

4. Benco, Ettahiri, and Loyet (2002) discuss bone tools and metalworking in medieval Morocco.

THE DOMESTIC DOG ASSEMBLAGE

While it is not unusual to find butchering and food debris, industrial debris, and the occasional discarded small animal carcass in abandonment contexts such as nonfunctioning wells or house ruins, the large number of domestic dog skeletons clearly came to be in the well by another mechanism. Their disposal in this one feature in such numbers—over 150 animals—is unique, and quite distinct from the few scattered and deliberate dog burials that have been found elsewhere in the Agora.[5]

In the well, the remains of domestic dogs were commingled throughout the 7 m of deposits that also contained the baby skeletons. Like the infants, these animals appear to have entered the well whole and articulated. Although the relative numbers of elements vary—larger limb bones being more commonly recovered than the smaller elements such as carpals, tarsals, and phalanges—all parts of the dog skeleton are represented. While old and healed injuries are apparent on a number of skulls and limb elements, there is no evidence of deliberate blows that might have killed the animals, nor were cut marks indicative of skinning, disarticulation, or meat removal found on any of the nearly 4,700 dog bones from the well.

Based on relative bone density and development, plus the known sequence of long-bone epiphyseal fusion, the minimum of 150 animals represented a range in age from fetal to aged adult. Rough age estimations can also be made based on the stage of tooth eruption in the mandibles. Since the permanent teeth of dogs are erupted by seven months of age, while all long-bone epiphyses are fused by 16 to 18 months of age, it is generally possible to divide an archaeological population into adult, juvenile, and newborn or pup components (Fig. 41).[6] In the well assemblage, approximately 65%–70% of the dogs represented were adults, 15% were subadults or juveniles, and 16%–18% were newborn or very young puppies (Fig. 42). This death assemblage stands in distinct contrast to the age distribution in the massive dog cemetery at Ashkelon,[7] where more than half of the burials were those of puppies less than one year of age. In fact, heavy puppy and aged adult deaths are common in a natural die-off, and a preponderance of these animals might be expected if the well deposit represented the disposal of unwanted carcasses resulting from random or natural deaths. The presence of so many adult, prime-age animals in the well suggests that these animals were deliberately chosen and put to death for a particular reason, after which their bodies were deposited in the well.

Among the adult animals, a range of sizes is represented (Figs. 41, 43, 44). By regression analysis based on long-bone lengths of modern animals of known height, the stature or shoulder height of the archaeological animals can be estimated.[8] Figure 45 presents a summary of the range of shoulder

5. For example, deposits R 10:3 (Thompson 1951, p. 52, pl. 26:a) and B 22:2 (Young 1951a, p. 268, pl. 83:c–e), of the Hellenistic period, and an unnumbered burial in Section N (notebook N 10, p. 1802). There are also instances of puppy bones in pots (burial? ritual?): e.g., deposit F 16:7 (Shear 1969, pp. 393–394; Miller 1974, pp. 195, 210 [n. 80], fig. 1 [with location marked by cross on plan], pl. 35; Jordan and Rotroff 1999, p. 148), 3rd century, and an unnumbered burial in an Early Byzantine amphora (P 26680) in Section ΠA, 9th–10th century A.D. See also Parlama and Stampolides 2000, pp. 157, 177, fig. 10, for dog burials, one dating to the 1st–2nd century A.D.

6. Silver 1969, pp. 285, 299.

7. Wapnish and Hesse 1993.

8. Lyman 2008, pp. 108–109.

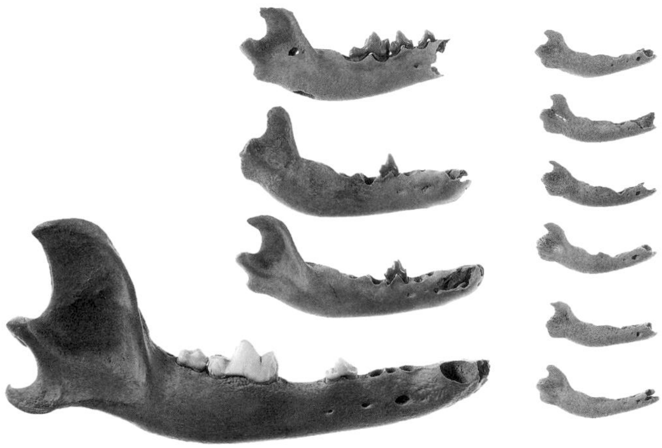

Figure 41. Representative sample of right mandibles of dogs, from adult (lower left), juvenile (upper left), and fetal/neonate (right) animals. Scale 1:2. Photo C. A. Mauzy

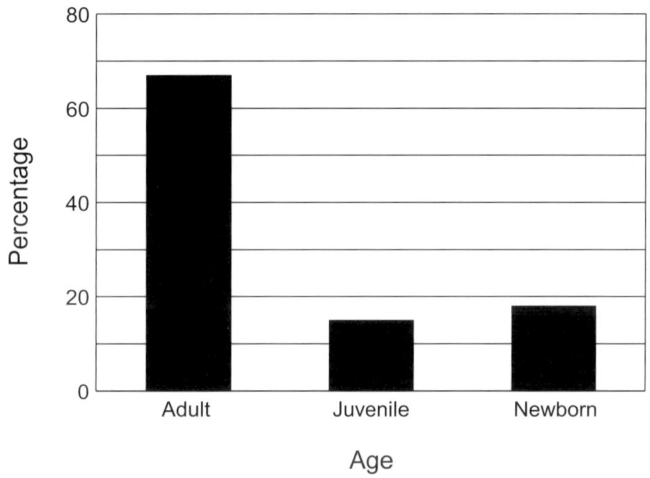

Figure 42. General age distribution of dogs, based on fusion data from 71 complete right femora

heights of adult animals in the well based on 71 complete right femora. The smallest animals were approximately 30 to 33 cm at the shoulder, although these small, perhaps terrier-like animals are relatively few in number. Four much larger animals, probably approaching 64 to 74 cm at the shoulder, also formed a small part of the assemblage. The skulls and other long bones that, based on size, probably belonged to these dogs suggest that they may have been large, relatively long-legged and heavy-bodied hunting hounds or guard dogs. The majority of animals, however, fall into a rather evenly spaced distribution between 33 and 49 cm, about the size of a beagle or small hound. This distribution shows that most of them were neither specially bred hunting or military hounds nor small pet or lap dogs. Rather, they may well have come from a living population of common urban mongrels or pariah dogs that inhabited the environs of Athens.

A second line of evidence indicating that these animals were not given special status before death is the number of pathologies present in the population. While few of the long bones show noticeable bowing or distortion of the long-bone shaft, indicative of under- or malnutrition, many animals show severe wear on one or more teeth and antemortem tooth loss, with associated evidence of periodontal disease and infection. At

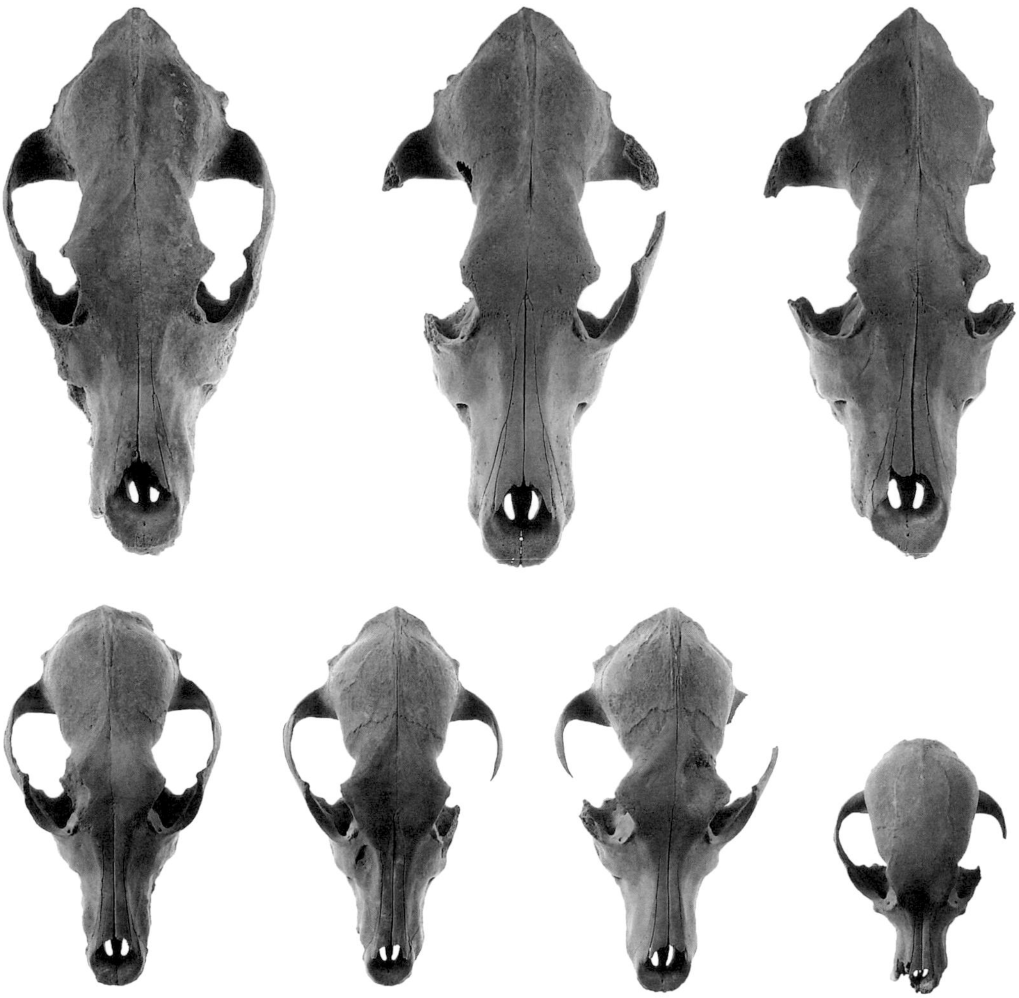

Figure 43. Representative sample of adult dog skulls, including those of large (top row), medium (lower left), and small (lower right) stature. Scale 1:3. Photo C. A. Mauzy

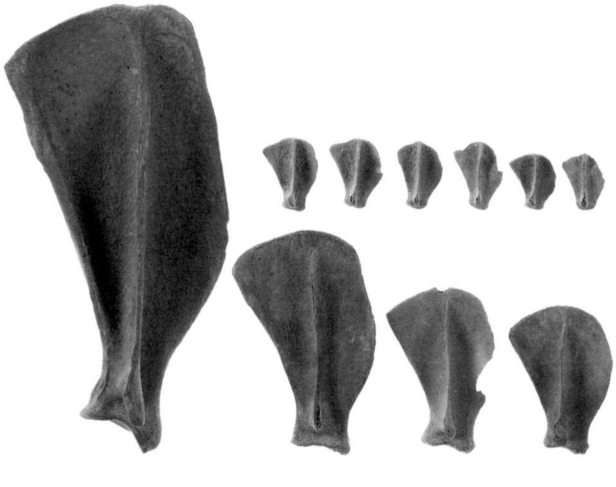

Figure 44. Representative sample of dog scapulae, from adult (left), juvenile (lower right), and fetal/neonate (upper right) animals. Scale 1:2. Photo C. A. Mauzy

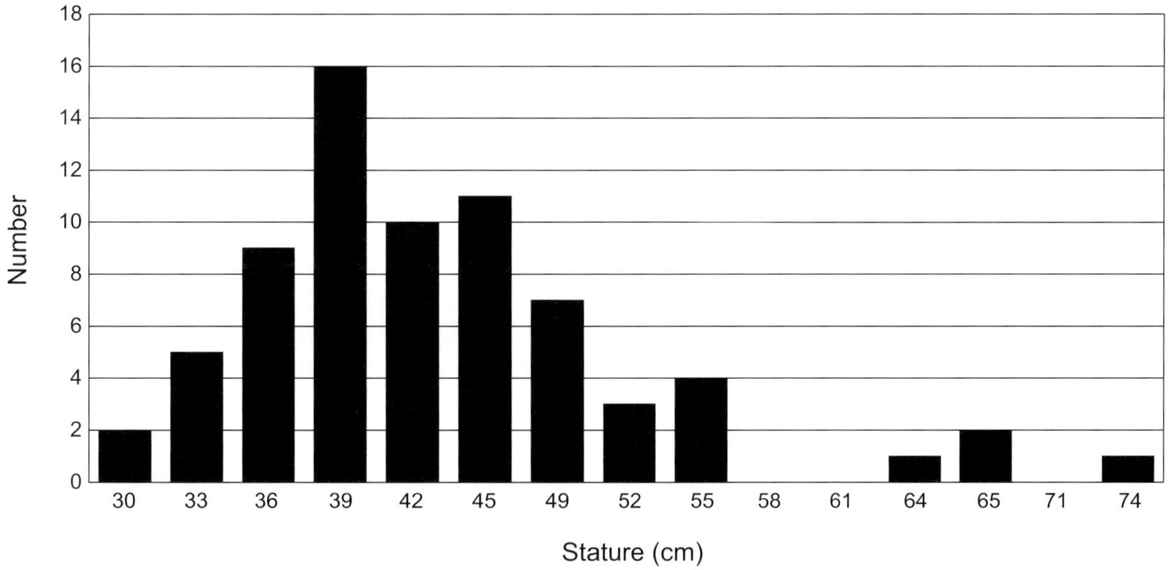

Figure 45. Relative distribution by stature of adult dogs, as represented by estimated shoulder heights based on the lengths of 71 adult right femora

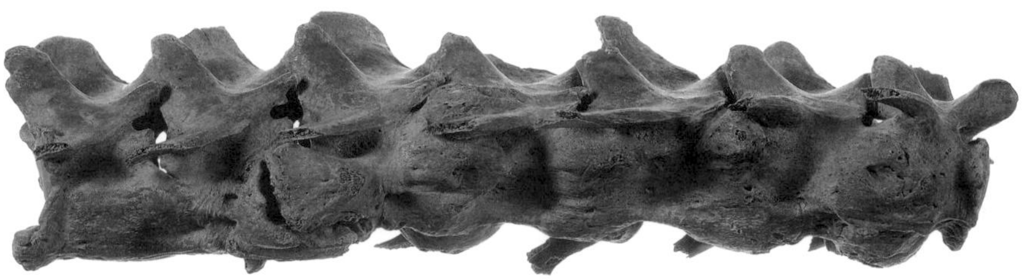

Figure 46. Fused vertebrae of one of the large dogs. Scale 1:2. Photo C. A. Mauzy

least one of the larger animals also probably experienced extreme pain and impairment of movement due to osteoarthritic lipping and eventual fusing of all lumbar vertebrae (Fig. 46). Broken and partially or completely reknit limb bones were also noted (Figs. 47, 48). These injuries were most often to the hind-limb bones, the femur or tibia, and might have been inflicted on animals who were slow in moving away from the kick of a human or horse. Depressed and healed fractures on a number of dog skulls (Fig. 49) are a further indication that many of these animals were probably free-roaming urban dogs, liable to injury through fighting, or more probably to blows by humans when they became a nuisance. Taken together, the pathologies, both infectious and traumatic, suggest that these were not dogs held in high esteem before their demise.

The sex of the animals in the well can also be tentatively determined. It has been suggested that the degree of development of the sagittal or nuchal crests along the top of the skull may distinguish male from female.[9] In addition, differences in morphology in the area of the basioccipital, perhaps based on differences in muscle development and the position in which the

9. The and Trouth 1976.

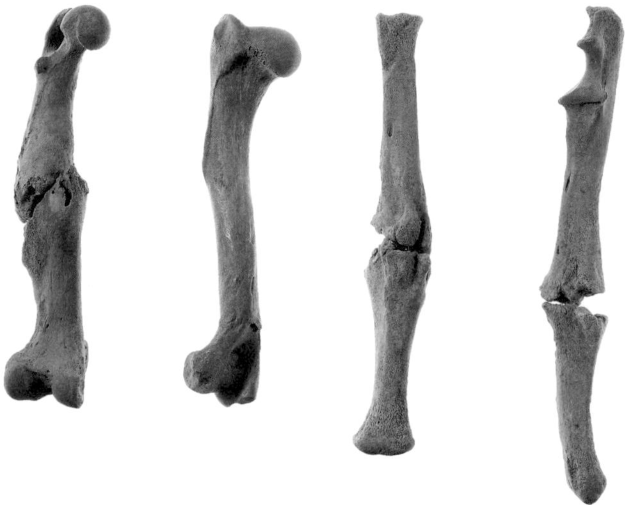

Figure 47. Canine femur, humerus, radius, and ulna, showing trauma. The femur and humerus (left) were broken and partially re-knit, and possibly are from the same adult animal. The radius and ulna (right) of a younger animal were broken and in the process of remodeling and re-knitting. Scale 1:2. Photo C. A. Mauzy

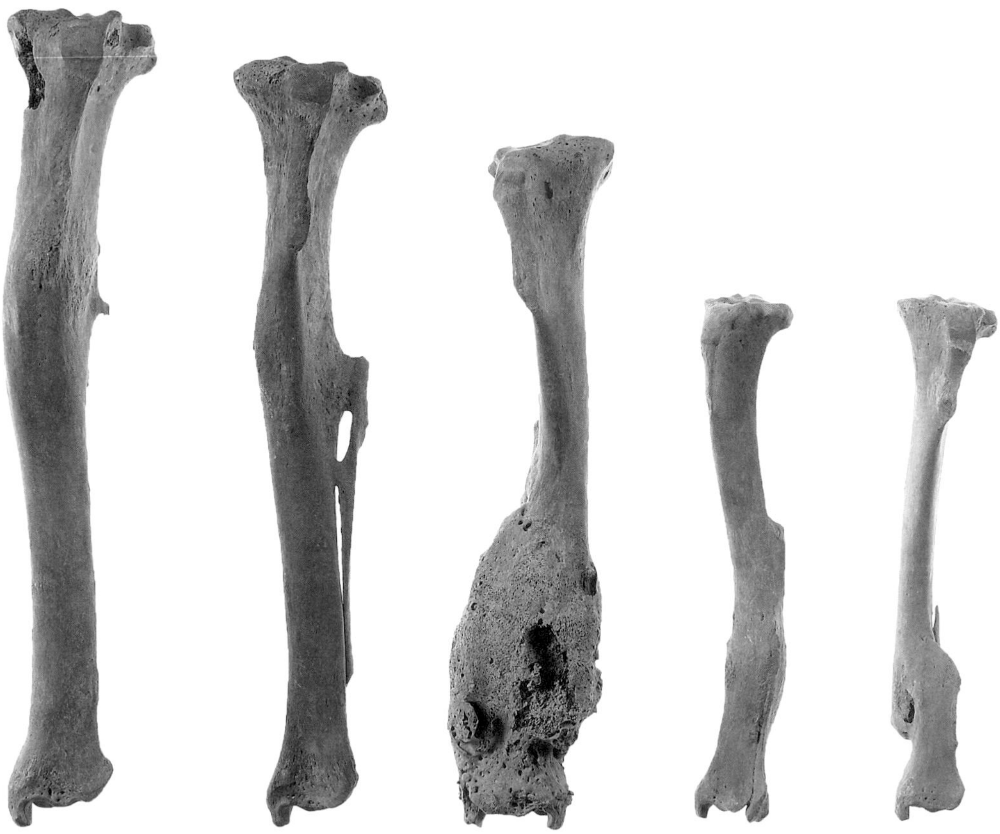

Figure 48. Tibiae of large through small adult dogs, all showing breakage and remodeling. The tibia in the middle shows extensive bony growth with associated infection. Scale 1:2. Photo C. A. Mauzy

head is held, may also be diagnostic of the sex of the animal.[10] Interpretation of these morphological characteristics can be highly subjective, however, as both tend to grade in expression and vary by breed. Nonetheless, based on these criteria, as applied to the more complete adult crania from the well, a ratio of 24 females to 34 males is indicated.

A more direct and unequivocal indicator of male dogs is the presence of the *os penis* or baculum, commonly known as the penis bone. These bones are present in a range of sizes and shapes in dogs and many other mammals, and are often diagnostic to species.[11] Dogs, however, are the only

10. Trouth et al. 1977.
11. Burt 1960, pp. 14–15.

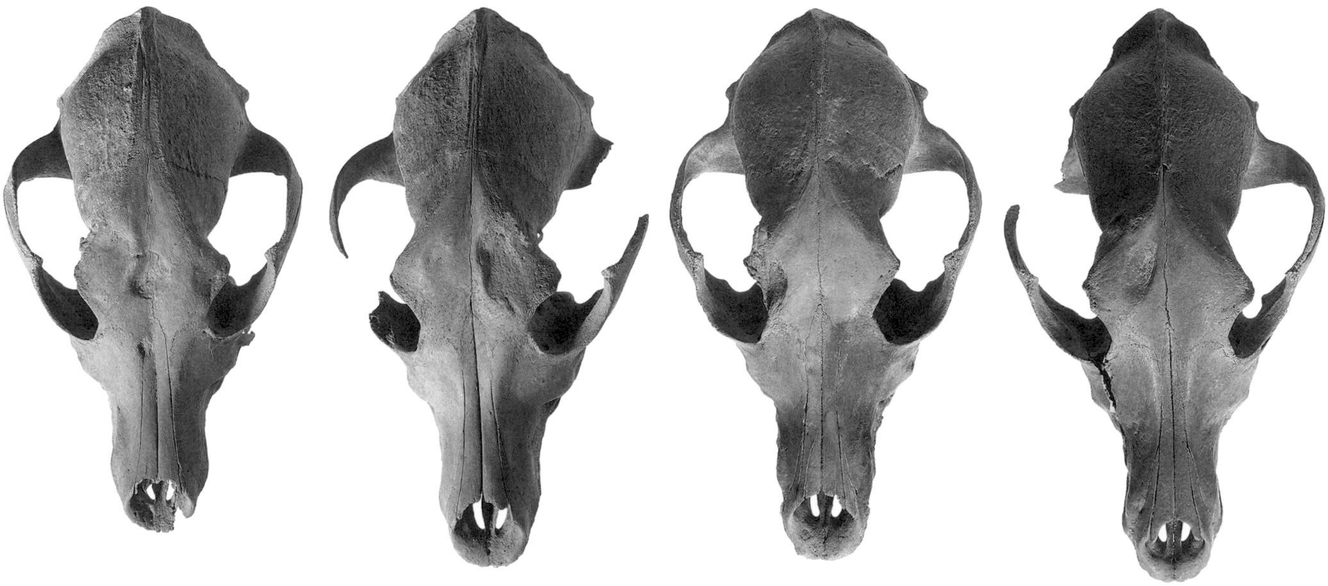

Figure 49. Four skulls of adult dogs showing one or more healed depressed fractures. Scale 1:2. Photo C. A. Mauzy

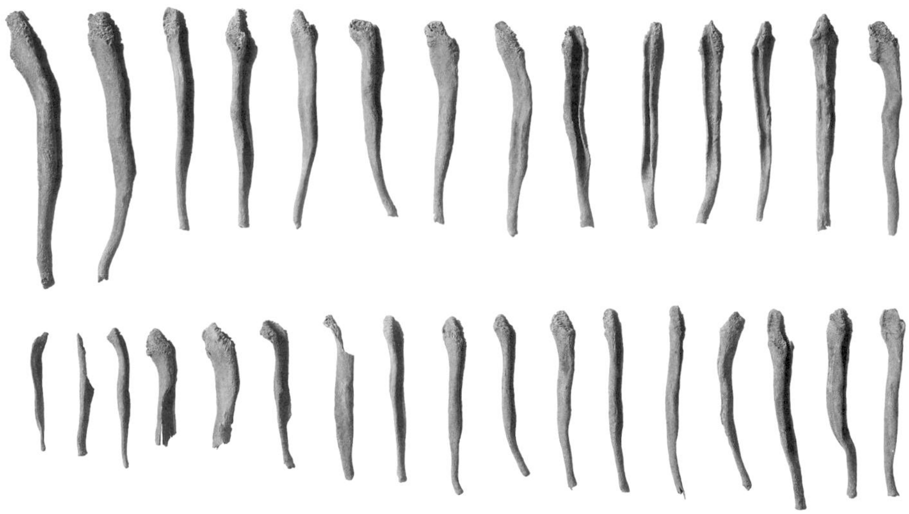

Figure 50. Bacula of dogs illustrating size and age variation in the male canid population represented in the deposit. Scale 1:3. Photo C. A. Mauzy

animal represented in the well that develops a baculum. Thus, by counting the number of complete and broken bacula recovered, a minimum number of male animals can be estimated. A total of 31 canid bacula are present in the assemblage (Fig. 50), representing at least 31 adult males. The sex of the very young animals and puppies is unknowable, due to the tiny size and undeveloped nature of their bones.

A minimum of 31 adult male dogs, as represented by bacula, compares well with the 34 males indicated by the more subjective analysis of skull morphology noted above. By either estimate, it is evident that both male and female dogs were deposited in the well; there was no selection for sex, whether male or female. Thus, neither sex, nor age, nor physical attributes, including size, seems to have played a major role in the selection of animals.

CHAPTER 4

Artifacts

RECOVERY, SORTING, AND CONSERVATION

The methods that were normally used in the 1930s for the excavation of a well and the subsequent treatment of the objects recovered has had an impact on the evidence that is available to us today. An attempt was doubtless made to retrieve every object from the Agora Bone Well, but recovery procedures were less exacting than they are now. Objects would be collected as they were encountered, but it was also the usual practice to save the excavated earth, allow it to dry, and then set a workman to dig through it again with a small pick, looking for items that had been missed. The earth was not sieved, and some small objects would inevitably be lost.

Complete objects would usually be inventoried as they were found or when the excavator had time to enter them in the notebooks. When excavation and the redigging of the dried fill were complete, fragmentary material would be spread out on tables for conservation. How thorough the mender or menders were in their search for joins would have depended on the press of work at any given time, and extant fragments might sometimes inadvertently be left out of the reconstructions. For these reasons, the absence of a few pieces from an otherwise complete pot from the Agora Bone Well need not be taken as an indication that it did not enter the well whole.

When mending had been completed, additional objects would be chosen for inventory; this selection usually included all complete or substantially complete items, along with any unusual or unique objects. In cases where multiple examples of a shape could be mended, one or two inventoried examples would probably suffice. At this point, some of the material that did not mend up would be discarded. No record of this procedure was kept, so we do not know what percentage of the whole was retained in any specific instance or how representative the remainder is of the deposit as found. The remaining uninventoried objects from the Agora Bone Well are stored in three boxes (two shallow wooden trays and one deeper one, measuring 37 × 76 × 8 or 16.50 cm deep) of combined fine and plain wares, and three tins (measuring 23 × 23 × 35 cm) of plain wares, three of transport amphoras, one of tiles, and one about half full of bronze waste (the latter now repacked and moved to the climate-controlled metals room at the Agora); there is also one tin of Byzantine material from the mouth of the well.[1] There are almost no fragments of vessel walls among this material; these were apparently removed, but some feature sherds may have been discarded as well, especially in cases where a shape was very well represented.

The manmade objects provide a date for the Agora Bone Well's contents and also throw light on the nature of the deposit and on activities that took place in the well's vicinity. Most of the objects fall into the category of pottery (including lamps), but there are also other items made of clay (loomweights, molds for a figurine and a lamp[?], a possible figurine fragment, and roof tiles) as well as a small marble herm, an ivory scabbard chape, and a large number of bronze fragments. One challenge is to divine which, if any, of these objects are directly related to the human remains in the well and which are not.

Over 290 vessels and lamps can be identified to shape and type, but about 180 of these are mere fragments and cannot come from vessels that entered the well whole or intact (see Tables 3–5 for a summary of the pottery and its state of preservation). Rather, they represent the scatter of ceramics that was to be found in any pile of earth in antiquity and were probably washed into the well by rain or thrown in with fill. Another 45 items represent less than half of a vessel; although some of these are substantial (for instance, the neck and handles of two Knidian amphoras, **72, 74**), most fall into the same category of chance debris, unrelated to the human remains in the well. Intact or only slightly damaged vessels that were still serviceable when discarded are the strongest candidates for close relevance to the human remains. Vessels that are broken but complete or substantially so may also be considered in this light, but there is no way of knowing whether they were broken before their discard (and hence fall into the category of rubbish) or broke as or after they fell into the well.

POTTERY AND OTHER CERAMIC OBJECTS

The pottery from the well provides the bulk of the evidence for the date of the deposit, so it is presented in some detail here. It also has the virtue of constituting a closely dated group of pottery typical of its time, and it is thus useful from the point of view of ceramic history and development.

Fine Ware

Fragments of over 150 fine-ware vessels were found in the well, of which only a small number are well preserved (Table 3). About one-fifth of this material is residual, dating from the Classical period to the 3rd century, and another 15–16 fine-ware items, most of them fragments, can be placed in the first quarter of the 2nd century (Table 4). The bulk of the material, however, amounting to over 100 pieces (although many are only fragments), forms a closely dated group within the second quarter of the 2nd century.

1. Lots ΛΛ 352–ΛΛ 361, ΛΛ 366.

TABLE 3. FINE-WARE VESSELS AND THEIR STATE OF PRESERVATION[1]

Shape (Catalogued Examples)	*Intact/ Serviceable*	*Whole or Little Missing*	*More than Half*	*Less than Half*	*Fragment*	*Total*
Vessels for Food						
Bowl with outturned rim (**1–6**)	1	1	5	7	15	29
Echinus bowl (**7–9**)	1			2	6	9
Bowl, beveled rim					1	1
Deep bowl, projecting rim (**10**)			1		1	2
Rolled-rim plate (**11**)				4	5	9
Rilled-rim plate (**12, 13**)	1	1	1	2	2	7
Fishplate					5	5
Saucer					9	9
Subtotal	*3*	*2*	*7*	*15*	*44*	*71*
Vessels for Drink						
Moldmade bowl (**14–18**)			4	1	30[2]	35
Two-handled cup (**19**)			1		1	2
Hemispherical West Slope cup (**20**)					2	2
West Slope kantharos					5	5
Hellenistic kantharos, black gloss?					1	1
West Slope amphora					2	2
Oinochoe					1	1
Olpe					1	1
Subtotal			*5*	*1*	*43*	*49*
Other Shapes						
Lug-handled krater (**21**)				1	2	3
Round-mouth jug (**22**)		1			1	2
Lekythos (**23**)				1		1
Canteen (**24, 25**)			1	1		2
Feeder (**26**)		1				1
Panathenaic amphora (**27**)					1	1
Pyxis					1	1
Hellenistic lamp (**28, 29**)	1			1	4	6
Subtotal	*1*	*2*	*1*	*4*	*9*	*17*
Early Pottery						
Classical lamp					6	6
Classical votive			2		1	3
Early fine ware					13	13
Subtotal			*2*		*20*	*22*
Total	***4***	***4***	***15***	***20***	***116***	***159***

[1] Counts are minima: e.g., if there are two fragments that could but do not necessarily have to come from two different vessels, they are counted as one.
[2] There are ca. 113 nonjoining sections of moldmade bowls; 30 is the estimated minimum number of bowls present.

TABLE 4. RESIDUAL POTTERY AND ITS STATE OF PRESERVATION

Shape (Catalogued Examples)	*More than Half*	*Less than Half*	*Fragment*	*Total*
3rd Century and Earlier				
Iron Age vessel			1	1
Figured or patterned ware			6	6
Classical black gloss			6	6
Rolled-rim plate, stamped			1	1
West Slope kantharos			5	5
West Slope amphora			1	1
Olpe			1	1
Lug-handled krater (**21**)		1	2	3
Classical lamp (types 22C, 23, 25)			6	6
Type 45C lamp (**28**)		1		1
Miniature votive	2			2
Votive lopadion			1	1
Early Knidian amphora (**71**)			1	1
Other transport amphora			3	3
Subtotal	*2*	*2*	*34*	*38*
First Quarter of 2nd Century				
Rolled-rim plate (**11**)		1		1
Moldmade bowl (**14**)	1?		10	10–11
Hemispherical cup (**20**)			2	2
West Slope amphora			1	1
Panathenaic amphora (**27**)			1	1
Unguentarium (**30**)			1	1
Koan amphora (**70**)	1			1
Other transport amphora			4	4
Subtotal	*1–2*	*1*	*19*	*21–22*
Total	*3–4*	*3*	*53*	*59–60*

Note: Items in the left column that span two of the time frames are tallied with their latest date, that is, the first quarter of the 2nd century.

Vessels for Food

Bowls (Figs. 51–53) are the most common shape, most frequently the bowl with outturned rim, which occurs in two forms and a range of sizes. The Classical form, which has a scraped groove at the base of the wall and usually bears stamped decoration on the floor,[2] is present in two well-preserved examples (**1**, **2**) and fragments of three or four more (including **3**). Most of the bowls, however, are of the plainer Hellenistic form (**4–6**), which exhibits neither of the ornaments described above.[3] Bowls with outturned rim outnumber echinus bowls by a factor of three to one, the standard

2. *Agora* XXIX, pp. 157–158.
3. *Agora* XXIX, pp. 158–159.

TABLE 5. PLAIN-WARE VESSELS AND THEIR STATE OF PRESERVATION

Shape (Catalogued Examples)	*Intact/Serviceable*	*Whole or Little Missing*	*More than Half*	*Less than Half*	*Fragment*	*Total*
Unguentaria						
Category 3 (**30**)				1		1
Category 4 (**31**)	1					1
Category 5 (**32–39**)	7	2	2	1	5	17
Subtotal	*8*	*2*	*2*	*2*	*5*	*19*
Household Ware, Open Shapes						
Lekane, form 1 (**40–42**)	1	1	1		4	7
Lekane, form 3 (**43**)			1		2	3
Lekane, form 4 (**44, 45**)		2		11	9	22
Deep bowl (**46, 47**)		1	1			2
Shallow bowl, large (**48, 49**)		1	1	1		3
Shallow bowl, small (**50–52**)			5	1		6
Krater (**53, 54**)			2	2	2	6
Mortar (**55**)			2	1		3
Beehive (**56**)				1		1
Pithos/vat?					1	1
Vat/amphora stand?					1	1
Lid					1	1
Subtotal	*1*	*5*	*13*	*17*	*20*	*56*
Household Ware, Closed Shapes						
Jug, form 2 (**57**)			1			1
Jug, form 4					2	2
Amphora, form 2 (**58**)				1		1
Lagynos (**59**)				1	1	2
Storage bin, form 1					2	2
Subtotal			*1*	*2*	*5*	*8*
Cooking Ware						
Chytra, form 1 (**60–63**)	3		2		3	8
Chytra, form 4 (**64**)			1	1		2
Chytra, form 10 (**65**)			1			1
Lopas, form 3 (**66**)				1		1
Lopas, form 4 (**67**)			1			1
Lid					2	2
Pan					1	1
Brazier (**68, 69**)					2	2
Subtotal	*3*		*5*	*2*	*8*	*18*
Transport Amphoras						
Koan (**70**)			1		4	5
Knidian (**71–75**)				2	9	11
Other					14	14
Subtotal			*1*	*2*	*27*	*30*
Total	***12***	***7***	***22***	***25***	***65***	***131***

Note: Names for the forms are those used in *Agora* XXXIII; even seemingly generic descriptions (e.g., "shallow bowl, large") refer to specific forms.

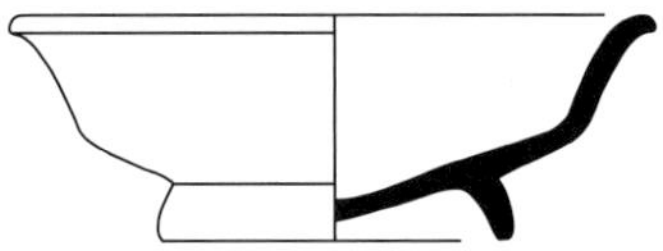

1

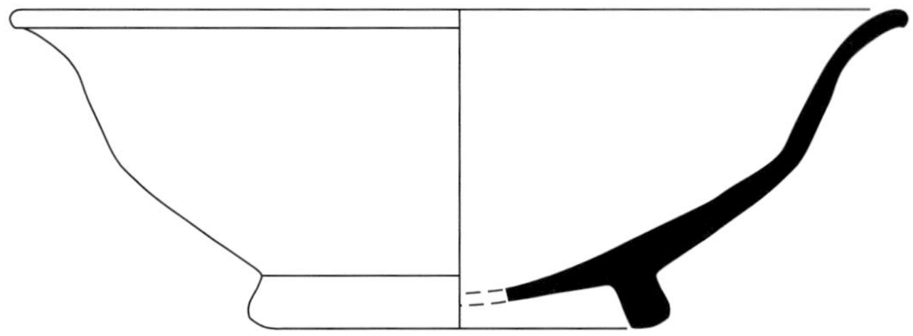

4

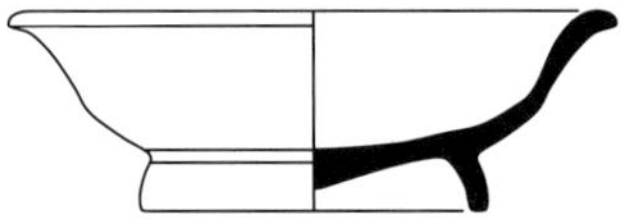

2

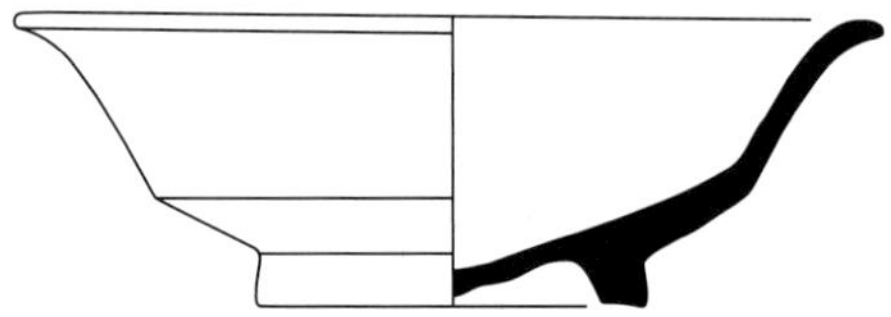

5

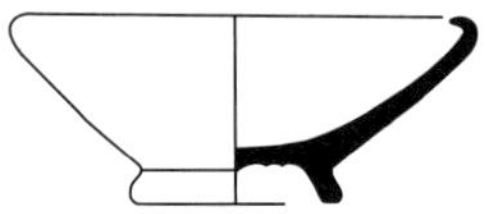

7

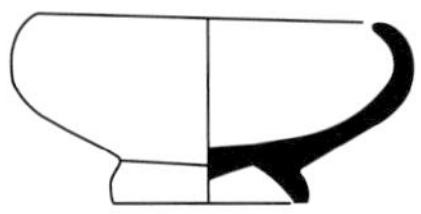

8

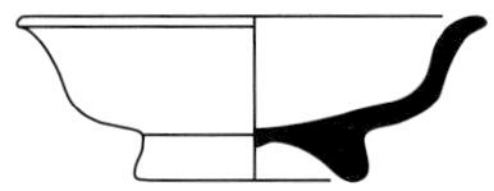

6

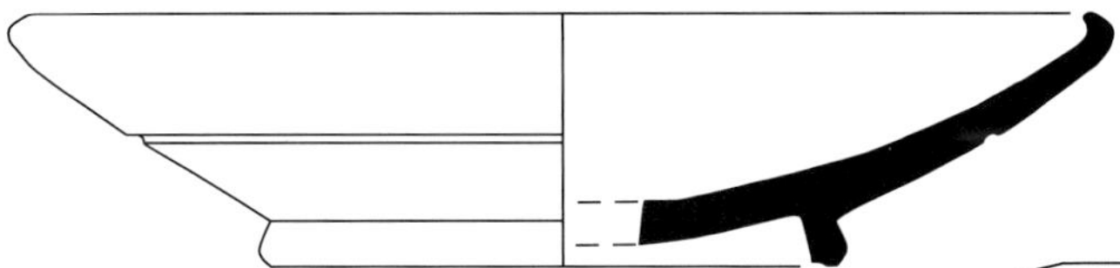

9

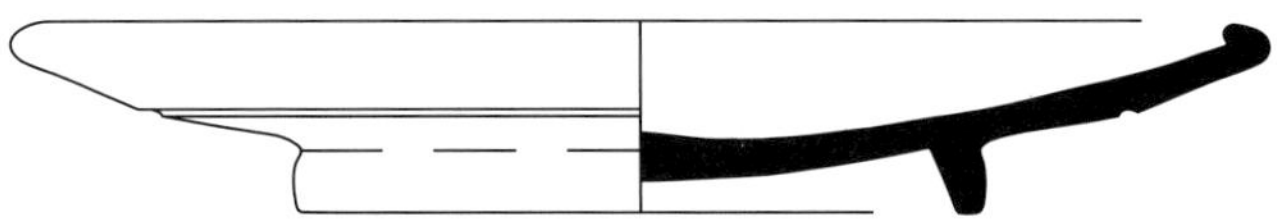

11

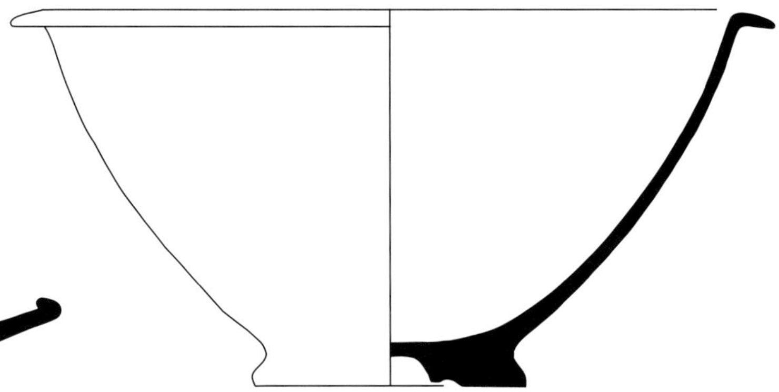

10

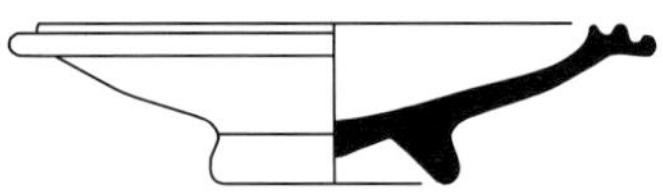

13

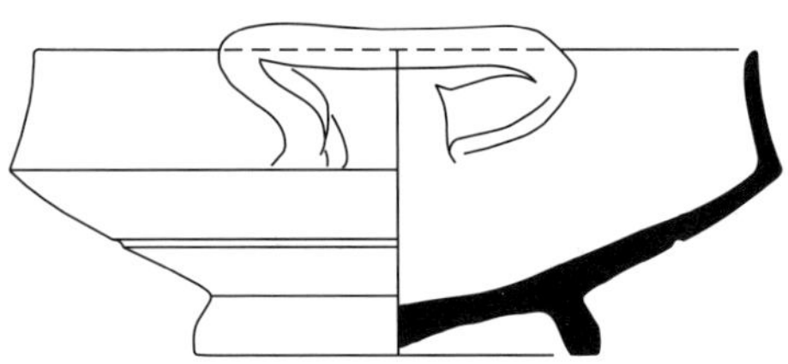

19

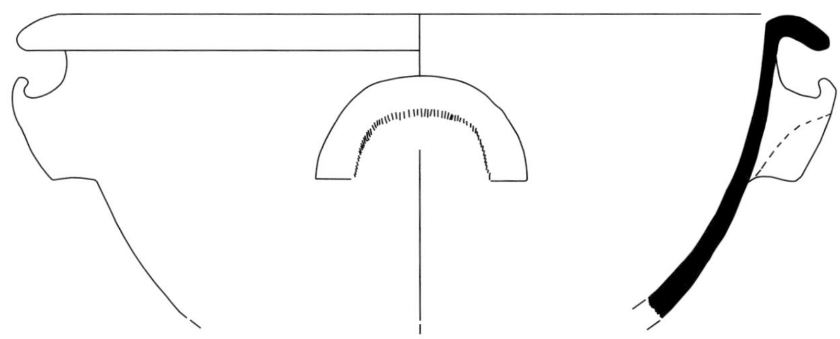

21

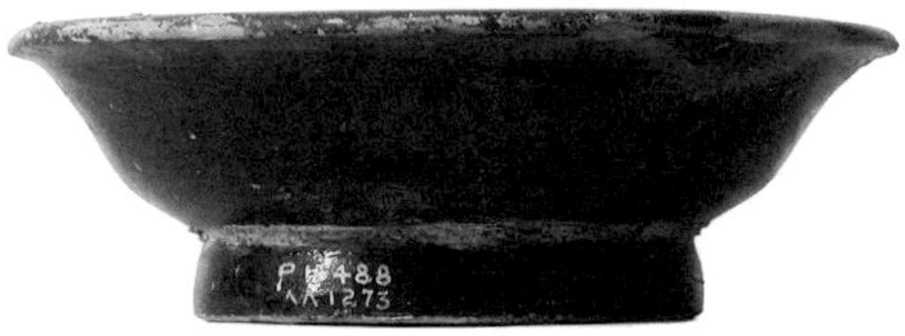

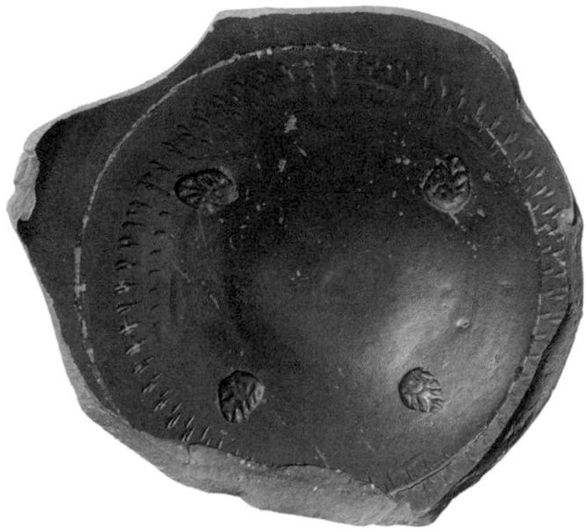

Figure 51 ***(opposite).*** **Fine ware, open shapes (1, 2, 4–11, 13, 19, 21).** Scale 1:3. Drawing S. I. Rotroff

Figure 52 ***(above, left).*** **Bowl with outturned rim (2).** Scale 1:2. Photo Agora Excavations

Figure 53 ***(above, right).*** **Bowl with stamped floor (3).** Scale 1:2. Photo C. A. Mauzy

proportion in 2nd-century Athens.[4] Of echinus bowls, only the small **8** is well preserved (one of the few intact vessels recovered); it is unusual in the pattern of the gloss, which covers only the interior and the upper exterior of the vessel (a fragment of another, slightly larger bowl with the same gloss pattern is uninventoried). This pattern is unknown in Attic pottery before the early 1st century,[5] and **8** is probably an import. The straight wall and nearly horizontal rim of **7** are typical for the second quarter of the 2nd century.[6] Three of the echinus bowls are remarkably large and decorated with a groove on the wall (e.g., **9**), a form that is extremely rare; a new review of the evidence suggests it was produced only in the second quarter of the 2nd century.[7] A rim fragment from the similar and also very rare beveled-rim bowl is also present.[8] A single deep bowl with a projecting rim was found, along with fragments of one or two others (see **10**).

Plates are a rarity (Fig. 51). Rolled-rim plates are present only in fragmentary examples (see **11**), and only one has stamped decoration: about one-quarter of the floor of a large plate bearing one linked stamp within rouletting (uninventoried). The stamp, which resembles those on bowls of the third quarter of the 3rd century,[9] marks the fragment as residual. Rilled-rim plates are represented by three well-preserved vessels and fragments of four more (see **12, 13**). Although the shape was put to ritual use in saucer pyres earlier in the Hellenistic period, it is also a common shape in domestic debris and does not necessarily have ritual overtones.[10] Fishplates are found only in fragments, and two of the five examples are very small—smaller than any other fishplates at the Agora. The saucer, a common shape at this period, is present only in fragments.

4. *Agora* XXIX, p. 156.

5. *Agora* XXIX, pp. 11–12.

6. *Agora* XXIX, p. 163; cf. p. 343, nos. 1022, 1024, fig. 63, pl. 77.

7. A date in the first quarter of the century (*Agora* XXIX, p. 164) now seems too early. The date is based on the few contexts in which the form is found: the Agora Bone Well, cistern F 5:1 (second quarter of the 2nd century), and the Middle Stoa building fill (H–K 12–14). The recent downdating of the closing of the Stoa fill from after ca. 183 to after ca. 170/168 makes a later date for the form seem likely. For this downdating, see p. 88, below.

8. See *Agora* XXIX, p. 164; cf. p. 344, nos. 1037, 1038, fig. 64, pl. 78.

9. Cf. *Agora* XXIX, pp. 331–332, nos. 885–888, pls. 144–146.

10. *Agora* XXIX, p. 151; for the shape in pyres, see Young 1951b; Rotroff 2013, pp. 27–28. It is probably these objects that Osanna (1988–1989, p. 89) terms *piatti sacrificali*.

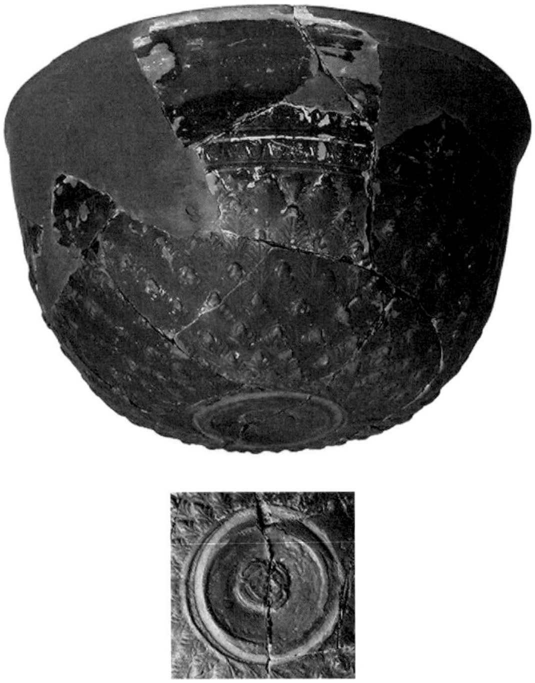

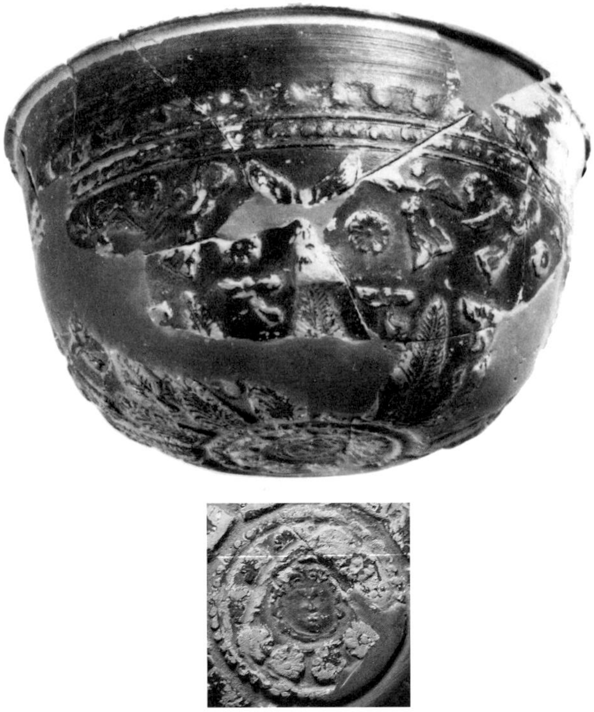

Figure 54 ***(left).*** **Imbricate moldmade bowl from Workshop A (14).** Scale 1:2. Photos S. I. Rotroff

Figure 55 ***(right).*** **Figured moldmade bowl, Class 1 (15).** Scale 1:2. Photos Agora Excavations, S. I. Rotroff

Vessels for Drink

Drinking cups are common in the ceramic assemblage throughout the Hellenistic world, reflecting both the human requirement for abundant liquid in a hot climate and the importance of the symposium in Greek culture. In the Agora Bone Well, however, only five substantially complete drinking vessels were found: four moldmade bowls (**14**, **15**, **17**, **18**, all of them missing several fragments; Figs. 54, 55, 57, 58) and a two-handled cup (**19**; Fig. 51). Less than half of a fifth moldmade bowl is preserved (**16**; Fig. 56). Fragments of West Slope kantharoi are residual, dating to the 3rd century. The same may be true of pieces of two West Slope hemispherical cups (see **20**; Fig. 59), a shape that enjoyed its greatest popularity in the 3rd century, although it continued to be made sporadically thereafter. Other vessels of the symposium assemblage are restricted to fragments of two West Slope amphoras and possibly one each of an oinochoe and an olpe. Fragments of three large lug-handled kraters (see **21**; Fig. 51) make an unusual concentration of this relatively rare, primarily 3rd-century shape; but despite its name, it is likely that this plain, black-gloss bowl was not commonly used in the context of symposium.[11] In any event, the shape was probably obsolete long before the well was filled. It seems clear that upscale drinking parties never took place on the north side of the Kolonos Agoraios.

The angular profile of the two-handled cup (**19**; Fig. 51) indicates a date after ca. 175,[12] but it can add little to the finer distinction of chronology. The moldmade bowls, however, provide important evidence for the narrowing of the date of the deposit. In addition to the five inventoried examples, there are about 113 nonjoining segments of bowls. The material is so fragmentary that it is difficult to estimate a minimum number of vessels, but at least 30 bowls are represented, and probably many more. The overall composition of this group is extremely uniform, which suggests that the deposit did not accumulate over a very long period of time.

11. *Agora* XXIX, p. 138.
12. *Agora* XXIX, p. 119.

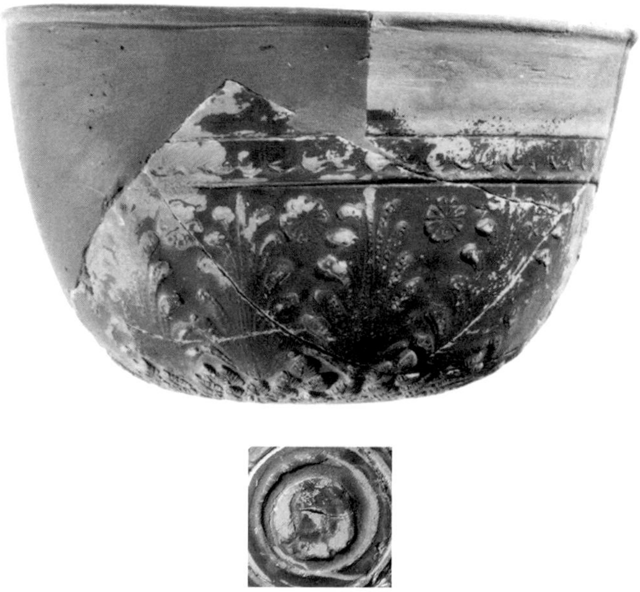

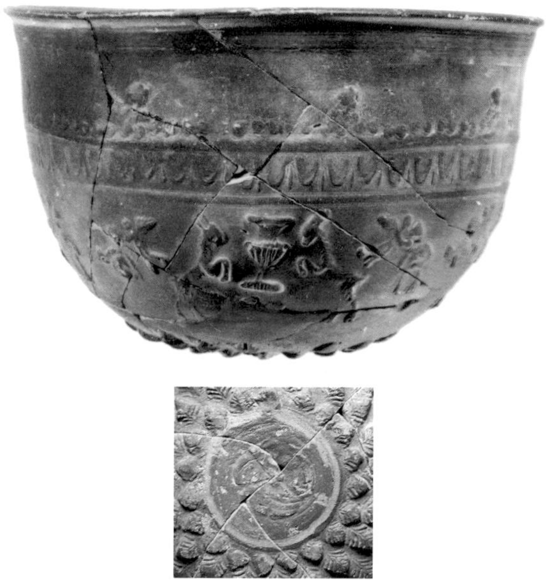

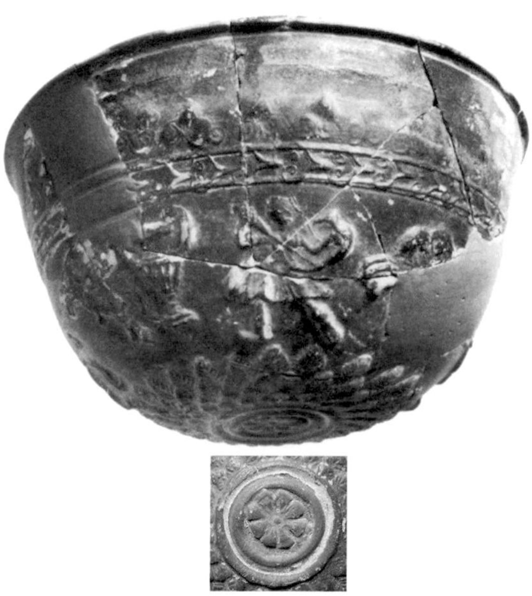

Figure 56 ***(left).*** **Floral moldmade bowl, Class 2 (16).** Scale 1:2. Photos Agora Excavations, S. I. Rotroff

Figure 57 ***(above, right).*** **Figured moldmade bowl, M Monogram Class (17).** Scale 1:2. Photos Agora Excavations, S. I. Rotroff

Figure 58 ***(right).*** **Figured moldmade bowl (18).** Scale 1:2. Photos Agora Excavations, S. I. Rotroff

Starting with the inventoried bowls, we may note that three of them can be associated with classes that find parallels within the second quarter of the 2nd century and not before: Class 1, Class 2, and the M Monogram Class (**15–17**; Figs. 55–57). All three of these classes are distinguished by simplified and rather small motifs, in higher relief than was usually the case in the earliest generations of production. Eleven examples of Class 1 are known from the Agora Excavations.[13] The earliest contexts in which they have been found have closing dates of around 160;[14] conversely, they do not occur in any of several large deposits, rich in moldmade bowls, that were laid down in the 170s.[15] The introduction of Class 1 can therefore be pinpointed in the decade 170–160. Only four examples of Class 2 have been identified at the Agora.[16] The earliest firm context there (other than the Agora Bone Well) is the building fill of the Stoa of Attalos, which was probably put in place around the middle of the 2nd century. Two further examples were recovered from *Abschnitten* VII and VIII of Dipylon Well B_1

13. Ten bowls and one mold; see *Agora* XXII, p. 30, with n. 68.

14. Cistern N 20:7 and well O 16:3; for the dates, see *Agora* XXXIII, pp. 368–369. Here and elsewhere, dates take into account Finkielsztejn's revisions to the Rhodian amphora chronology (Finkielsztejn 2001). See below, p. 88.

15. F 17:4, M 21:1, the middle fill of N 21:4, and P 21:4; for the current dating of these deposits, see *Agora* XXXIII, pp. 357, 365–366, 369, 371–372.

16. See *Agora* XXII, pp. 30–31.

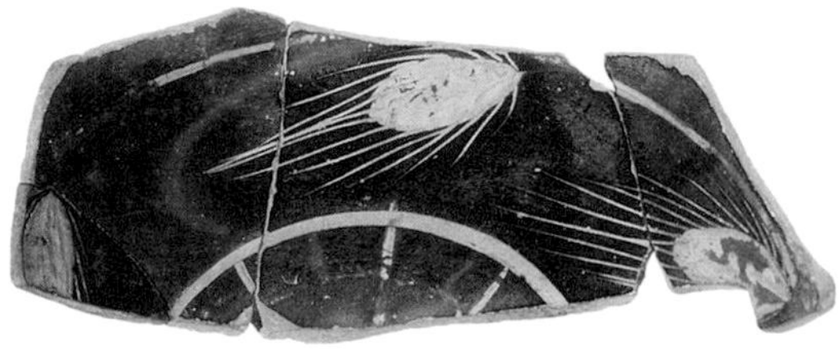

Figure 59. Hemispherical West Slope drinking cup (20). Scale 1:2. Photo Agora Excavations

at the Kerameikos, deposited in the 170s or later.[17] The fact that no bowls of Class 2 occur in the large Agora deposits of the first 30 years of the 2nd century mentioned above urges an initial date later than ca. 170. These early deposits also lack examples of the M Monogram Class, a monotonous series of bowls almost always decorated with rampant goats and dramatic masks. Although only a few have been inventoried, many have been recognized in context pottery.[18] Two fragments have been found in the large fills that lay under the Middle Stoa (H–K 12–14) and over the Square Peristyle Building at the northeast corner of the Agora (Q 8–9), with material largely from the first third of the 2nd century, but most come from deposits that were laid down no earlier than ca. 160. A fourth bowl (**18**; Fig. 58), although not attributed to a class, shares the high relief of the others, and through its stamps can be linked to bowls from deposits of the second quarter of the century.[19] The only bowl that may be earlier is **14** (Fig. 54), an imbricate bowl that can be attributed to Workshop A, a shop that was active from the earliest years of the production of moldmade bowls, in the later 3rd century. The rim pattern of this bowl, however, lacks the fine detail of the shop's earlier products, so it is possible that it, too, dates to the second quarter of the 2nd century.

A restricted time frame emerges even more clearly from an analysis of the fragments. Most share the late characteristics of the bowls discussed above—small stamps, high relief—as well as other indicators, such as manufacture in very worn molds. Only 15 fragments come from bowls with the crisp decoration characteristic of the first 50 years of production.[20] Bowls of this sort are the staple of the deposits laid down in the 170s; their limited representation in the Agora Bone Well suggests that this material went into the well considerably later than that, when even fragments of these

17. Braun 1970, pp. 150–151, 154, nos. 150, 174, fig. 24, pls. 65, 66, 68, 70. A *terminus post quem* for the deposit of the lower of those two levels (*Abschnitt* VII) is furnished by a Rhodian amphora handle with the eponym Archidamos (Braun 1970, p. 152, no. 159, pl. 66), dated to ca. 180/178 (Finkielsztejn 2001, p. 192, table 19).

18. For a list of contexts in which they occur, see *Agora* XXII, p. 29, n. 67.

19. The same amazon stamp appears on P 23039 (*Agora* XXII, p. 73, no. 235, pls. 45, 84, from the fill of South Stoa II, deposited ca. 150 [see *Agora* XXIX, p. 462, under M–N 15:1]), which is further linked to a bowl in Group C by a stamp of a hoplite (P 4101, Thompson 1934, p. 353, no. C 20, fig. 38; for the deposit date of Group C, ca. 165, see *Agora* XXII, p. 109, and *Agora* XXIX, pp. 452–453, under G 6:2). Note, however, that Group C is dated on the basis of its moldmade bowls, so it can hardly be used in turn to date them.

20. Two small floral fragments, possibly from a single bowl; one fragment of an imbricate bowl probably from Workshop A (cf. *Agora* XXII, p. 48, no. 30, pl. 5); four figured fragments from Workshop A, all perhaps from the same bowl (rampant goats; cf. *Agora* XXII, p. 57, no. 108, pl. 19); two small calyx fragments perhaps from Workshop A; four figured fragments from the Workshop of Bion (cocks: cf. *Agora* XXII, p. 60, nos. 134, 136, pl. 25; biga, eros on goat: cf. *Agora* XXII, p. 62, no. 153, pl. 28, 78; erotes between fronds: cf. *Agora* XXII, p. 64, no. 171, pls. 31, 79; ovolo rim pattern: cf. *Agora* XXII, p. 64, no. 170, pls. 31); and two small calyx fragments, perhaps from the Workshop of Bion (cf. *Agora* XXII, pp. 56, 74, nos. 106, 242, pls. 18, 47) and possibly from the same bowls as some of the figured fragments.

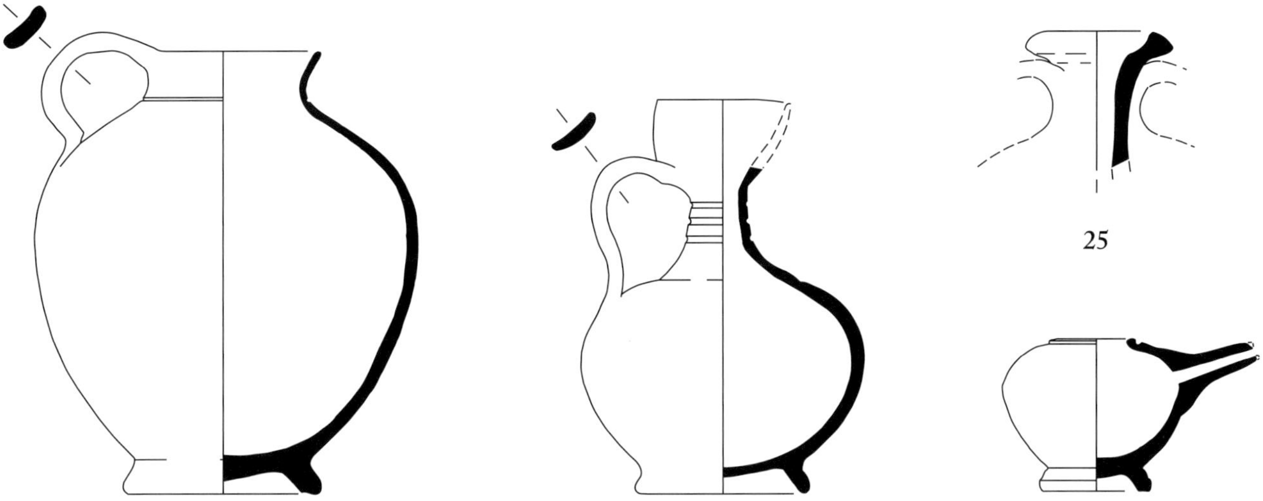

Figure 60. Fine ware, closed shapes (22, 23, 25, 26). Scale 1:3. Drawing S. I. Rotroff

types were no longer entering the archaeological record: ca. 165 or later. Since long-petal bowls, introduced close to 150, are lacking, the period of accumulation will have been short, probably no more than 15 years.

Other Shapes

Substantially complete closed shapes (Figs. 60–62) are limited to three vessels: a round-mouth jug (**22**), a canteen (**24**), and a feeder (**26**). There is also a lekythos (less than half preserved, **23**), a small oil vessel suitable for use at the table and in the kitchen. The plainness of the round-mouth jug suggests use with water rather than wine; the shape may also have served as an informal measure,[21] and as such would have been useful in either household or workshop. About 50 canteens are known from Athens, ranging in date from the early 3rd to the mid-2nd century.[22] There are two in the well: one substantially complete (**24**; Fig. 61), the other preserved only in fragments (**25**; Fig. 60). Both were stamped with a maker's name: Dorotheos on **24**, a different but illegible name on **25**. Dorotheos's stamp closely resembles the stamp of a fabricant of Rhodian amphoras whose career apparently spanned the years ca. 182–140.[23] If the canteen was made in the same workshop, a date somewhat later than the span 190–175 assigned to **24** in *Agora* XXIX is probable.[24] The feeder (**26**; Figs. 60, 62) is an extraordinarily rare shape, known in only two other Hellenistic examples at the Agora and only a few published examples of Hellenistic date elsewhere.[25]

21. For the use of the shape as a measure, see *Agora* XXIX, p. 132; *Agora* XXXIII, p. 79; Rotroff 2011a.

22. *Agora* XXIX, pp. 183–187.

23. Jöhrens 1999, p. 69, no. 180. He is associated with the eponyms Kleonymos and Aristogeitos, whose terms Finkielsztejn (2001, pp. 192, 195, tables 19, 21) places in ca. 182 and 140.

24. *Agora* XXIX, p. 359, no. 1206. Note also that, if it was made in this workshop, it is probably a Rhodian import, not Attic. For this issue, see *Agora* XXIX, pp. 186–187.

25. For the other examples from the *Agora*, see *Agora* XXIX, p. 358, nos. 1194, 1196, fig. 73, pl. 87. See n. 110, below, for other Hellenistic feeders.

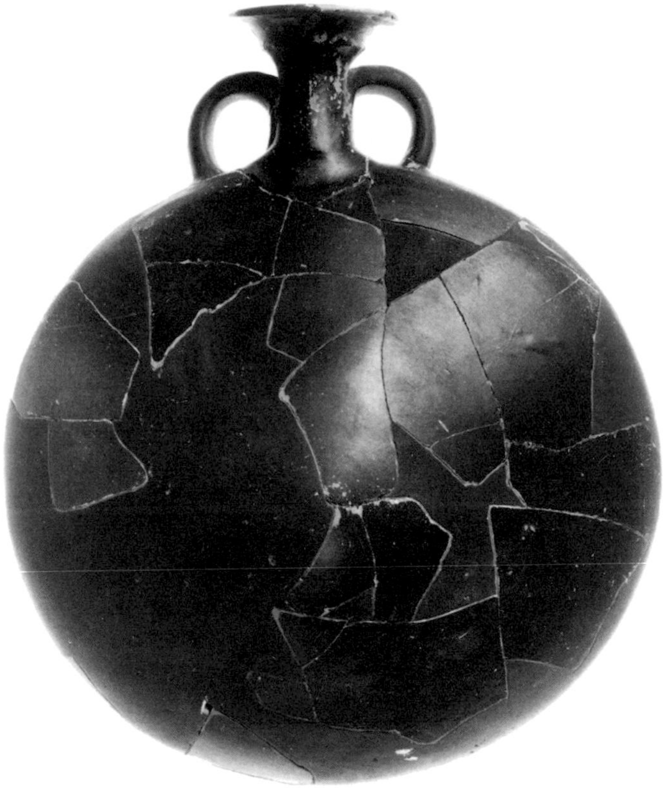

Figure 61. Canteen (24). Scale 1:3. Photo Agora Excavations

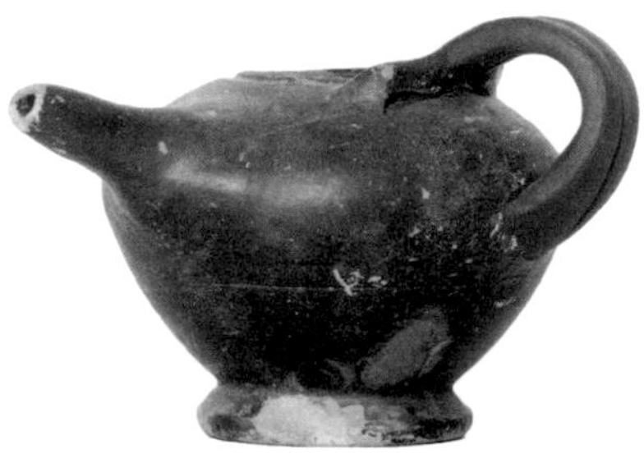

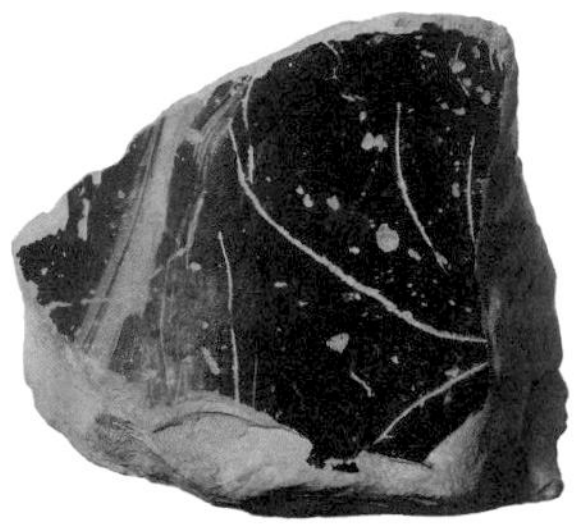

Figure 62 *(left)*. Feeder (26). Scale 1:2. Photo Agora Excavations

Figure 63 *(right)*. Fragment of a Panathenaic amphora, showing part of helmet and face of Athena (27). Scale 1:2. Photo C. A. Mauzy

Generally similar vessels were made at many other times and places as well—for example, in Roman Gaul and in prehistoric Egypt[26]—and there has been much discussion of their purpose. Although use as a lamp filler, breast pump, or invalid feeder has been proposed, most scholars have accepted an identification as a feeding bottle for infants or small children,[27] and chemical analysis of Roman examples has confirmed that they once held milk (whether human or otherwise has not been determined).[28]

Although it is only a small fragment, the Panathenaic amphora (**27**; Fig. 63) is of interest in connection with the ultimate source of the material in the well. G. Roger Edwards, noting a concentration of Panathenaics of the 3rd and early 2nd century on the Kolonos Agoraios, suggested that

26. For discussions of the Roman examples, see Rouquet 2003. For an Egyptian example, see Murail et al. 2004, p. 274, fig. 9.

27. For bibliography and discussion, see *Agora* XII, pp. 161–162; Rouquet 2003; Centlivres Challet 2016.

28. Huttmann et al. 1989. They analyzed 38 feeders of glass and clay, mostly probably from graves of the 2nd to 4th centuries A.D. in Germany.

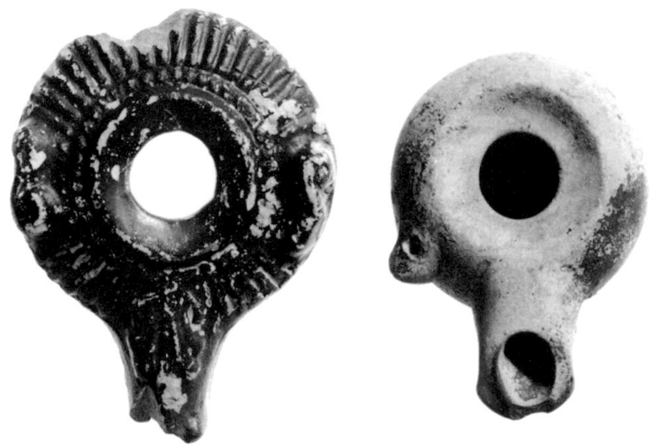

28 29

Figure 64. Lamps (28, 29). Scale 1:2.
Photo Agora Excavations

during this period the collection of prize oil became the duty of the military treasurer, and that Panathenaics were stored in the Arsenal, located to the south and up the hill from the well.[29] This, then, may be the source of our fragment.

Two miniatures—an unglazed two-handled cup and a small closed vessel (an oinochoe?) covered with black gloss—are probably votives (both uninventoried). The cup is of a type documented only in the 4th and 3rd centuries and must be residual; its source may be the same as that of the hundreds of similar cups found in the Cave Cistern, about 30 m to the south of the Agora Bone Well.[30] An uninventoried fragment of a lopadion, a small version of the lopas that is found almost exclusively in ritual pyres,[31] is also of votive character. Its form and gritty cooking fabric date it to the late 5th or 4th century and hence mark it too as residual.

The only complete lamp is a plain wheelmade one of Howland's type 33A (**29**; Fig. 64), a type that was made from the late 3rd to the middle of the 2nd century.[32] A large moldmade lamp of type 45C (**28**; Fig. 64), with crisp details though less than half preserved, finds its closest parallel in a lamp from a context no later than ca. 200 and probably dates to the 3rd century. Ten more lamps are documented by small fragments. Four may be contemporary with the deposit (fragments of one type 43D and three of perhaps type 33 or 34); the others are residual, ranging in date from the 5th to the mid-3rd century.

29. Edwards 1957, pp. 333–337; see also Pounder 1983, pp. 249–250.

30. Rotroff 1983, pp. 268, 270, 289, no. 46, pl. 55. Votive cups of this type were very common in the Late Classical and Early Hellenistic periods but had disappeared from the archaeological record by ca. 175 (*Agora* XXIX, p. 209). The form of the example from the Agora Bone Well (with well-developed handles) suggests a date in the 4th century. We know of no Hellenistic parallel for the other miniature.

31. *Agora* XXIX, p. 216; Rotroff 2013, pp. 20–22.

32. *Agora* IV, p. 103, no. 440, pls. 15, 42, with its closest parallels in deposits of the first half of the 2nd century: cf. *Agora* IV, p. 103, no. 439, pls. 15, 42, from the building fill of the Stoa of Attalos, and L 4572 (unpublished) from the lower fill of deposit D 17:4 (see *Agora* XXXIII, p. 439).

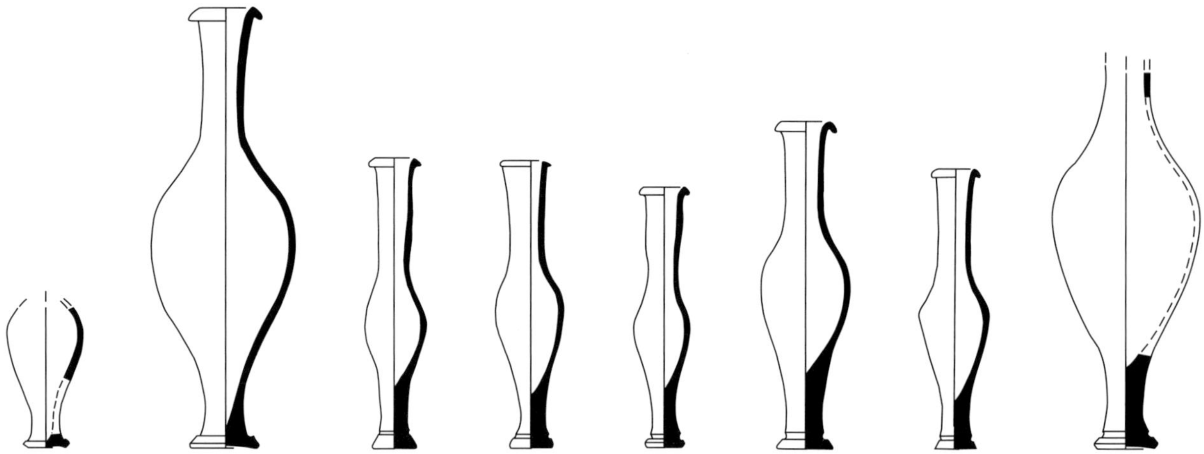

Figure 65. Unguentaria (30–34, 36, 38, 39). Scale 1:3. Drawing S. I. Rotroff

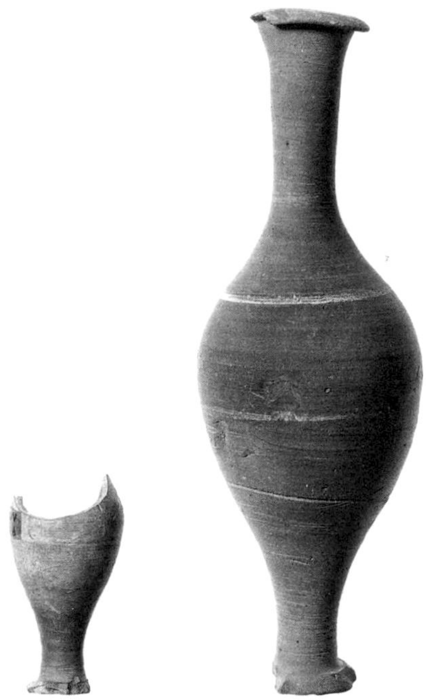

Figure 66. Unguentaria (30, 31). Scale 1:2. Photo Agora Excavations

Plain Ware

Unguentaria

Nineteen unguentaria (containers for perfumed oil) are represented in the Agora Bone Well, most of them probably contemporary with the bone deposit (Figs. 65, 66; Table 5). The fragmentary **30**, with a hollow stem and tooled foot, belongs to category 3 and is probably residual from the first quarter of the 2nd century.[33] The well-worked foot and largely hollow stem of **31** assign it to category 4, a type that ranges from the late 3rd to the mid-2nd century. The rest, seven of which are intact or lack only minor chips and two whole but broken, belong to category 5 (see **32–39**); here the

33. For the classification of gray unguentaria and their dates, see *Agora* XXXIII, pp. 150–156.

stem is completely solid and the foot indicated by a simple groove. Such unguentaria were made from about 180 until the end of the 2nd century.

Household Ware, Open Shapes

Over 60 vessels of household ware (not including transport amphoras) are documented from the well, almost all of them large open shapes (Table 5). The greatest proportion belongs to two-handled basins (lekanai), present in at least 32 examples, six of them well preserved (Figs. 67, 69). It is unlikely that repetitive examples of these bulky items would have been mended and inventoried during the original processing of the finds. What now remains among the context pottery consists almost exclusively of rim and wall fragments with handles attached, some quite large and preserving complete profiles; we may assume that wall, foot, floor, and handleless rim fragments were discarded as insufficiently diagnostic, and that the total count of substantially complete vessels was once higher.

The most common type in the well is a broad, shallow vessel with a straight wall and an overhanging rim, with handles that have been pressed into the rim by the potter's thumb (lekane, form 4; see **44**, **45**; Figs. 67, 93).[34] This form was introduced around 200 and grew to become the commonest type of basin in the remainder of the Hellenistic period. At least 22 are documented in the well; some have a flat bottom (see **45**), a variant that is first found around 160. A smaller, more delicate basin with a profiled rim and upturned handles, an invention of the Early Hellenistic period, is present in three well-preserved examples (one intact except for chips), along with fragments of four more (lekane, form 1; see **40–42**; Figs. 67, 93).[35] There is one largely complete deep lekane with horizontal handles, a long-lived form with a Classical ancestry (lekane, form 3; **43**; Fig. 67);[36] handles of two more are present. Similar to this, but lacking handles, are two deep bowls (**46**, **47**; Figs. 67, 68, 93).[37] Despite its simplicity, this form is unknown earlier in the Hellenistic period; these two are the earliest documented at the Agora. A broader and shallower but still capacious bowl, preserved in three examples (see **48**, **49**; Figs. 67, 69), is a much commoner form and was made from the Late Classical period through the first half of the 2nd century.[38] Smaller bowls of the same shape occur in five largely complete examples and slightly less than half of a sixth (see **50–52**; Figs. 67, 69). This shape is known in only a few other instances, all of them found with material discarded between 175 and 125.[39] The heavy concentration of this rather uncommon shape in the well is surprising but difficult to interpret.

In addition to the lekanai and bowls described above, there are two well-preserved kraters and fragments of four others (see **53**, **54**; Figs. 70, 93).[40] Introduced somewhat before the middle of the 3rd century, the household-ware krater was made throughout the Hellenistic period at

34. *Agora* XXXIII, pp. 112–113.
35. *Agora* XXXIII, pp. 109–110.
36. *Agora* XXXIII, pp. 111–112.
37. *Agora* XXXIII, p. 114.
38. *Agora* XXXIII, pp. 114–115.
39. The other inventoried examples are P 8581, P 11670 (*Agora* XXXIII, p. 277, no. 302, fig. 52, pl. 41), P 14310, and P 27365; they are from deposits E 6:2 (lower fill, deposited ca. 125), M 20:4 (deposited ca. 175), and N 20:7 (deposited ca. 160). For these deposits, see *Agora* XXXIII, pp. 351, 365, 368–369.
40. *Agora* XXXIII, pp. 105–107.

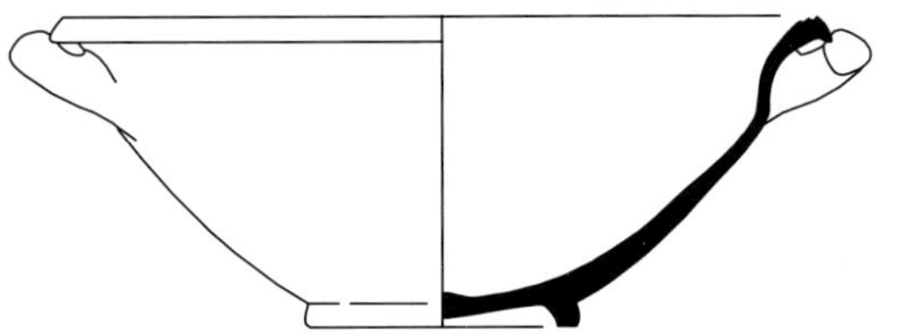

40

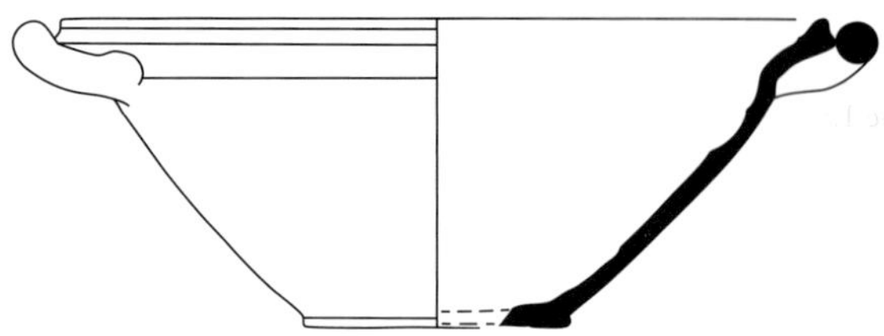

42

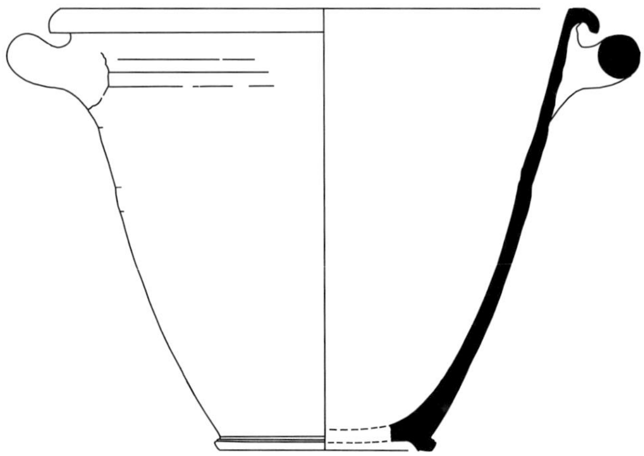

43

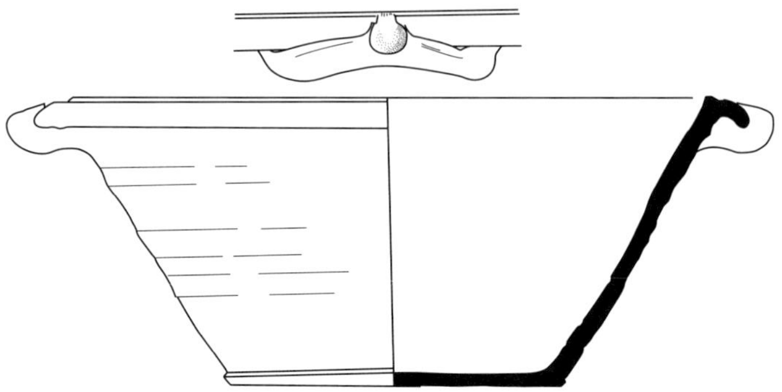

44

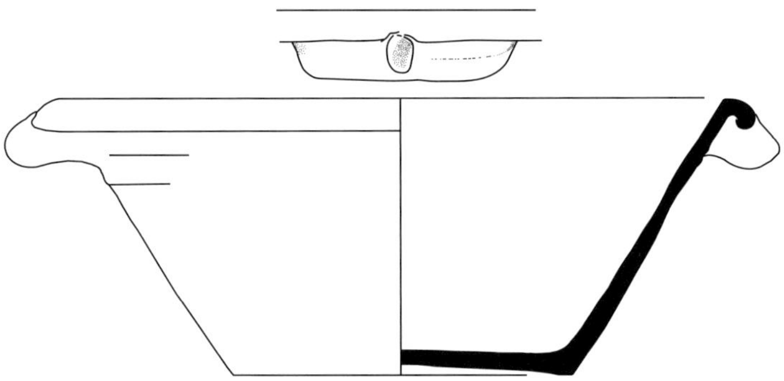

45

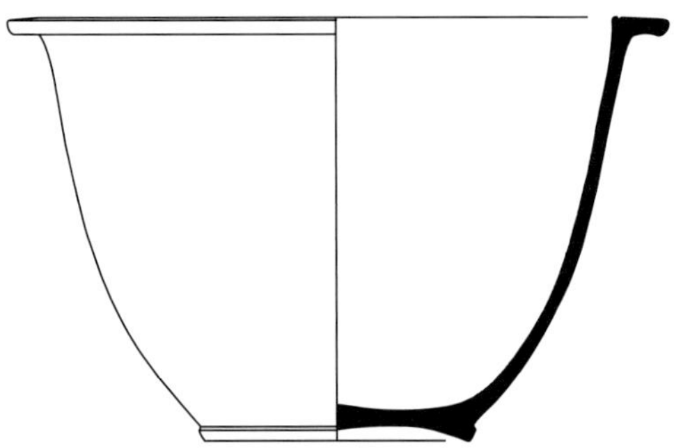

46

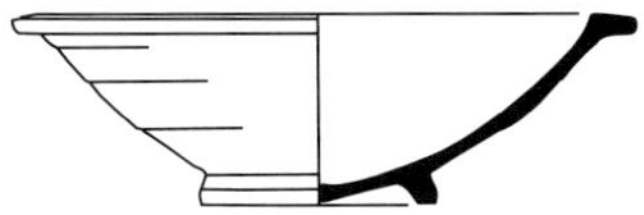

50

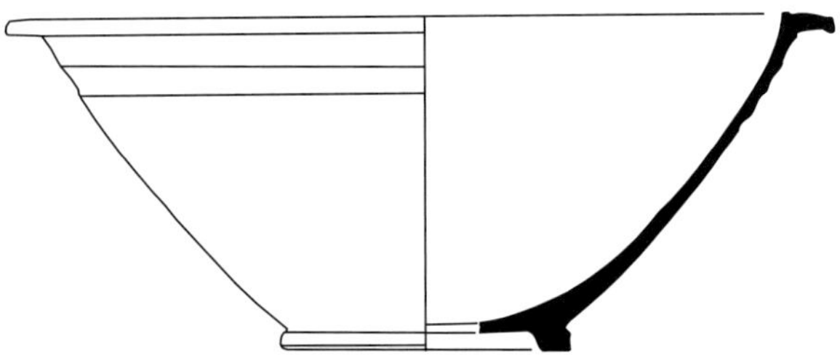

49

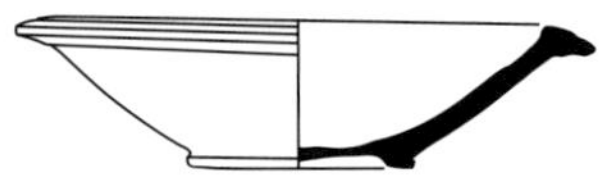

52

Figure 67 *(opposite)*. **Household-ware lekanai and bowls (40, 42–46, 49, 50, 52).** Scale 1:5. Drawings A. Hooton, S. I. Rotroff

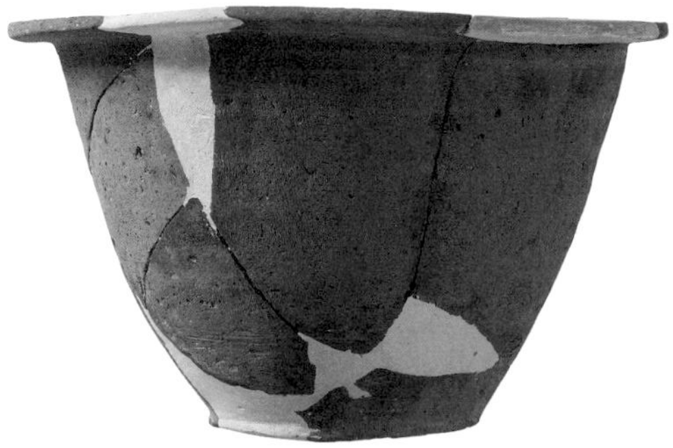

Figure 68 *(right)*. **Household-ware deep bowl (47).** Scale 1:4. Photo C. A. Mauzy

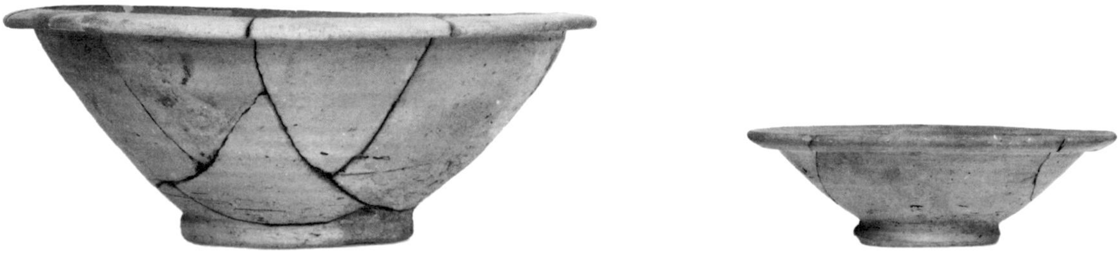

48 **51**

Figure 69. Household-ware bowls (48, 51). Scale 1:4. Photo Agora Excavations

Athens. Its function, however, remains obscure. It resembles the fine-ware column krater of earlier times and carries simple painted decoration, but its coarse fabric seems to preclude use as a table vessel. There are two well-preserved mortars and a large portion of a third (see **55**; Fig. 70). These are of the typical Hellenistic variety, with a spout, a downcurved rim, and piecrust handles, which remained a common shape throughout the period.[41] The vessel could be used for grinding vegetables, greens, herbs, spices, and the like. There is also the lower part of a beehive (**56**; Fig. 71), identified by the characteristic scoring on the interior;[42] this vessel had been broken and mended with lead clamps in antiquity. A final miscellany includes a small fragment from the rim of a pithos or vat, a very large foot (of a vat or perhaps an amphora stand), and the knob of a lid.

Household Ware, Closed Shapes

Closed household shapes are almost completely lacking. A single large jug with a cylindrical neck, a profiled rim, and a thick round handle is the only well-preserved example (form 2: **57**; Fig. 70).[43] The shape occurs throughout the Hellenistic period at Athens and has a Classical ancestry at Corinth. No jugs of this shape have been found in the period-of-use fills of Agora wells, so it was apparently not used for the drawing of water, perhaps being considered too large for this task. Two rim fragments may come from jugs of form 4, a shape that was probably more commonly used as a measure than a water vessel.[44] The absence or minimal representation of jugs is not unparalleled in Agora deposits, but here it underlines the

41. *Agora* XXXIII, pp. 100–102.
42. *Agora* XXXIII, pp. 124–128.
43. *Agora* XXXIII, pp. 76–77.
44. *Agora* XXXIII, pp. 78–79; Rotroff 2011a, pp. 702–703.

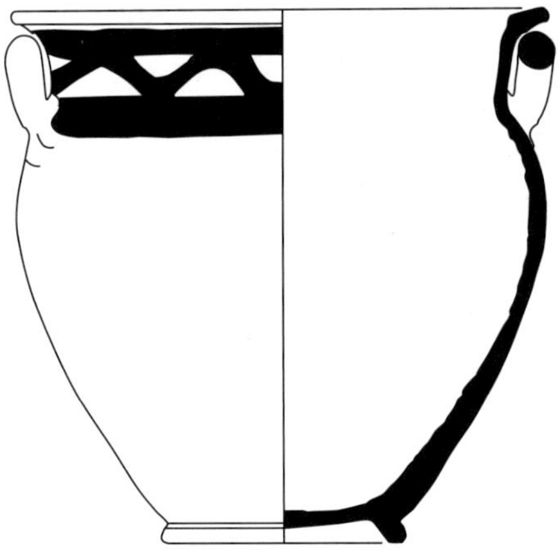

53

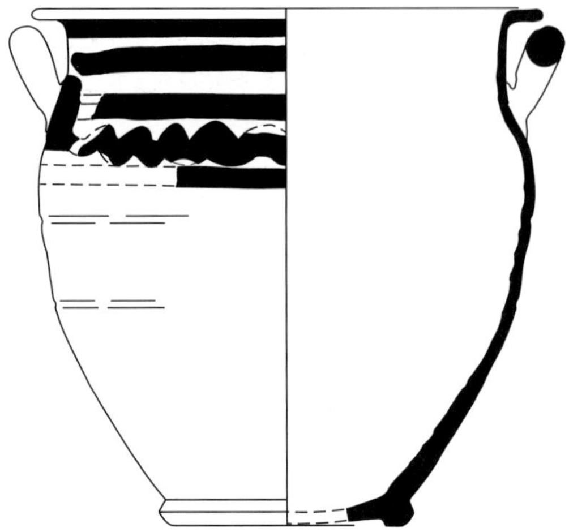

54

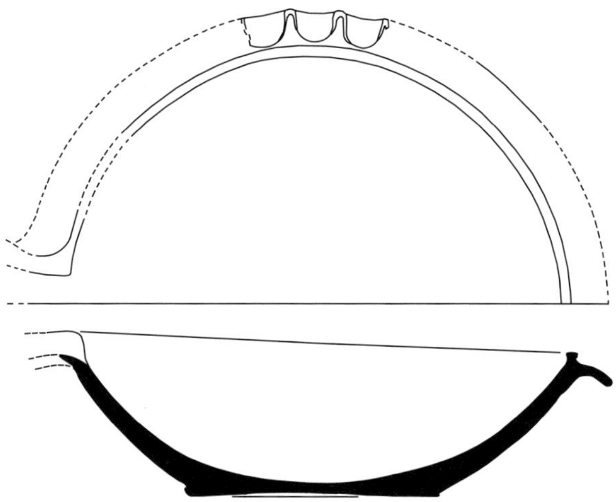

55

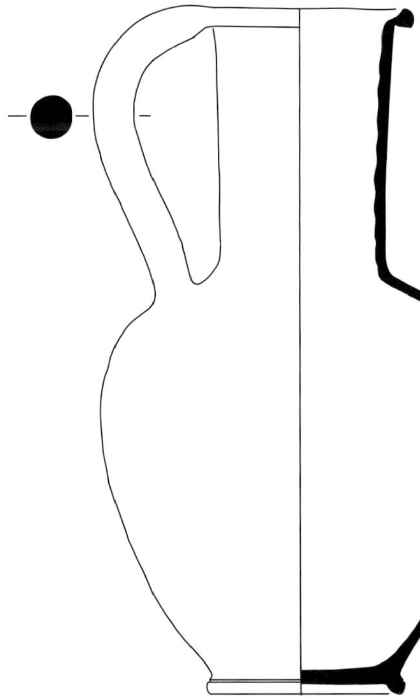

57

Figure 70. Kraters (53, 54), mortar (55), and jug (57). Scale 1:5. Drawings A. Hooton, S. I. Rotroff

obvious fact that this well was not being used as a source of water during the time documented by the deposit. The upper part of a narrow-necked amphora survives, a local imitation of an imported form, made of the Pink temper fabric characteristic of 2nd-century Athens (**58**; Fig. 72).[45] Parts of two lagynoi (see **59**; Fig. 73), imported thin-necked jugs brought to Athens for their contents, are also present.[46] Storage bins are attested by two rim fragments.[47]

45. See *Agora* XXXIII, pp. 86–87 (for the shape), 23–28 (for Pink temper fabric).

46. *Agora* XXXIII, pp. 82–84.

47. Form 1; see *Agora* XXXIII, p. 94.

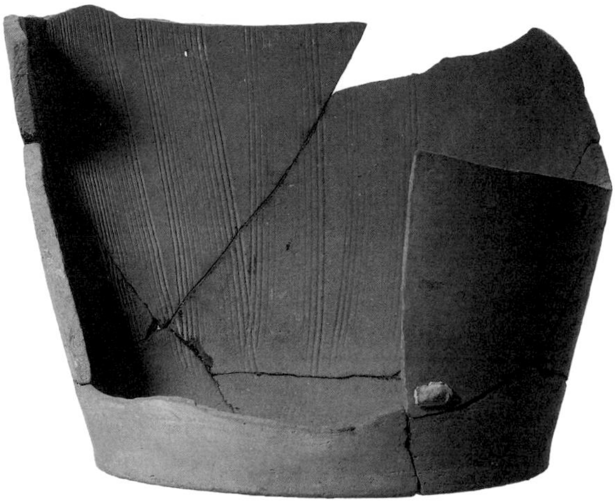

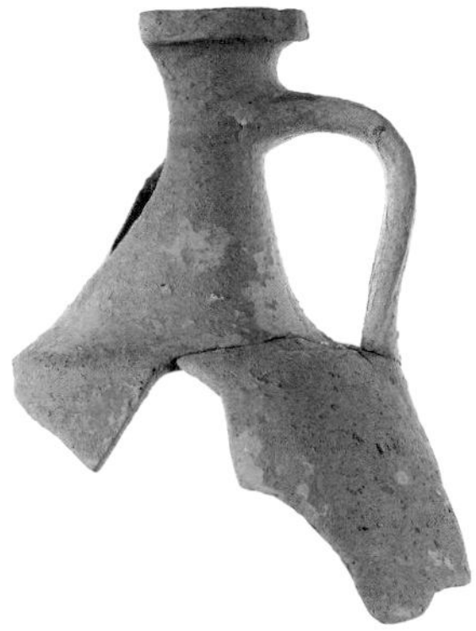

Figure 71 ***(left)*****. Beehive (56).**
Scale 1:4. Photo Agora Excavations

Figure 72 ***(right)*****. Amphora (58).**
Scale 1:3. Photo Agora Excavations

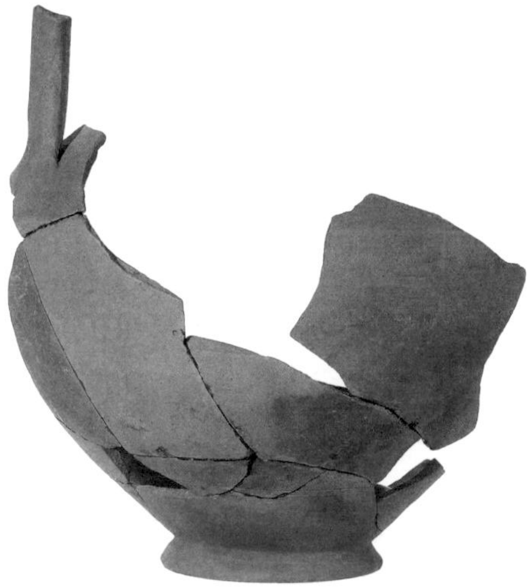

Figure 73. Lagynos (59). Scale 1:4.
Photo Agora Excavations

Cooking Ware

The well's assemblage of cooking ware (the remnants of 20 vessels) is somewhat unusual (Fig. 74; Table 5). While the lopas dominates Hellenistic Athenian cooking equipment, it is substantially outnumbered by the chytra here. Three forms of chytra are represented. The simple, one-handled, lidless form 1 (**60**–**63**; Figs. 74, 75, 92)[48] occurs in three intact examples, two that are over half preserved, and three fragments. They are uniformly small, with complete examples measuring between 0.10 and 0.12 m in height. This is in accord with the development of the shape, for although large chytrai are the rule in the 3rd century, form 1 chytrai from deposits laid down after ca. 170 are generally of this smaller size, inadequate for the stewing of even pot-sized pieces of meat. Their function remains mysterious—quickly heating water when only a small amount was called for?—but sooting on their exteriors shows that they had seen use. Only three large chytrai are represented. One is a two-handled vessel with a grooved, vertical rim (**64**; Fig. 74), a variant of form 4,[49] and one of the largest chytrai of any form found at the Agora.

48. *Agora* XXXIII, pp. 167–169.
49. *Agora* XXXIII, pp. 172–173.

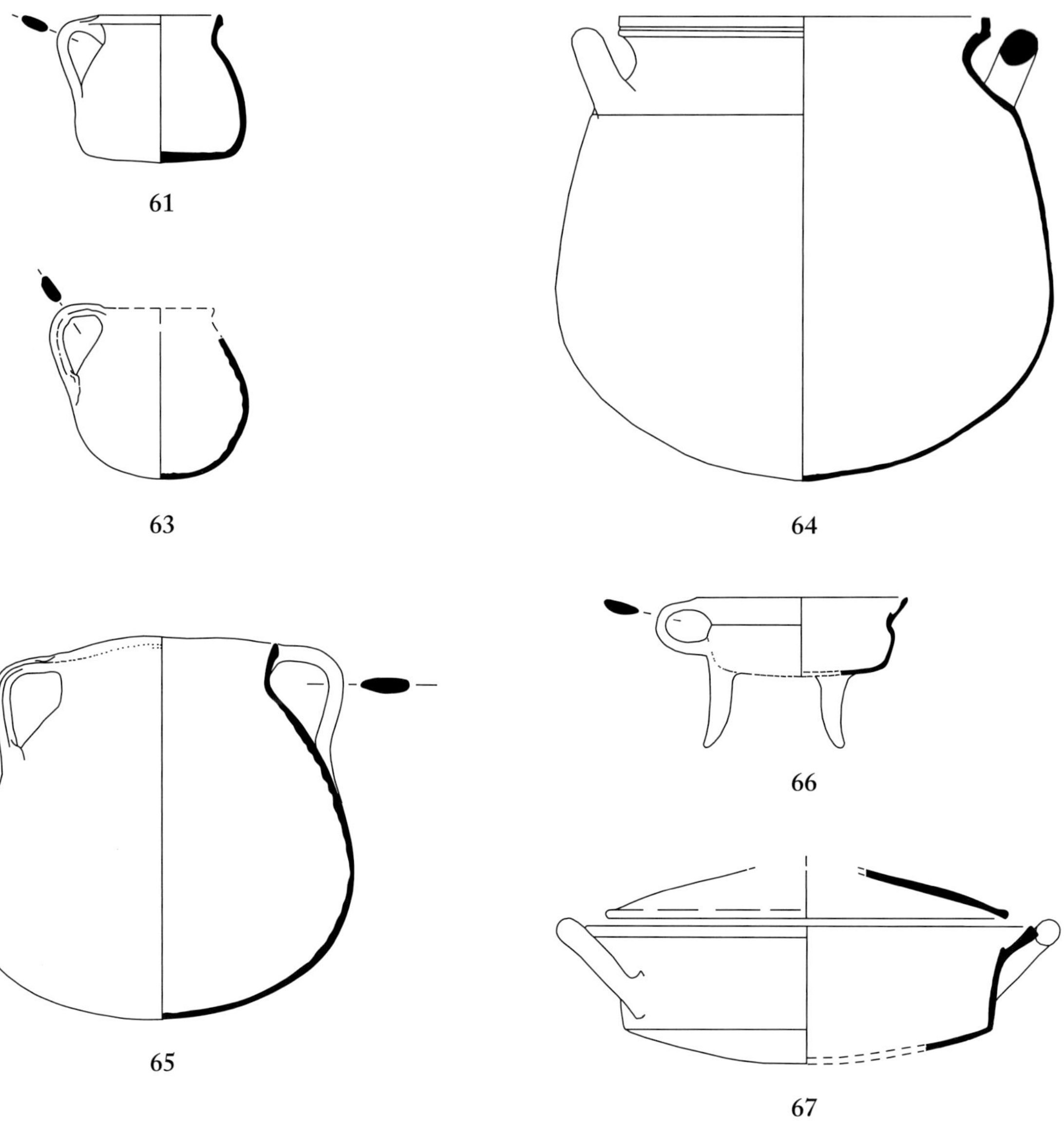

Figure 74. Cooking ware (61, 63–67). Scale 1:5. Drawing S. I. Rotroff

Its gritty, ochre fabric marks it as an import;[50] the fabric is found in only four examples at the Agora, all from deposits of the second quarter of the 2nd century. Fragments of a second, identical vessel bore a thick, calcareous deposit with a remarkably high lead content on its floor, the remnant of some craft or industrial activity.[51] A single two-handled chytra with a baggy body (form 10: **65**; Fig. 74), a local shape that was introduced in the 2nd century,[52] is one of the two earliest certain examples of the shape.

The lopas is present in only two examples. One (**66**; Fig. 74), more than half of which is restored, represents an unusual variant on the most common Attic lopas of the Hellenistic period (form 3).[53] The shape is characterized by a flat bottom, a nearly vertical wall, and an offset rim with a slight flange on the interior to receive a lid. Usually there are two horizontal handles; in this case, however, there is a single vertical one, and the vessel has been equipped with three tripod legs. These are arranged so that it is easy to tip up the vessel with the handle, and it was probably designed for that purpose. The other lopas (**67**; Fig. 74) is an import and

50. For this fabric, see *Agora* XXXIII, p. 47.

51. Rotroff 2011c, p. 124, where it is suggested that this material might be lead putty.

52. *Agora* XXXIII, pp. 177–178.

53. *Agora* XXXIII, pp. 180–182.

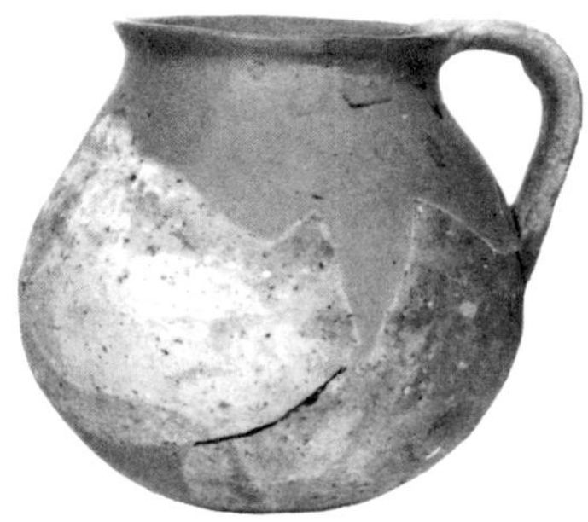

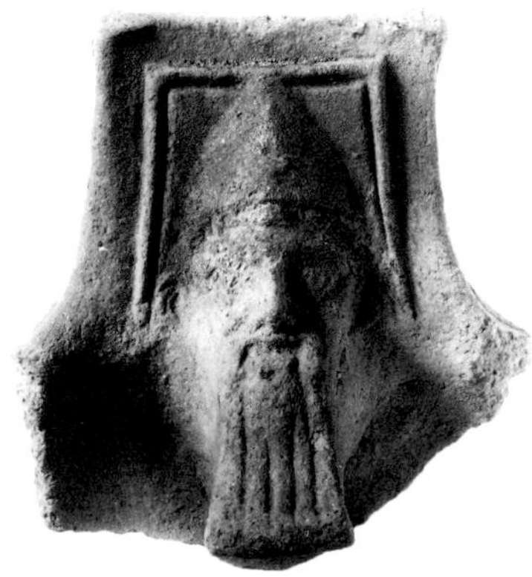

Figure 75 ***(left)*****. Chytra (63).** Scale 1:3. Photo Agora Excavations

Figure 76 ***(right)*****. Brazier lug (68).** Scale 1:2. Photo Agora Excavations

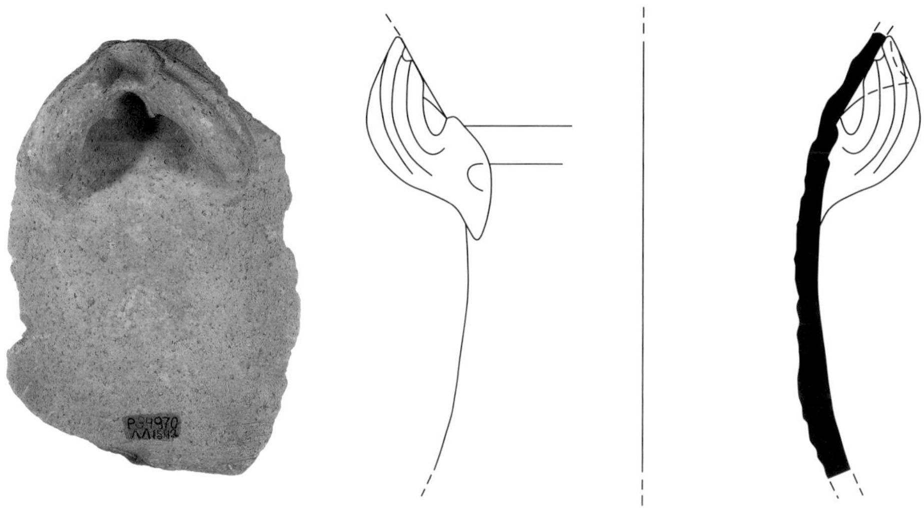

Figure 77. Brazier stand (69). Scale 1:4. Photo Agora Excavations; drawing S. I. Rotroff

belongs to form 4,[54] characterized by a rounded bottom that meets the vertical wall at an angle, an outturned rim with a flange at its inner edge, and diagonally canted horizontal handles. Fragments of its conical lid were found as well. The type began to be imported to Athens around the end of the first quarter of the 2nd century. Two button knobs from cooking-pot lids are present,[55] probably of the type usually associated either with lopades of form 3 (like **66**) or lidded chytrai of form 5 (of which no examples are present in the well). A single fragment of a pan is of the plain, pie-pan shape, either form 1 or 2,[56] and is probably an import.

The well contained two fragments of braziers. This widespread Hellenistic form combines a hollow stand with a fire bowl equipped with three moldmade supports, usually decorated with a bearded head: the beard served to support the pot over a charcoal fire.[57] Braziers began to be imported to Athens around 175 and were soon imitated locally. These early imports are represented in the well by a support (**68**; Fig. 76) from a brazier brought to Athens from somewhere in the eastern Aegean;[58] it represents a man wearing a pilos, a standard image on these devices. The other fragment (**69**; Fig. 77), preserving part of the stand and one handle, is also an import; the ware appears to be shell-tempered, the earmark of braziers made in Cyrenaica.[59] Only two other fragments from this region have been identified at the Agora.[60]

54. *Agora* XXXIII, pp. 183–186.
55. Cf. *Agora* XXXIII, pp. 196–197, forms 2, 3.
56. *Agora* XXXIII, pp. 188–190.
57. For a recent study of braziers, with further bibliography, see *Agora* XXXIII, pp. 199–222.
58. Didelot 1997, p. 381 (type égéen); *Agora* XXXIII, pp. 43–45, 216–217 (Quartz cooking fabric).
59. See Riley 1979, pp. 94–95, Benghazi local fabric 1.
60. *Agora* XXXIII, p. 333, no. 814, pl. 84, and the unpublished P 34502.

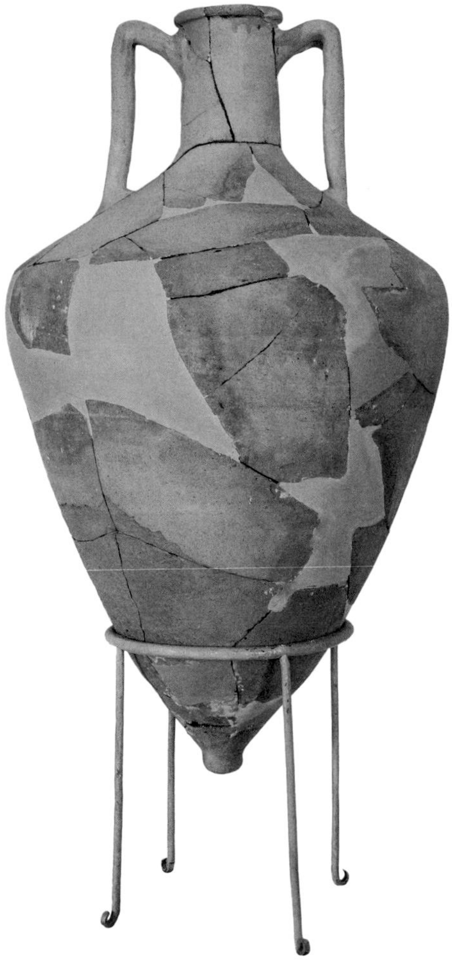

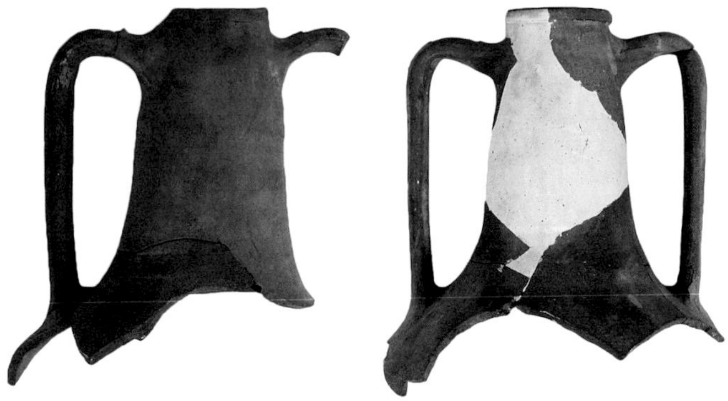

Figure 78 *(left)*. **Koan transport amphora (70).** Scale 1:8. Photo Agora Excavations

Figure 79 *(right)*. **Knidian transport amphoras (72, 74).** Scale 1:8. Photo S. I. Rotroff

Transport Amphoras

The fill contained one broken but largely complete jar and fragments of others, including six stamped handles, the latter of special significance for the dating of the deposit. Dorothy Thompson recorded two stamped amphora handles on June 9, 1938 (**73, 75**), giving the depth at which they were found as 13.00 m, the very top of the bone deposit or slightly above it. No depth is given for the four other inventoried amphoras and stamps (**70–72, 74**), but from their higher inventory numbers we can safely assume they were found later, and therefore deeper in the well, most likely below 14.70 m, the point at which large amounts of coarse pottery were first recorded.

A Koan amphora (**70**; Fig. 78) bearing a single stamp that reads [Ἀ]σκλη̣(–) may be the earliest largely complete object in the well. Grace tentatively suggested a date of about 200 for this jar;[61] more recently, a date simply in the first half of the 2nd century has been cited.[62] In terms of its shape, it falls between P 6353, from deposit E 14:1, where most of the material dates before 200, and SS 14082, found in deposit O 16:3, which was laid down ca. 165.[63] It is possible, then, that the date is somewhat after 200, probably in the first quarter of the 2nd century, but it is still earlier than

61. Grace 1949, p. 186, no. 8.

62. Whitbread 1995, p. 82, pl. 4:15.

63. For P 6353, see Grace 1979, fig. 56, the first jar on the left. SS 14082, bearing the retrograde stamp Διονυσίας, is unpublished. For the dates of these deposits, see *Agora* XXXIII, pp. 352, 369. Note also that the height:diameter ratio of the amphora from the Agora Bone Well is 1.74, considerably lower than Finkielsztejn's estimated norm (1.9) for Koan amphoras of the middle of the century (Finkielsztejn 2004, p. 156).

the bulk of the deposit. Fragments of at least four more Koan amphoras are stored with the context pottery.

As is to be expected at this period, Knidian amphoras dominate the deposit. The total count of jars of this type is 11, including three stamped handles (**71**, **73**, **75**) and two necks with stamped handles attached (**72**, **74**; Fig. 79), along with the characteristic toes. An anepigraphic handle with an incuse fishhook device (**71**) is early Knidian, and hence residual in the deposit.[64] The other Knidian stamps date in Grace's period IV A (see below for the dating of this period), earmarked by the appearance of an official called the *phrourarchos* on the stamps, sometimes in company with an ordinary eponym.[65] At least one amphora, a neck with both handles (**72**), names the eponym Sokrates, who probably served early in this span.[66] Two other eponyms (Aristarchos and Asklepiodoros, on **74** and **75**) have been placed later in the period. The dating of the fifth handle (**73**), stamped by Euphragoras as eponym, is problematical. Grace placed this official in the subsequent period IV B (currently dated 167–146), and toward its end: "perhaps a year or two after the middle of the century, but not far, because of name connections."[67] Her date provided a comfortably firm mid-2nd-century *terminus post quem* for the deposit, which has been quoted repeatedly in earlier discussions.[68] Euphragoras has now, however, been found on a handle in association with the phrourarch Philtatos and the fabricant Demetrios, who was active in periods III and IV A,[69] details that suggest a date in the early part of period IV A, along with Sokrates. His association with later fabricants remains unexplained, but it seems likely that Euphragoras is to be dated earlier than Grace thought.

The latest stamps in the well, then, are **74** and **75**, which fall in the later part of period IV A. Grace identified the phrourarchs as garrison commanders and associated them with the period 188–167, during which Rhodes maintained control of some of the mainland sites of Asia Minor. This association provided a date (188) for the beginning of the new stamping practice, with phrourarchs at first countersigning the stamps of ordinary eponyms but then taking over as the sole eponyms. This historical connection, however, is not entirely secure. The nature of the phrourach's office, attested at Knidos only on the stamps, remains unknown, and it is not necessarily related to the Rhodian occupation.[70] In addition, there are now indications that Grace's dates may need to be revised downwards. In 2001, Gérald Finkielsztejn

64. Early Knidian stamps are currently assigned to the span ca. 240–220; see Börker and Burow 1998, p. 56.

65. Grace 1985, pp. 13–14; Jefremow 1995, p. 68.

66. Sokrates is paired with a phrourarch, a feature probably limited to the first seven or more years of the period (Grace 1985, p. 15). Note, however, that Jefremow (1995, p. 69) divorces Sokrates from this earliest group.

67. We quote Grace's unpublished analysis of the amphora stamps from the well, dated April 27, 1959, on file in the excavation archives. See also Grace and Savvatianou-Petropoulakou 1970, p. 335, under no. E 102. The "name connections" Grace refers to are presumably the fabricants with whom Euphragoras is associated. According to her lists, now housed in the archives of the American School of Classical Studies at Athens, some of these fabricants are attested throughout period IV, but others only in period IV B (Alkinos, Hermippos, Hippokritos, Kleandros, Philotas, Theudotos, and Xenokritos), and one of them only in periods IV B and V A (Charmokrates). For published partial lists of the fabricants associated with Euphragoras, see Jefremow 1995, pp. 125–131, table X, and Jöhrens 1999, p. 151, under no. 457.

68. *Agora* XXII, p. 100; *Agora* XXXIII, p. 358; Rotroff 1999; 2014, p. 518; Liston and Rotroff 2013a, p. 65.

69. Empereur and Garlan 1987, p. 90.

70. See Jefremow (1995, pp. 54–58) for a discussion of this office and an alternative hypothesis as to its nature; see also Koehler and Matheson 2004.

proposed a new chronology for Rhodian amphoras, establishing dates at least 11 years later for stamps contemporary with Knidian period IV A.[71] The Rhodian and Knidian chronologies are closely intertwined, as the two types are found together in several large deposits that are foundational for their dating. Although the Knidian sequence has yet to be reviewed, the Rhodian revisions will surely have an impact on the Knidian chronology.[72] For example, hundreds of both Rhodian and Knidian amphora stamps have been found in the building fill of the Middle Stoa at the Agora. Grace dated the latest Rhodian stamps in the fill to ca. 183; Finkielsztejn revised this to 170/168,[73] with the effect of moving the probable terminal date of this deposit from ca. 180 to ca. 165. In the Knidian stamps from the same fill, Grace found examples from about five years after the beginning of the phrourarch period, bringing her again to the year 183.[74] If the two series are indeed closely interlocked, the year would instead be close to 170. We might then suggest a date in the 170s for **72** and **73**, stamped by eponyms of the early phrourarch period. The eponyms Aristarchos and Asklepiodoros (**75**, found at the top of the deposit, and **74**, deeper within it), belonging to the period's more developed phase, would date in the 160s. Whether such a revision can be reconciled with the evidence for earlier and later Knidian periods remains to be seen.

The well also contained fragments of one Mendaean, one Erythraean, three Thasian, one Chian, one Corinthian/northern Peloponnesian, one Rhodian, two Greco-Italic, and four unidentified amphoras. Where datable, they are residual, that is, earlier than the second quarter of the 2nd century (see the Catalogue for dates).

Other Objects Made of Clay

Two molds attest to the craft activities that took place on the hill: a fragment of a mold taken from the upper body of a heavily draped, probably female figurine (**76**; Fig. 80), and a small fragment of a mold perhaps for a lamp (**77**; Fig. 81). A single small lump of fired clay may represent the heavily worn head of a figurine. There are ten biconical loomweights, most of them intact or nearly so (see **78**; Fig. 82); a single pyramidal weight is probably residual.[75] A large part of a Laconian pan tile (**79**; Fig. 83) was reconstituted from fragments in the well (four more fragments exist in the context pottery). Seven small fragments of large, square-edged tiles of Corinthian fabric are also stored there. One fragmentary object may be an opaion tile.

71. Finkielsztejn 2001, p. 192, table 19, shows Grace's dates and Finkielsztejn's revisions for Rhodian amphoras of periods IIId–IVa, contemporaneous with Knidian period IV A. These revisions have been taken into account in recent studies of Hellenistic pottery at the Agora (and in the dating of material in the Agora Bone Well), resulting in adjusted deposit dates for some contexts in which Rhodian amphoras are found. See *Agora* XXXIII, pp. 7–8, 342, and compare the deposit dates of contexts of the late 3rd and first half of the 2nd century in the deposit summaries there (pp. 343–376) with those given in earlier *Agora* volumes (*Agora* XXII, pp. 96–106; *Agora* XXIX, pp. 433–473).

72. For preliminary comments, see Lawall 2002, p. 319, urging revision downwards, and Koehler and Matheson 2004, presenting arguments against it.

73. Grace (1985, pp. 8–10) suggested Athenadotos as the latest Rhodian eponym in the fill; for Finkielsztejn's date, see Finkielsztejn 2001, p. 192, table 19.

74. Grace 1985, p. 15.

75. Davidson restricts pyramidal weights at Corinth to the Classical period (*Corinth* XII, p. 162).

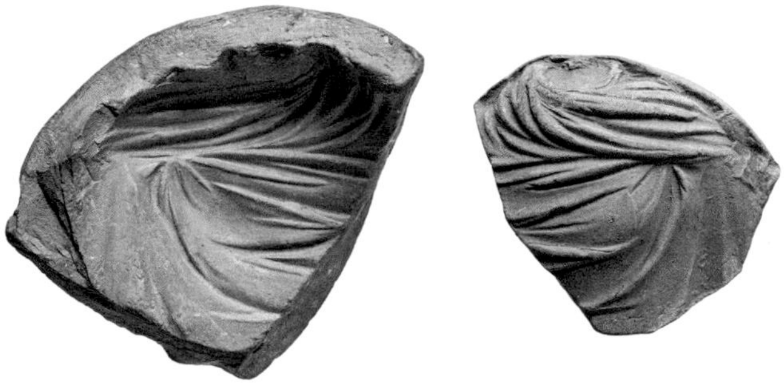

Figure 80. Mold for a terracotta figurine (76, left) with cast (right). Scale 2:3. Photo Agora Excavations

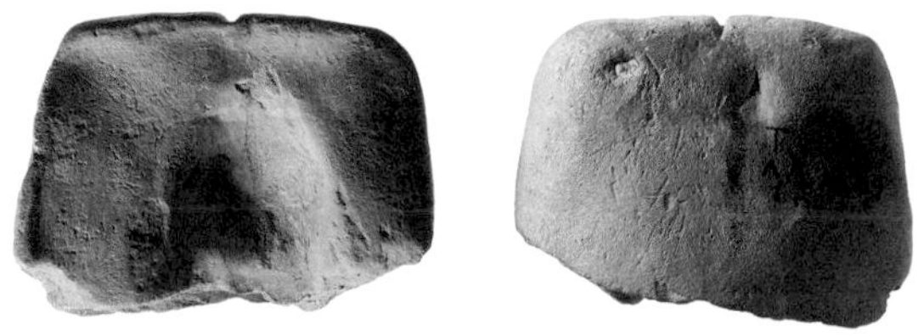

Figure 81. Mold for a lamp(?) (77), interior and exterior. Scale 2:3. Photo C. A. Mauzy

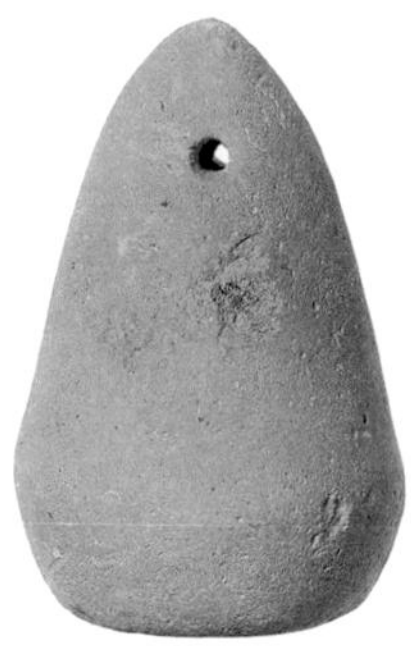

Figure 82. Biconical loomweight (78). Scale 1:2. Photo Agora Excavations

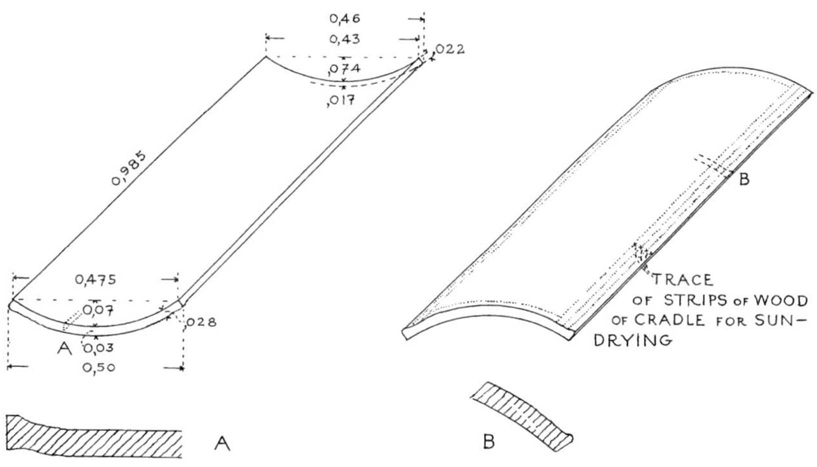

Figure 83. Laconian pan tile (79). Drawing G. P. Stevens

THE HERM

The female herm (**80**; Fig. 84) is one of the most unusual objects in the fill and has garnered more attention than any other.[76] Since its discovery in 1938 and publication a year later by T. Leslie Shear Sr.,[77] and despite its extraordinarily specific, even unique context, its elucidation has been bedeviled by Pausanias's note (1.14.7) that a shrine of Aphrodite Ourania and its cult statue by Pheidias stood somewhere in the northwest corner of the Agora, and his later description of her image in her other sanctuary by the Ilissos as "square like the images of Hermes" (1.19.2). This comment, in turn, prompted the theory that the herm found in the well is either a replica of Pheidias's Aphrodite Ourania in the Agora, if this was herm-like also, or a support for such a replica, if it was not. Yet the top of its head is modeled, not broken across or chiseled flat, showing that it supported nothing, and the supposed shrine of Aphrodite Ourania on the Kolonos Agoraios is a phantom.[78]

Moreover, in June 2008, Greek archaeologists discovered a fragment of a Pentelic marble relief built into a modern house wall at 5 Areos Street in Plaka, east of the Agora. Only just over 0.20 m high and broken on three sides, it shows three female herms bordered above by a battered entablature. Its architrave is inscribed [- - -]ΣΠΙΚΗΕΙΛ[- - -], evidently a dedication by a woman from Thespiai, [- - - ΘΕ]ΣΠΙΚΗ, to Eil[eithyia]. The right-hand pair of herms is joined at the arms; the leftmost one is too battered to tell. All three have the same broad faces, petite mouths, and coiffures as **80**, but now wear *poloi* and have the usual rectangular "arms." The relief's type and letter forms date it to the 4th century B.C.[79]

The earliest mention of an Athenian shrine to Eileithyia occurs in a speech by the 4th-century orator Isaios.[80] Pausanias tells us that it stood near the Temple of Serapis and housed three *xoana* of the goddess, draped down to the feet.[81] Erysichthon had brought the first one to Athens from Delos, and Phaidra later brought the other two from Crete. So it may also be no coincidence that on the relief, the leftmost herm's *polos* is distinctly taller than the other two. Although this trio is not obviously draped, their clothing could have been painted on the relief or simply added to the *xoana* themselves at some time between the 4th century and Pausanias's visit half a millennium later. The progressive elaboration of the Athena Polias in the Erechtheion offers a good parallel.[82]

Although the Serapeion and thus this shrine of Eileithyia apparently stood somewhere near Athens's cathedral, about 400 m east of the Agora, an inscribed lease from the Agora mentions a second shrine to her in the

76. This section was authored by Andrew Stewart. The herm is treated among similar pieces of Hellenistic sculpture in Stewart 2017, pp. 118–123, and the aspects most relevant to this discussion of the Agora Bone Well are reproduced here for the benefit of the reader.

77. Shear 1939, p. 238, fig. 37.

78. See p. 21, above, and Stewart 2017, pp. 120–121, 123.

79. Library of Hadrian, apotheke ΠΛ 2328; Sourlas 2017, pp. 164–174. I thank Dimitris Sourlas for alerting me to this find, allowing me to examine and discuss it, and kindly sending me a photograph and a copy of his study in advance of its publication.

80. Isae. 5.39; Pingiatoglou 1981, pp. 42, 146, no. L.26.

81. Paus. 1.18.5: μόνοις δὲ Ἀθηναίοις τῆς Εἰλειθυίας κεκάλυπται τὰ ξόανα ἐς ἄκρους τοὺς πόδας. τὰ μὲν δὴ δύο εἶναι Κρητικὰ καὶ Φαίδρας ἀναθήματα ἔλεγον αἱ γυναῖκες, τὸ δὲ ἀρχαιότατον Ἐρυσίχθονα ἐκ Δήλου κομίσαι; Pingiatoglou 1981, pp. 42–44, 81, 149, no. L.56; *LIMC* III.1, 1986, p. 694, no. 94:a, s.v. Eileithyia (R. Olmos); Donohue 1988, pp. 141, 365, no. 188. On Pausanias's consistent use of *xoana* to mean wooden cult images, see Donohue 1988, pp. 1–8, 140–141, with pp. 141–143 on the Athenian Eileithyiai and others.

82. See Kroll 1982.

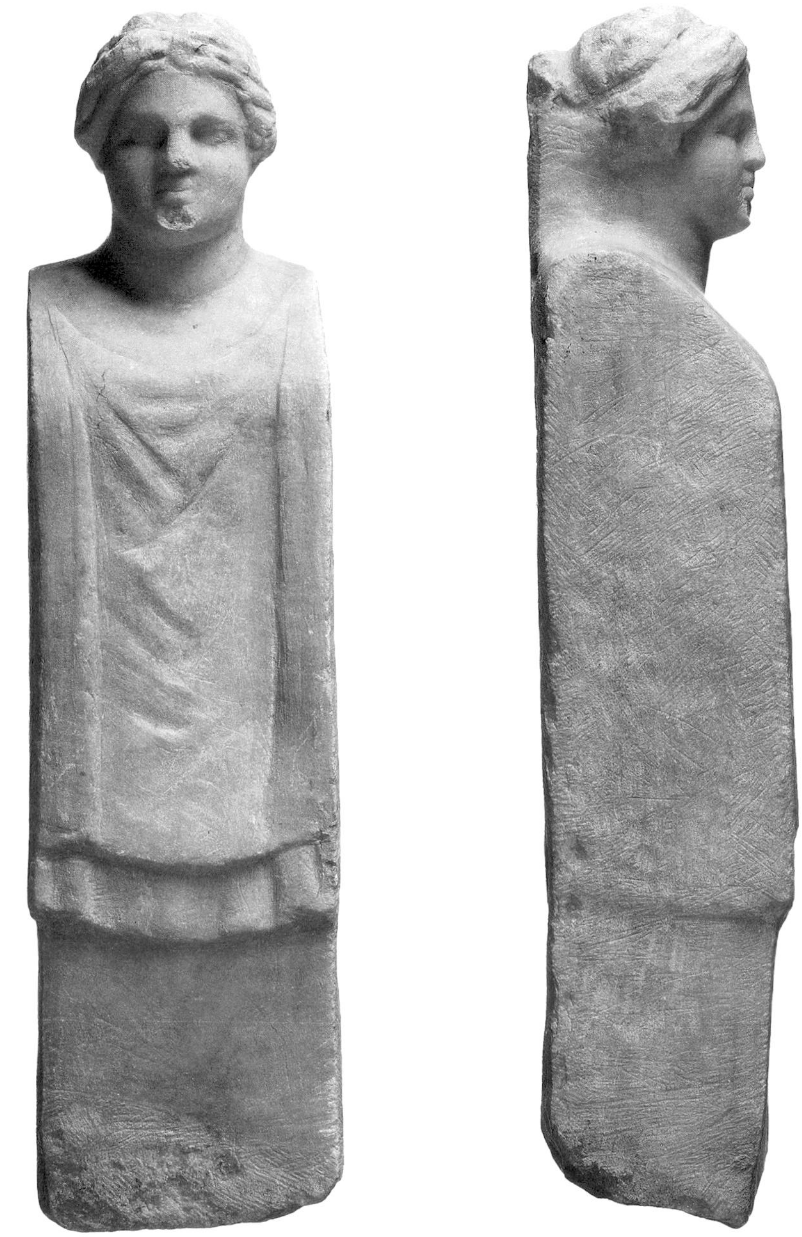

Figure 84. Small marble herm of Eileithyia (80), front and profile views. Scale 1:2. Photo Agora Excavations

deme of Kollytos, roughly between the Areopagus and Kolonos Agoraios and including the Agora's Industrial District.[83] In addition, in 1981 Semele Pingiatoglou collected seven widely scattered Athenian dedications to Eileithyia; another Agora lease published more recently mentions her sanctuary in Kollytos, and an unpublished Late Hellenistic/Early Roman dedication to her in the Agora completes the current epigraphical roster.[84]

83. Serapeia: Greco 2011, p. 534 (M. C. Monaco); Lalonde 2006. I thank Kathleen Lynch for this reference.

84. Pingiatoglou 1981, pp. 42–44, with a catalogue of inscriptions on pp. 158–160 (nos. E.38–E.44). For the Agora base I 5016 (Pingiatoglou's no. E.43), see now *Agora* XVIII, pp. 310–311, no. V594. On Kollytos, Agora I 7117, see *Agora* XIX, p. 182, no. L6, lines 97–98. For the second lease, Agora I 4732, see Walbank 2013, pp. 314–315, no. 9. The unpublished inscription is a dedication by Axiothea, daughter of Isidoros of Xypete, of a statue of her baby son, Kleon, Agora I 7576, found built into the south wall of room 1:c of the Library of Pantainos, catalogued August 1992 (Section PP, notebook PP 12, p. 2347). I thank John Camp for alerting me to this inscription.

Although Pausanias's description, the relief, and **80** do not exactly match, the obvious explanation is that the Agora herm represents the goddess herself, not the cult *xoana* that Pausanias saw. As for the sculpture's hermaic form, presumably it was chosen because Eileithyia had to be represented as always available and thus as immobile.[85] Compare Hera's spiteful and ultimately vain attempt to keep her from attending poor Leto, "racked nine days and nine nights with pangs beyond wont," and what happened when Iris alerted her to this:

> As soon as Eileithyia the goddess of sore travail (μογοστόκος) set foot on Delos, the birth pangs seized Leto, and she longed to bring forth; so she cast her arms about a palm tree and knelt on the soft meadow while the earth [of Delos] laughed for joy beneath. Then the child leapt forth into the light, and all the goddesses raised a cry.[86]

Like Hermes in this format, Eileithyia too was a liminal goddess, potent only in those critical moments at the threshold of life. To keep her around was vital; everything else (arms, clothes, *polos*) was secondary and thus dispensable. Moreover, being "indispensable to every family,"[87] kindly and a "savior" (σωτήρ), she smiles. Two Agora terracotta molds for female herms (Fig. 85), differing from **80** only in that they both wear *poloi* and omit the lower chiton folds, confirm all this and indicate that such hermaic images of the goddess were far from unknown in Late Classical and Hellenistic Athenian households.[88]

To explain why the herm was tossed down the Agora Bone Well, however, is harder. Because of its small size and pristine surface, it must have been made for domestic cult, and because apparently it is a unique example of the type in marble, perhaps it belonged not to an ordinary family but to a midwife. If so, one may imagine that she would have prayed or even sacrificed to it before setting out to do her job, which included not only assisting at births, but also helping to care for newborns and disposing of them if they died.[89] Although broken away from its base, presumably accidentally, the herm has not been ritually "killed" by decapitation. Since it was found about two-thirds of the way down the deposit of bones and Hellenistic pottery in the well, it is reasonable to hazard that after it broke, its owner decided to drop it down there as a propitiatory offering to the goddess. By this means Eileithyia could be thanked for all the live births in the deposit whatever their eventual fates.

THE CHAPE

An ivory chape (**81**; Fig. 86)—the upper termination of a scabbard for a sword—was found at a depth of 16.85 m, together with a concentration of bronze and a sheet of lead, as well as the usual bones and pottery. The chape is approximately rectangular, but the sides angle outward toward the bottom. The lower edges are not horizontal, but rise toward the center, where there is a projection to which the sheath (probably of wood) would have been attached. In the lower corners on both sides of the chape is a teardrop-shaped area that had been decorated with an anthemion inlaid in

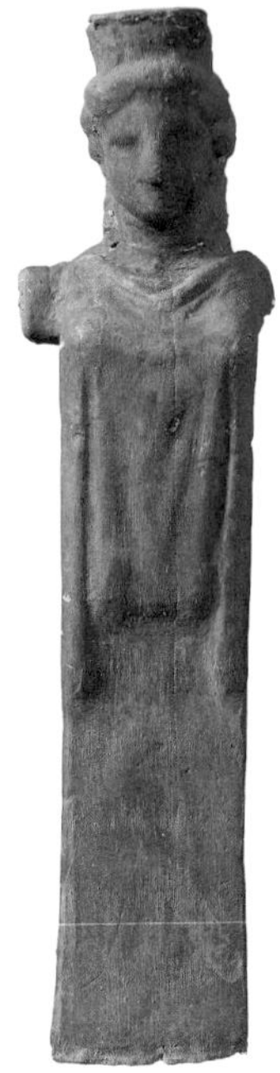

Figure 85. Cast taken from a mold for a terracotta female herm (T 1828). Scale 1:2. Photo C. A. Mauzy

85. Cf. Paus. 3.15.7 on the chained Ares at Sparta and wingless [Athena] Nike at Athens.

86. *Hymn. Hom. Ap.* 115–119; trans. H. G. Evelyn-White, Cambridge, Mass., 1936, adapted.

87. Burkert 1985, p. 170.

88. Agora T 1828, from deposit S 19:2, the mostly 2nd-century fill of a cistern (for the date, see *Agora* XXIX, pp. 471–472): Gawlinski 2014, p. 179; and T 4005, from an Early Hellenistic underfloor fill in Roman house ε at Q/4–6/12 (lot BΔ 323). Susan Rotroff also kindly draws my attention to Kerameikos 11479, a headless female herm in ivory from the 4th-century Building Z3, probably a brothel (*Kerameikos* XVII, p. 216, no. 846, pl. 131).

89. Pl. *Tht.* 151C; discussion, Liston and Rotroff 2013a, pp. 76–77.

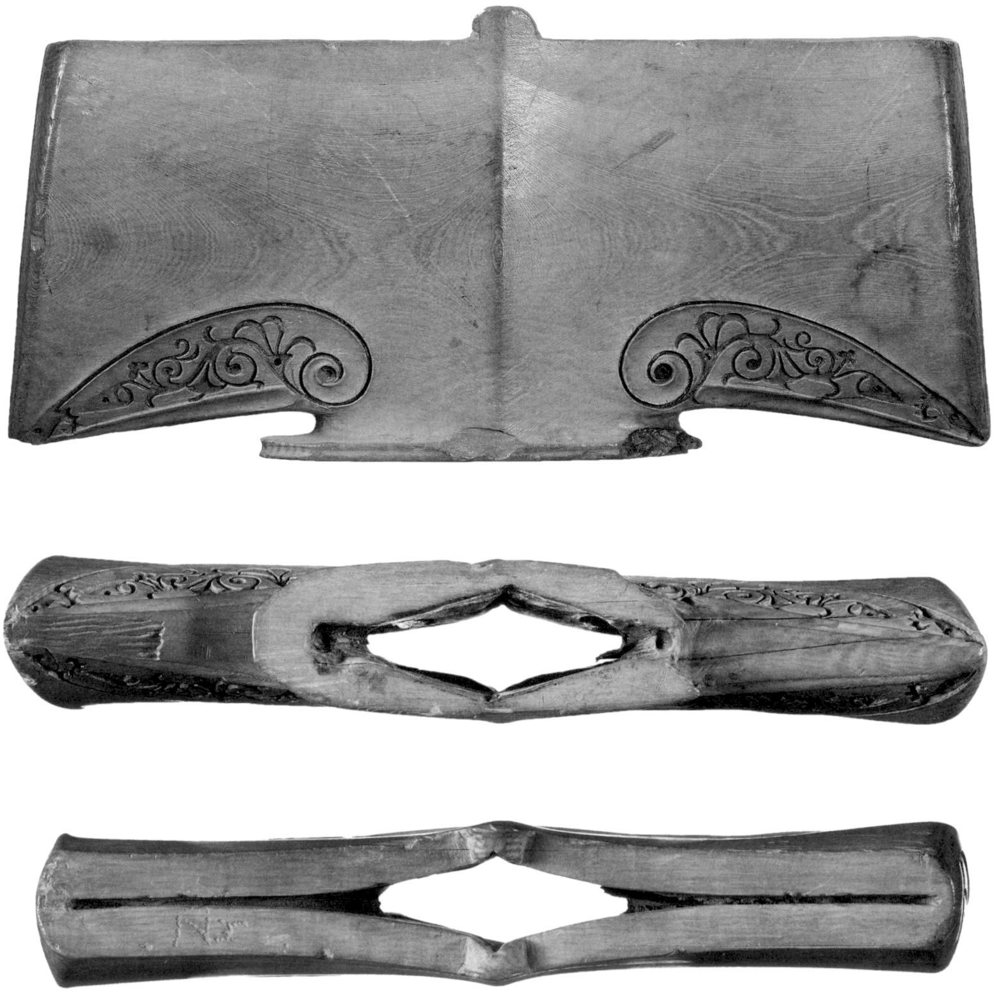

Figure 86. Ivory chape from the scabbard of a sword (81): face, bottom, and top (with inscription). Scale 1:1. Photos Agora Excavations

gold. Traces of the metal are visible in the cuttings under high magnification; it had been attached with six small nails. The opening through the chape has a minimum width of 0.048 m but widens out at the top to nearly the edge of the chape to accommodate the spreading root of the blade.[90] A projecting button in the middle of the top surface of the chape would have fit into an answering notch in the handguard of the sword.

The chape was cut from a tusk at least 0.104 m in diameter and probably larger; on this basis, Gejvall, who examined it along with the animal bone when it was found, suggested that the material was mammoth rather than elephant ivory. More recent research has shown that elephant and mammoth ivory can be distinguished reliably on the basis of the intersecting Schreger lines,[91] which appear clearly in the polished ends of the chape. Edgard Espinoza, who developed these criteria, was kind enough to examine a photograph of the object; in his opinion, it is made of elephant ivory (probably from an African elephant), though from a remarkably large tusk.[92]

An inscription picked into the top surface of the chape has so far eluded interpretation. An owner might well have wanted to identify such a valuable item as personal property, but the letters do not suggest an

90. See Touratsoglou 1986, pp. 618, 620, for illustrations of the details of this arrangement, and passim for a thorough discussion of swords of this variety.

91. Espinoza and Mann 2000, pp. 9–12; the assistance of conservator Amandina Anastassiades was invaluable in this investigation.

92. Pers. comm. It is mostly the inner Schreger lines that are visible on the chape, and these have acute angles; as one approaches the outer part of the tusk, the angles become larger. This is the measurement that, according to Espinoza, is critical in the identification.

abbreviated name. Their picked style resembles that of weight inscriptions on silver plate,[93] so possibly the inscription represents a weight or valuation of some sort.[94] This further suggests that the chape may at one time have been part of a curated treasure or collection of some sort.

Chapes very much like this one have been associated with a type of sword that was probably developed sometime in the 6th century.[95] Numerous red-figure vases show swords and their scabbards. The chapes are approximately the same shape as the Agora example; they sometimes show decoration, and even the detail of the interlocking button on the chape and notch on the handguard may be illustrated.[96] An ivory chape from Olympia is much smaller and simpler than our example, but it shares the wide cutting for the root of the blade and the projecting button.[97] Weaponry of this type is particularly well documented in Macedonia, both by actual weapons from warrior graves and by images, especially in the late 4th and early 3rd centuries. The swords were buried in their scabbards, which have largely disintegrated; some, however, preserve traces of a bone or ivory chape, though none can compare with the Agora chape for preservation.[98] The hunters in the lion- and stag-hunt mosaics from Pella wield similar weapons, as does Alexander the Great on the eponymous mosaic.[99] Such swords appear in Macedonian funerary painting as well.[100] Sculpted swords also provide comparanda; a fragmentary sword from a bronze statue recovered from the Antikythera wreck provides the closest parallel. Its shape is identical to that of the Agora chape, there are traces of a teardrop-shaped ornament in its lower corners, and the lower projection to which the sheath was attached has the same form as that of the Agora chape.[101] On stylistic grounds, Peter Bol suggests a date in the first half of the 2nd century for this object; if this is correct, it is about contemporary with the Agora chape.

93. E.g., Gill 2008, pp. 337–338, fig. 1.

94. Parallels for weight inscriptions on ivory may be found in the Hellenistic Delian inventories (Hamilton 2000, p. 128, Apollo treasure B, no. 60c, and p. 398, Hieropoion/Andrians treasure D, no. 46).

95. Remouchamps 1926, pp. 36–39, type 15.

96. For example, on an amphora by the Kleophrades Painter (Munich 2305, *CVA,* Munich 4 [Germany 12], pl. 175 [553]:1) and a cup by Douris (Vienna 3694, *CVA,* Vienna 1 [Austria 1], pl. 10 [10]).

97. Hampe and Jantzen 1937, p. 51, figs. 21, 22.

98. Vergina, tomb II (Andronikos 1984, p. 145): an ivory chape with gold decoration; a projecting button notches into the handguard of the sword. Kozani (*Treasures of Ancient Macedonia,* p. 41, no. 43, pl. 9): a bone chape partially preserved; the notch in the handguard is clearly visible. The North Cemetery of Pydna (Makriyalos; Pandermalis 2004, p. 56, no. 7): part of an ivory chape preserved. Veroia (Touratsoglou 1986, pp. 612–628): only traces of an ivory chape are preserved, but note the notch in the handguard of the sword to accept the projecting "button" of the chape. Earlier swords of this type (from the first quarter of the 5th century and the third quarter of the 4th century) were buried with men at Vitsa (Vokotopoulou 1986, p. 293, nos. 4, 5, fig. 86, pls. 11, 32); another, of the last quarter of the 4th century, still retains part of the knob-like attachment at the lower end of the scabbard (made of bone), although no trace of the chape remains (Vokotopoulou 1986, p. 193, no. 6, fig. 87, pl. 299). For a carved ivory scabbard knob, see Barnett 1982, p. 65, pl. 70:c.

99. Charbonneaux, Martin, and Villard 1973, pp. 109–110, 116, figs. 105–107, 115.

100. E.g., on the sarcophagus from Aidonochori (Koukouli-Chrysanthaki 1983, p. 136, fig. 32a) and in the Lefkadia-Naoussa tomb (Petsas 1966, p. 114, n. 2, pl. ΣΤ). There is also a fine one on a Hadra vase from the Chatby Necropolis at Alexandria (Breccia 1912, p. 34, no. 53, figs. 25, 26); an actual sword of the same type was also found there, but without its scabbard (p. 172, no. 544, fig. 98).

101. Bol 1972, pp. 37–38, fig. 2, pls. 18:3, 19:1; Kaltsas, Vlachogianni, and Bouyia 2012, p. 101, no. 47. See also the statue of Demetrios Poliorketes from the Agora (Shear 1973a, pp. 165–168, pl. 36), where, however, no details are preserved.

The chape was found together with a large mass of bronze debris, none of which, however, is weaponry. A possible source for the object is the Arsenal, up the hill from the Agora Bone Well, in which weapons must have been stored. The use of luxury materials, however, hints that this would have been a prized private possession rather than government-issue weaponry. In any event, it had clearly gone out of use by the time it was discarded, since the gold had been carefully picked out of the inlay. Perhaps it ended its life as part of a craftsman's stock, awaiting recycling into another form. It is difficult to explain why this valuable raw material was discarded, unless by mistake.

THE BRONZE

A heavy concentration of bronze at a depth of 16.00–16.85 m stained many of the bones green, and, as noted above, the antibacterial effects of the metal probably contributed to their preservation. The bronze at first received little attention; it was not until a decade after excavation that five representative pieces were cleaned and inventoried (**82**, **84–87**; Figs. 87, 89).[102] They were by then in a very poor state of preservation, and one (**84**) may not have survived cleaning. A substantial amount of bronze was then returned to the tins, where it remained until its transfer to climate-controlled storage in the Agora metals room in the early 2000s. The total amount of bronze that was saved, including the extant inventoried objects, amounts to over 8 kg, making this a highly unusual concentration of metal in an Athenian well.

The bronze is now thoroughly corroded, and although forms can be made out, they often consist only of corrosion product; cleaning is not an option. Several different classes of objects are represented here: corner edging, bead-and-reel ornament, rods, twisted rods, and a heavy bronze knob. The largest group is the edging (**82–85**; Figs. 87, 88), which accounts for more than half of the bronze by weight. These are reinforcements for angles; one of the two faces has a scalloped edge and there are holes in the plain face for rivets (sometimes with rivets in place) for attachment to another element, probably sheet bronze. They represent several different forms: **82** and **83** are straight, sometimes with a corner preserved, and **84** and **85** reflect various sorts of curves. On most, the scalloped face is at right angles to the plain one, but in one series the angle of the two faces is oblique. There are also differences in the measurements and in the design of the scalloping, but the repeated scallop pattern—a gentle convex curve alternating with a pointed tooth—suggests that all of these fragments are related, possibly from a single object. The total preserved length of the fragments amounts to close to 7 m, however, so a single object would have been of considerable size, not to mention complexity. Traces of woven organic material are preserved on **83** (Fig. 88), two pieces of straight edging corroded together; a trace of scallop pattern shows that it belongs to the same series as the others. Strips of organic material adhere to the longest piece of edging. They are about 0.025 m wide but have separated into narrower widths, suggesting some kind of plant fiber. The strips lie in a woven

102. A marginal note in Homer Thompson's hand reads: "from depth 16 to 16.85 come many fragments of bronze, samples of which have been catalogued . . . the hopeless rubbish discarded. May, 1948" (notebook ΛΛ 8, p. 1488). The fragments with woven organic material (**83**) were still stored in the tin when this study was undertaken.

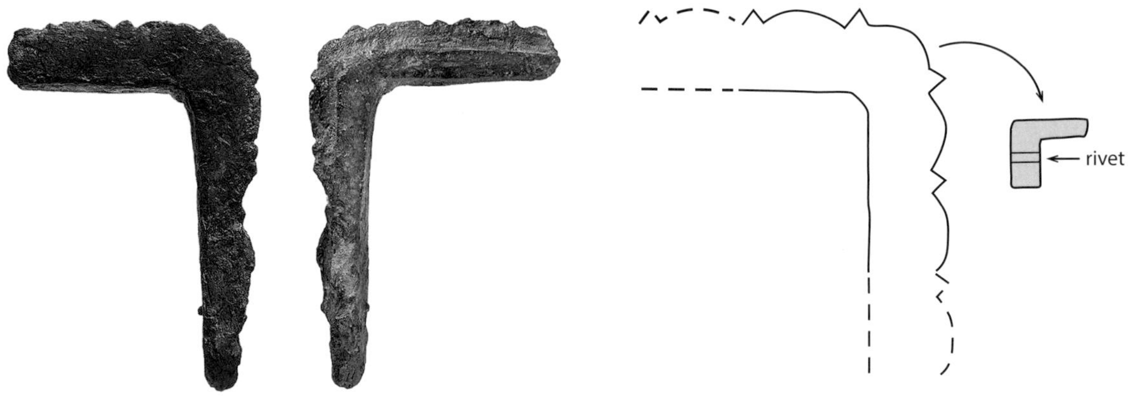

82

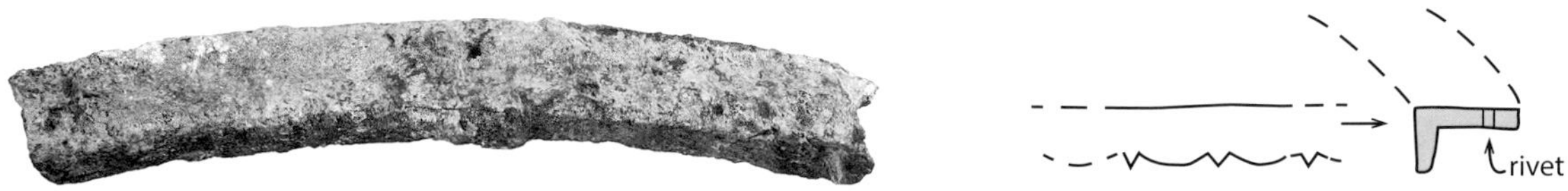

84

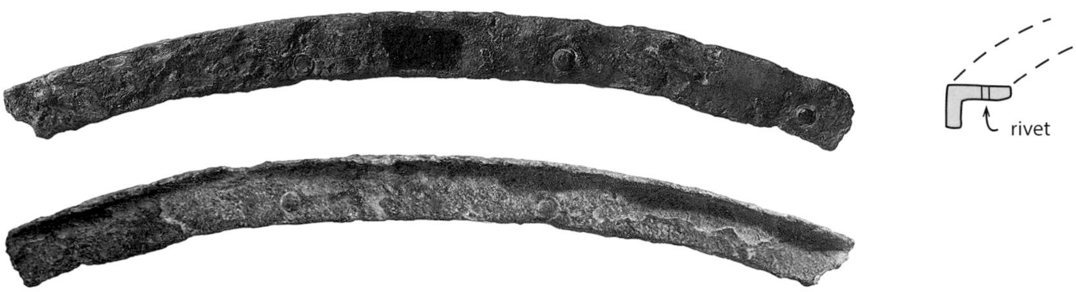

85

Figure 87. Bronze edging with scallop pattern: straight (82, top and bottom views) and curved (84, from above, and 85, top and bottom views). Scale 1:2. Photos Agora Excavations, C. A. Mauzy; drawing S. I. Rotroff, based on sketches in notebook ΛΛ 10, pp. 1823–1824, made by H. A. Thompson at a scale of 1:2 when the items were inventoried

pattern at right angles to one another. That they are integral to the bronze edging, and did not simply come to rest against it by chance, is suggested by their orientation at 45 degrees to the edging. Possibly the object was a chair, stool, or bed, and the organic material its webbing.[103] If so, it is hard to understand the scalloped ornament, which would have been obscured by the webbing wrapped around it.

Other fragments represent bead-and-reel ornament (**86**; Fig. 89), with a flattened edge indicating it was once attached to something; a length of ca. 0.75 m is preserved, again indicating a large object, possibly a chest. Fragments of twisted rods (**87**; Fig. 89) may represent drill bits; two of the uninventoried pieces appear to come to a point (unless this is simply an artifact of corrosion). Bronze is a relatively soft material for this purpose, however, so they may come from tools of another sort. An intriguing parallel, though made of iron, has recently come to light at Pistiros, in Thrace: a

103. For chairs with the seats woven on the diagonal, see Richter 1966, figs. 181, 646; a woven chair back appears to be represented by lead miniatures from Stageira (Andrianou 2009, p. 25, nos. 3, 4, figs. 4, 5; see pp. 22–50 for the limited surviving instances of Greek seats and beds).

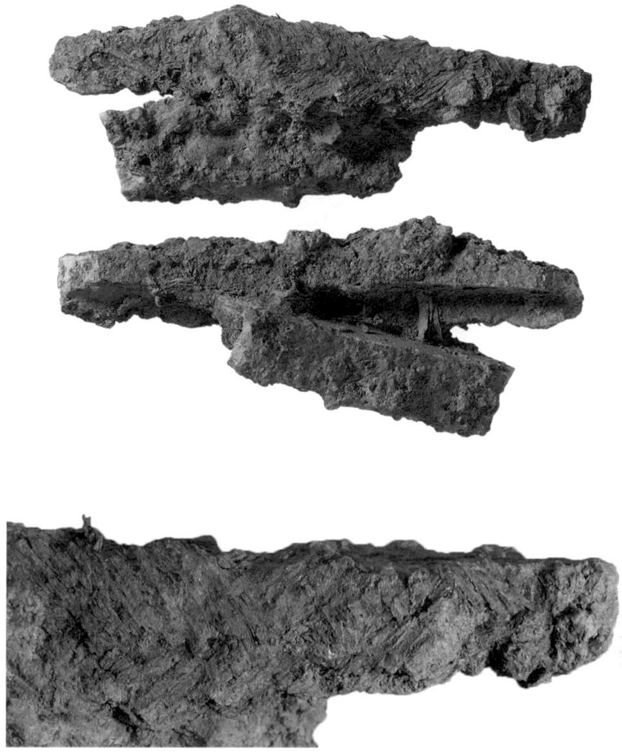

Figure 88. Two pieces of bronze edging corroded together, with woven organic material (83). Above: two views. The scalloped edge is visible in the lower view, at the right end of the upper rod. Below: detail of organic material. Scale 1:2; detail not to scale. Photos C. A. Mauzy, S. I. Rotroff

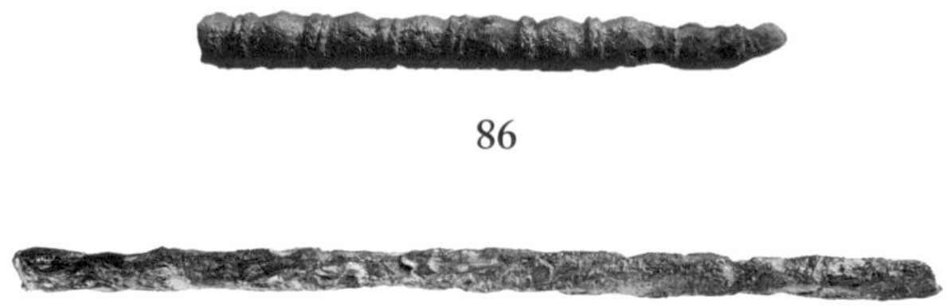

Figure 89. Bronze bead-and-reel appliqué (86) and twisted bronze rod (87). Scale 1:2. Photo Agora Excavations

small triangular blade with a long, thin, twisted handle, identified as a hearth or furnace rake.[104] Given the evidence of bronzeworking on the Kolonos Agoraios, the presence of such a tool would not be surprising. Among the uninventoried fragments are several more bronze rods, approximately square in section. Three are very heavy and might have functioned as the legs of a piece of furniture; the others are much lighter and may be tools or part of a scale. There is also a single large, heavy, vertically pierced knob or finial with a molded profile.

The presence of the bronze here remains without explanation. If it is scrap or a damaged object, it still would constitute a significant amount of valuable metal, presumably worth recycling; and yet it was discarded. If it was part of the stock of the bronzecasters who had abandoned the nearby houses, it is hard to understand why anyone took the trouble to throw it into the well, unless, perhaps, to effectively "bury" a body discarded here. But it is equally hard to imagine why anyone would haul it here from elsewhere, only to throw it away.

104. Andonova 2013, pp. 239, 245, fig. N 2:4.

OBJECTS FROM THE UPPERMOST FILLS

Few items are recorded from the upper 13 m of the well. The only objects inventoried from the deep fill that closed the well in ancient times (from ca. 2.15 to 13 m) are a fragment of a 4th-century broad-based bowl, inventoried because of the owner's mark ΔA on its underside (**88**), an early Rhodian amphora handle (**89**), and a coin of the late 4th or early 3rd century.[105] A fill in the uppermost 2 m, presumably introduced to counter settling in the ancient fill, included a mixture of Byzantine and ancient material: five Byzantine bowls, a plate, and a lamp,[106] as well as a nearly complete marble triglyph (visible in Fig. 7) and a 2nd-century Knidian amphora handle (see p. 157).

THE ARTIFACTS AND THE BONES

The objects in the well—human bone, animal bone, and artifacts—together pose an important question: to what extent is this a disparate and uncoordinated collection of random items, on the one hand, or, on the other, an internally cohesive assemblage? Given their numbers, if nothing else, it is clear that the human beings and dogs were brought from elsewhere, possibly some distance away, and we will argue below that some of the artifacts were brought with them. But what of the remains of butchering, the roughly worked bone tools, bronze fragments, and other artifacts that have no apparent connection with the bone deposit? They cannot have originated in Building 3 or 4, the stratigraphy of which indicates that they were not occupied during the time when human and animal bodies were being disposed of in the well. Assuming that people did not go further than necessary to dump unwanted trash, we must conclude that the butchering debris, worked bone, and bronze waste came from not too far afield, a place where food preparation and industrial activities continued after Buildings 3 and 4 were abandoned: that is, the well had gained a reputation as a convenient dumping place for a variety of unwanted materials, a useful feature in the days before regular waste removal. In the following section, we attempt to distinguish between those items that are connected to the bones and those that are not.

A number of items can be identified with greater or lesser confidence as grave gifts. The clearest example is the feeder (**26**). By far the most common context for this shape, both in Classical Athens and elsewhere, is the grave, usually the grave of a child. Nine 5th-century graves in the Südhügel cemetery at the Kerameikos included feeders among their furnishings; in all cases they can be confirmed on the basis of skeletal material or grave

105. ΛΛ-562: Megara, prow left/two dolphins in circle. See *BMC (Attica)*, p. 120, no. 25, pl. 21; cf. *Agora* XXVI, pp. 216–217, variety 643.

106. Although the date on their inventory cards reads June 23, 1937, by that date a depth of 11 m had been reached and excavation had been terminated for the year. The cards describe the objects as coming from the "mouth," so "June 23" must refer to the date on which the objects were inventoried rather than the date of excavation.

type (amphora or larnax) as the interments of children.[107] In the five cases where the skeleton is preserved, it is that of a child, not a newborn. Four 4th-century graves in the Eridanos cemetery were furnished with feeders; in two, the skeletal remains are described as those of small children (not newborns).[108] Fourteen of the 15 feeders reported from Olynthos were found in the cemeteries, 11 of them within graves, mostly the graves of children (apparently not infants).[109] This association can also be documented, though less fully, in the Hellenistic period.[110] From the ages of those with whom feeders were buried, it appears that the vessel was most commonly used in the care of older children rather than small babies; indeed, in the unsanitary conditions that prevailed in antiquity, bottle feeding a newborn would almost certainly have proven fatal.[111] A 5th-century terracotta figurine from Boiotia shows a woman using such a vessel to feed a child, a hefty little boy who already has a full head of hair.[112] The few ancient testimonia that can be mined for information about the weaning process suggest it was not completed until fairly late, perhaps when the child was two or older.[113] Evidence tends to be anecdotal; one of the most touching instances can be found in Plutarch's letter of consolation to his wife on

107. *Kerameikos* IX, pp. 125–126, 133, 141, 143, 148–149, 150, 152–153, graves 152, 194, 226, 229, 239, 242, 276, 284, 295. For two more graves with feeders, excavated in 1932 (E44, E52), there is no information about grave type or age of the deceased.

108. Schlörb-Vierneisel 1966, pp. 54, 68–69, 89–90, 91, nos. 106, 129, 155, 158. The adult graves are puzzling. Schlörb-Vierneisel (1966, pp. 89–90) postulated that one (no. 155) was a double burial originally containing a child whose bones have completely disappeared; the other instance (no. 159) is a supposed cremation from which, however, no bones at all were recovered. Two feeders from the late-5th-century cemetery at Syntagma Square (Charitonides 1958, p. 62, no. 2, fig. 104; p. 79, no. 3, fig. 137) probably come from the graves of children, although confirmation from skeletal material is not forthcoming, and one of them is apparently a cremation. Both were found with other grave gifts suitable for children (a terracotta doll in one case, a small chytra in another).

109. *Olynthus* V, pp. 258–259, nos. 1080–1083, pl. 193; *Olynthus* XIII, pp. 264–268, nos. 477–487, pls. 178–179. The graves are described in *Olynthus* XI; see the discussion there on p. 191. Eleven feeders were found within ten graves (an additional three were found in the cemetery but are not certainly associated with a particular grave; for another, no information is provided). In nine cases, these are documented as the graves of small children either by skeletal remains (four cases, all described as "child" rather than "infant") or by the size of the grave (five cases). The only feeder found near an adult grave lay above tile grave 343 (*Olynthus* XI, p. 106); Robinson speculates that it belongs to a later, superposed grave where the skeleton has completely disappeared.

110. For feeders from Hellenistic graves at Athens, see Schlörb-Vierneisel 1966, pp. 89–90, no. 155:2, pl. 58:2 (Athens, Eridanos cemetery, ca. 300); Charitonides 1979, p. 178, no. 5, fig. 4:θ, pl. 45:α (Athens, 3rd century). For feeders elsewhere in the Greek world, see Breccia 1912, p. 60, no. 151, pl. LI:95 (one of eight from the Chatby cemetery at Alexandria, Early Hellenistic); Pagenstecher 1913, pp. 141–142, figs. 148, 149:f, h (Alexandria); Adriani 1940, p. 117, fig. 53:49 (Alexandria); Petsas 1963, p. 223, grave H, pl. 261:δ (Vergina, Early Hellenistic); Bucovală 1967, p. 103, no. 63:a (Hellenistic cemetery at Tomis, late 2nd to early 1st century); Andreiomenou 1972, p. 177, pl. 62:γ (children's cemetery at Chalkis, 4th century); Graepler 1997, pp. 175–176 (Taranto); Krstić 2004, p. 589, pl. 294:b (Budva, probably from children's graves, 2nd and 1st centuries).

111. Sally Kevill-Davies (1991, p. 40) cites the grim statistics of the Dublin Foundling Hospital, where, in the late 18th century, only 45 of over 10,000 hand-fed babies survived (a mortality rate of 99.6%). Her discussion (pp. 40–42) of the dangers of the procedure in the 18th and 19th centuries holds true for antiquity as well. See also Centlivres Challet 2016, pp. 171–174.

112. Gourevitch and Chamay 1992. See also Berlin Antikensammlung F2395, a red-figure hydria of ca. 430 where Eriphyle breast-feeds a well-grown Alkmaion (*CVA*, Berlin 9 [Germany 74], pl. 26 [3716]:5).

113. Gourevitch and Chamay 1992, p. 79. Terms of nursing contracts preserved in Roman Egypt range from six months to three years (sources are collected in Bradley 1980, p. 322, n. 5). Study of stable isotopes in a population of infants at the Dakhleh Oasis in Egypt in the 3rd century A.D. suggests that weaning there began at six months and was complete by the age of three years (Dupras, Schwarcz, and Fairgrieve 2001). This is approximately the same as the regime suggested by Soranus (*Gyn.* 2.21.46–47: solid food after six months, then the gradual elimination of breast-feeding in the third or fourth semester). See also Centlivres Challet 2016, pp. 166–167.

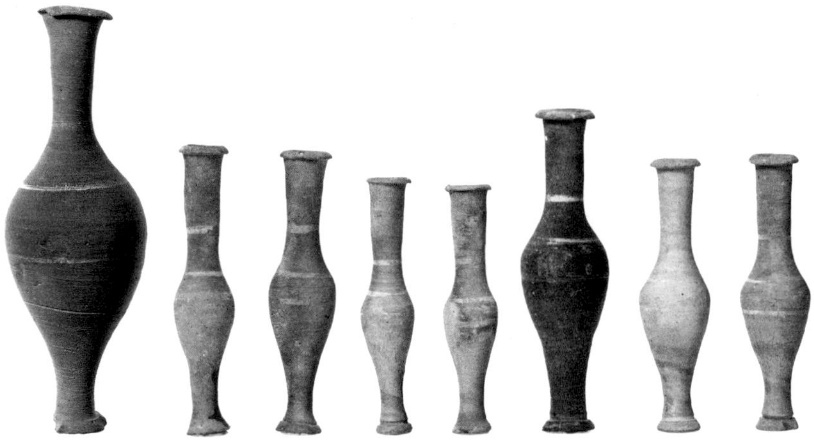

Figure 90. Unguentaria that are intact (32, 34, 35, 37) or chipped (31, 33, 36, 38). Scale 1:3. Photo Agora Excavations

the death of their small daughter (*Mor.* 608d). He illustrates the generous character of the child by the fact that she often offered the breast on which she was suckling to other children, not the gesture of a tiny baby. The feeder, then, may have been a weaning cup, used to accustom children to food other than mother's milk, and its high profile as a grave gift for young children is a reminder that weaning, like birth, was a dangerous time in the life of a young child.[114] And yet, the rarity of the feeder in the archaeological record overall indicates that it cannot have been used regularly in the weaning process. It may be, then, that the feeder was pressed into service primarily for older infants with some handicap or deficiency.[115] The link between the feeder and the grave, and between the feeder and children, is so strong that it seems certain that the feeder entered the well as a grave gift, probably for one of the older infants. It could be one more indication of the concern of caregivers for the hydrocephalic child AA 26b.

Unguentaria are the most common, and in many cases the exclusive, grave gift of Hellenistic Athens. Eight of the unguentaria from the well are intact or only slightly chipped (**31–38**; Fig. 90) and two more are whole, though broken, suggesting the possibility that they entered the deposit as grave gifts. Unguentaria were used in daily life as well, however, and are commonly found in deposits of household debris. Comparison with other deposits is made difficult by the fact that in all cases their contents were sorted shortly after excavation and much was discarded, and consequently the original proportions of the objects within the deposits have been lost. In what remains, however, only four Agora deposits have more unguentaria than the Agora Bone Well. These, however, are much larger groups, with from 535 to 995 identifiable vessels.[116] Three deposits have a larger percentage of unguentaria than the Agora Bone Well,[117] but the percentage of *complete* unguentaria in the Agora Bone Well is substantially greater than is the case in any other deposit.[118] The fact that four unguentaria that look very much like two pairs (**32–35**) were found within the same one-meter segment of the well (perhaps together?) may also provide support for their identity as more than chance rubbish.

114. Goodman and Armelagos 1989, p. 227; Scott 1999, p. 32. See Katzenberg, Herring, and Saunders 1996, pp. 178–181, 193–194, for the relationship of weaning to infant mortality and discussion of the "weanling's dilemma": the choice between new foods contaminated with pathogens and faltering growth if exclusively breast-feeding continues for too long.

115. As recently stressed by Sneed (2018).

116. E 14:1, M 21:1, P 21:4, and E 14:3, with 39, 35, 24, and 23 unguentaria respectively; these deposits contain approximately 730, 535, 995, and 389 identified vessels, respectively.

117. D 17:4, 11 unguentaria out of 87 vessels (12.6%); E 15:4, 18 out of ca. 230 vessels (7.8%); and Homer Thompson's Group C, 11 out of 152 vessels (7.2%). Compare these to 19 out of 282 vessels (6.7%) in the Agora Bone Well.

118. Half of the Agora Bone Well unguentaria are intact or substantially whole, in comparison to a quarter or less in the deposits cited in nn. 116, 117.

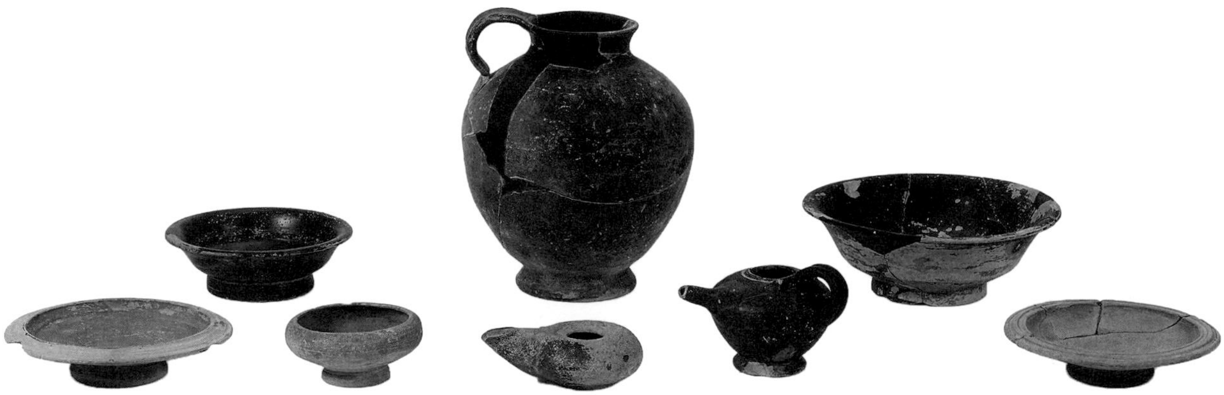

Figure 91. Fine-ware vessels that are intact (8), chipped (2, 12, 29), or missing only small fragments (5, 13, 22, 26). Back row: 2, 22, 5. Front row: 12, 8, 29, 26, 13. Photo C. A. Mauzy

Other possible grave gifts may be sought among objects that were, or may have been, serviceable when they entered the well. Fine-ware vessels found intact or nearly so (Fig. 91) include a bowl with outturned rim, an echinus bowl, a rilled-rim plate, and a lamp (**2, 8, 12, 29**). Another bowl and plate are broken, but nearly complete (**5, 13**), as is a round-mouth jug (**22**). These are common shapes and, with the possible exception of the rilled-rim plate, have no marked connection with ritual. Lamps and small bowls occur in the graves of children of the Classical period,[119] but there is no way of knowing if these items continued to be considered appropriate accompaniments for the infant dead, since infant graves are absent from the archaeological record of Hellenistic Athens. The rilled-rim plate seems to have been an exclusively ritual shape at its beginnings, in the 5th and 4th centuries, when it was commonly deposited in graves, graveside pyres, and saucer pyres within the city.[120] It continued to occur in saucer pyres down into the 2nd century,[121] so must have retained some ritual associations, but the form also appears in large numbers in domestic dumps, so the case for a sacred connotation in the Agora Bone Well is not very strong. The workaday jug **22** finds no parallels in ritual or funerary contexts, but the three nearly identical and well-preserved chytrai (**60–62**; Fig. 92) constitute a noteworthy concentration of this shape and call to mind the even smaller chytrai in the graves of Classical infants and children.[122] Loomweights, too, are occasionally found in graves, even infants' graves,[123] so some of those in the deposit (**78**, along with nine more that are intact or only chipped) might also have accompanied an infant into the well.

The two canteens (**24, 25**), although not grave gifts, may have a special relevance to childbirth. The most common purpose of this unusual shape was probably the same as that of the modern canteen—furnishing water to

119. E.g., Schlörb-Vierneisel 1966, pp. 34, 35, 49, nos. 60, 62, 99, Beil. 27, 38 (5th century); *Kerameikos* XIV, p. 58, no. 56, pl. 44 (amphora grave, 360/350).

120. Rotroff 2013, pp. 27–28.

121. Eleftheratou 1996–1997, pp. 102–110, figs. 2, 3, pls. 37–40; Parlama and Stampolides 2000, pp. 100–103.

122. E.g., Schlörb-Vierneisel 1966, pp. 89–90, 106, nos. 155 (the grave of an adult, but with a feeder, suggesting a newborn was also buried there, 330/320), 194 (amphora grave, early 3rd century), Beil. 58, 61; *Kerameikos* XIV, p. 58, no. 56, pl. 44 (amphora grave, 360/350).

123. Schlörb-Vierneisel 1966, p. 106, no. 194, Beil. 61 (amphora grave, early 3rd century).

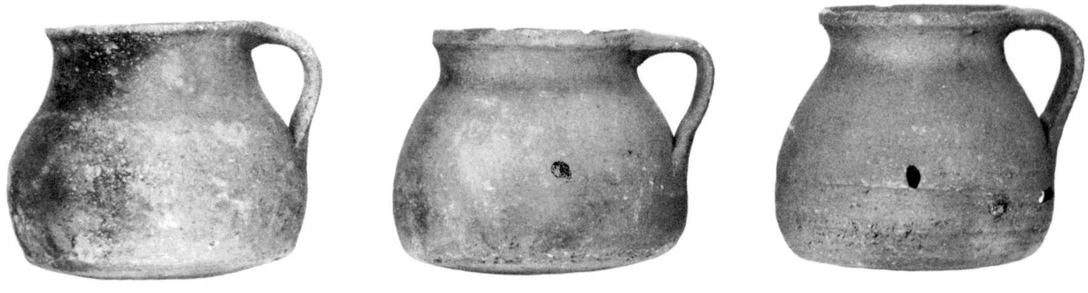

60 61 62

Figure 92. Three small chytrai, intact (60) or chipped (61, 62). Scale 1:3. Photo Agora Excavations

travelers. A medical usage as a hot-water bottle, however, is also attested. Soranus of Ephesos, a physician of the 2nd century A.D., recommends that bladders filled with warm oil be placed on the woman's sides to ease labor (*Gyn.* 2.3.4), and canteens could serve the same purpose.[124] In a case where the child did not survive, the fragments of a canteen used in childbirth might be discarded, polluted by their association with this unfortunate event.

The one feature that most clearly sets this assemblage of pottery apart from the usual run of household debris, however, is the number of large, open household-ware vessels: lekanai, large bowls, kraters, and mortars (Figs. 67–70, 93). The number of lekanai of form 4 is particularly striking: two substantially whole examples (**44, 45**) and fragments from at least 20 more. No other deposit in the Agora even comes close to such a concentration of this shape.[125] A wide variety of purposes are documented for lekanai in the kitchen, dining room, laundry room, workshop, and building site,[126] but the heavy concentration here prompts one to ask whether they could have anything to do with the infants. The fact that two of the form 4 lekanai are nearly whole suggests that they did not go into the well as secondary garbage, and the excavator and early students of the well wondered if the basins might have served as biers for the newborns' bodies. It would have been convenient and respectful to carry the remains of the deceased (and perhaps accompanying afterbirth) in a container of some kind. A basin may have been ready to hand; although no source specifies basins among the equipment necessary for a birth, Soranus (*Gyn.* 2.2.2) lists warm water and sponges, and a basin would have been useful for catching the afterbirth and for bathing the newborn child.[127] If the birth did not go well, the same basin could have been used to carry the corpse to its place of disposal. If this was the function of the lekanai (or some of them), we should also look at other shapes in the well that could have done the same job. These include lekanai of forms 1 and 3 (**40–43**), large bowls (**46–49**), kraters (**53, 54**), mortars (e.g., **55**), and a beehive (**56**) (Figs. 67–71, 93). One of these is

124. For later canteens (late 1st century B.C. and 1st century A.D.) specifically crafted to fit the afflicted parts of the body, see Nicolaou 1989, pp. 310–318. Medical advice preserved in the Oxyrhynchus papyri prescribes the use of a ceramic hot-water bottle for fever patients (*POxy.* VIII 1088, lines 46–47).

125. The next largest concentration is in cistern E 14:1: eight lekanai of form 4 in a collection of over 700 identified vessels.

126. See Lüdorf 2000 for the ancient sources on the functions of the lekane.

127. Soranus's instructions on cleansing the newborn infant (*Gyn.* 2.8.13) include bathing with lukewarm water, a process in which a basin would be essential.

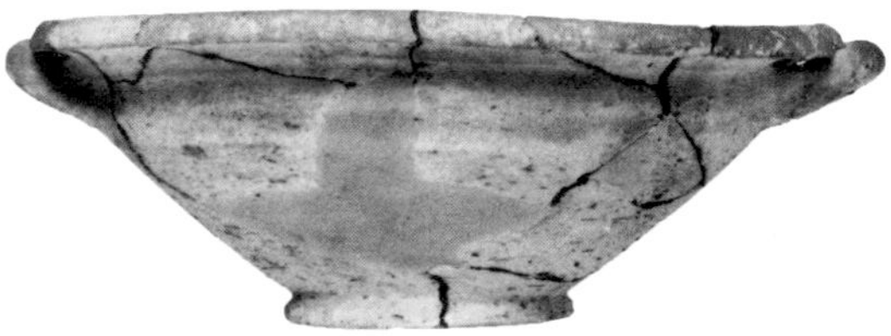

41

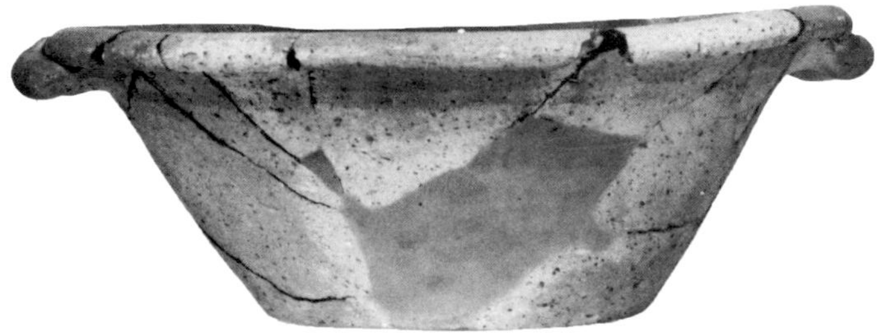

45

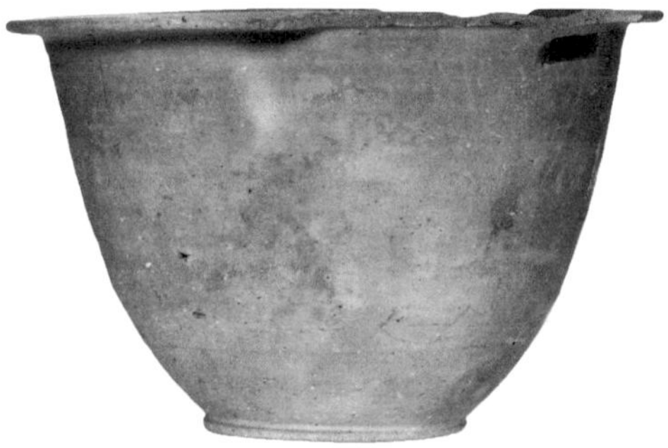

46

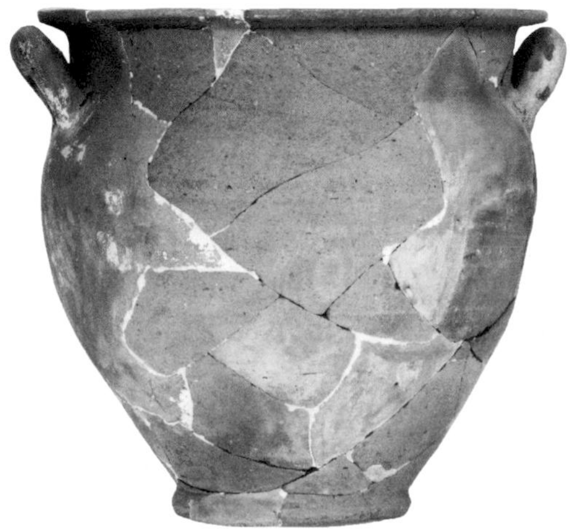

54

Figure 93. Two forms of lekane (41, 45), a deep bowl (46), and a krater (54). Scale 1:5. Photo Agora Excavations

intact save for chips, three are substantially complete, and another eight are more than half preserved (see Table 5), indications that they may have gone into the well whole or nearly so. Together these capacious open household containers account for 80% of the household pottery, a truly remarkable concentration. Among the fine ware, a deep bowl (**10**) and a segment of a lugged krater (**21**) might have served a similar purpose, as could the two large chytrai (**64, 65**), and perhaps roof-tile fragments as well (**79**).

In this connection it is well to remember that in Archaic and Classical Athens pots often served as containers for infant burials. These were most commonly amphoras, but other shapes were employed as well: kraters, pithoi, kadoi, hydriai, and lekanai are documented in the Südhügel cemetery,[128] and chytrai were used as containers for two graves in the Eridanos cemetery.[129] A complete lekane of form 4 came to light in the Kerameikos, near the grave of Hipparete;[130] although it cannot be associated with a grave, its complete state suggests that such is its provenience.

Given that the small female herm (**80**) can now be recognized as the birth goddess Eileithyia, there can be little doubt of its relevance to the bone deposit, though precisely what role it played and where it originated remain guesswork.[131] The break at the bottom suggests it was not purchased new as some sort of grave gift, but the image shows no sign of weathering and cannot have stood for any time in the open air. Herms were displayed

128. *Kerameikos* IX, pp. 25–29.

129. Knigge 1966, p. 122, grave 217; Schlörb-Vierneisel 1966, p. 27, grave 44. See also *Kerameikos* XIV, p. 45, grave 40, in precinct VIII. The grave is reported to have contained the burned bones of a newborn; this raises some doubts, however, since newborns were almost never cremated.

130. Brückner 1909, p. 120; Lüdorf 2000, p. 87, no. L 22, pl. 16.

131. For a review of the goddess's mythology, cult, and character, see Pingiatoglou 1981.

in sanctuaries, and in theory this one might have stood in a roofed area within a temenos. The archaeological remains—casting pits, houses with industrial installations immediately to the south—make it clear, however, that the Agora Bone Well cannot have been located within the boundaries of such a sanctuary. So if a sanctuary was the herm's source, someone had removed it from its sacred setting. Yet dedications were the property of the divinity and, except in times of war, they remained within the shrine; even if damaged, they were buried there, not thrown out, and it is difficult to imagine the removal of a dedication from an active shrine in order to make a private offering elsewhere. It is more likely, then, that this herm stood in a private setting, probably a home.[132] The molds for much smaller female terracotta herms, probably also of Eileithyia,[133] show that such items were cheap and mass-produced, possibly as talismans for pregnant women. Any expectant mother of some means might install a larger marble herm in her *gynaikonitis,* then discard it after an unsuccessful birth, but as Andrew Stewart argues above, a midwife is the most likely person to look particularly and repeatedly to the goddess for assistance, and it may be she who added the herm to the deposit.

132. For the evidence for herms within houses, see Wrede 1985, pp. 49–50; he notes in particular the use of small herms of various divinities in Delian houses. A small female herm oversees marriage preparations in the *gynaikonitis,* or women's quarters, on a 4th-century Attic red-figure lekanis lid (St. Petersburg, Hermitage St. 1858; see Metzger 1965, p. 86, no. 32, pl. XXXVII). Delivorrias lists it as a herm of Aphrodite (*LIMC* II, 1984, p. 11, no. 15, s.v. Aphrodite).

133. See n. 88 above.

CHAPTER 5

The Wider Archaeological and Cultural Context of the Well

The archaeologists who excavated the Agora Bone Well thought that they had come upon physical evidence of an extraordinary event or a major crisis. In his preliminary publication, Shear postulated that the newborns had died natural deaths but were dedicated to the goddess Aphrodite Ourania "as a symbolic sacrifice and a token survival of the original oriental ritual."[1] This scenario was rejected early on. Angel, writing in 1945, postulated starvation or plague as the most likely explanation for such a large concentration of bone, both animal and human,[2] and he associated the deposit with the Sullan sack of 86. Evelyn Harrison, who discussed the deposit briefly in the context of her publication of the herm (**80**), gave notice of Roger Edwards's redating of the deposit to the middle of the 2nd century and invoked an unrecorded epidemic as the source of the deposit.[3] She added the attractive hypothesis that the dogs may have served as purification sacrifices, a possibility we explore further below. The connection with Aphrodite Ourania has subsequently been revived and more thoroughly investigated by Osanna,[4] who argues that the well was located in the sanctuary of the goddess—although, as we have seen, the topography of the hill rules this out. The large collection of infant bones, in Osanna's view, may be connected either with an epidemic or with ritual ("aspetti rituali"). In what follows, we pursue these and other possibilities, calling on archaeological parallels and the literary record to help decode the deposit.

THE INFANTS: ARCHAEOLOGICAL PARALLELS

Differential treatment of the infant dead is a widespread phenomenon. Ethnographic and archaeological instances of special burial practices for children under a particular age abound, and we can observe them in our own time as well.[5] A 1965 survey of the ethnographic literature collected 70 examples from all over the world.[6] In a more up-to-date approach, a Google Scholar search for articles including "infant burial practices" yields over 68,000 hits with examples spanning human history,[7] and the eHRAF (electronic Human Relations Area Files) World Cultures database provides 99 accounts in 74 ethnographically documented cultures.[8] Special status

1. Shear 1939, p. 239.
2. Angel 1945, pp. 311–312.
3. *Agora* XI, pp. 168–169.
4. Osanna 1988–1989.
5. Surveyed briefly in Scott 1999, pp. 26–27.
6. Schwidetzky 1965, pp. 233–237. See also Ucko 1969, pp. 270–271.
7. The search was performed on scholar.google.com on July 13, 2014, using the phrase "infant burial practices."
8. The search was performed on ehrafworldcultures.yale.edu/ehrafe/ on July 14, 2014, using the phrase "infant burial practices."

may be accorded to individuals on the basis of their age or size, their developmental state (for example, before the appearance of teeth), or whether or not they have undergone a certain ceremony, such as baptism or naming. Unusual circumstances involving the mother or infant, including multiple births, also may result in differential or non-normative burials. The different procedures could involve burial in a different place (for example, in a children's cemetery, or within a settlement) or according to a different ritual (for example, placement in trees rather than burial, or burial rather than cremation). In a few cases, it is even documented that very young children were simply set out—in the bush, the woods—or thrown into a river. Some of these solutions leave no archaeological trace, but infant cemeteries, burials within houses and settlements, and a preference for burial rather than cremation for infants are amply documented in the archaeological literature.[9] We can safely conclude that, at many times and places, it was normal to treat infants differently from adults in death.

While the Agora Bone Well is unusual in the number of individuals involved and their ages, the archaeological record elsewhere has produced parallel cases where infants have been disposed of in an unusual way. In what follows, examples of three forms of differential disposal of very young children are discussed: infants found in wells or sewers along with ordinary domestic debris, infant burials within settlements, and infant cemeteries. Our aim here is not to make an exhaustive survey of these practices, but rather to point out some of the closest parallels to the Agora Bone Well, to review the interpretations that have been assigned to them, and to examine the reasons for those interpretations. In turn, our analysis of the Agora material challenges some of these interpretations and suggests that other possibilities should be considered as well.

Infants in Wells, Pits, and Sewers

Although infant bones have been reported in pits and wells singly or in small numbers from time to time,[10] we are aware of only four significant concentrations of individuals in such contexts in the Mediterranean world: in two wells at Eretria (one 3rd-century B.C., the other Roman), in a 3rd- to 2nd-century-B.C. well at Messene, and in a Late Roman sewer at Ashkelon.

9. Scott 1999 provides an exhaustive study of the phenomenon.

10. Soren and Soren (1999, p. 486) report that the discovery of infants in refuse pits is "not uncommon in the Roman world." Hooper (1975, p. 376) makes a similar general statement: "pits full of the normal detritus of the Roman household do sometimes contain the skeletons of infants," alluding in particular to an unpublished instance of six infants in a pit at Radwinter, Essex. Portchester provides another example, where the remains of over a dozen fetuses and infants up to the age of ca. 18 weeks were found in refuse pits (Hooper 1975; for the pits, see Cunliffe 1975, pp. 81–172). Previously unrecognized bones from two infants were identified by Snyder and Little while sorting through the animal bone in the Hellenistic fill of well J 5:1, beside the Panathenaic Way, on the north side of the Agora (for the stratigraphy of the well, see *Agora* XXIX, p. 458), and Liston has identified an infant and young child in a Geometric well (J 3:8) north of the Agora. The reconstruction of the human behavior behind such instances is deeply intertwined with the particular social, cultural, and historical context to which the find belongs; see, for instance, a discussion of two infants found in an 18th-century pit in Philadelphia (Burnston 1982, 1997), where access to substantial historical documentation makes it possible to decide plausibly between abortion, normal burial procedure, poverty of the mother, or infanticide as an explanation.

Eretria

The 3rd-century well, excavated in 1997, is located on the north side of the main east–west thoroughfare on the lower southern slopes of the acropolis of Eretria. It is 1.20 m in diameter and about 5.00 m deep, and was situated, apparently in public ground, at the intersection of two streets.[11] At the very bottom was found a hoard of 338 silver and 16 bronze coins, probably hidden in the well for safekeeping. The latest coin, a silver tetradrachm of Antiochos I (r. 281–261) or II (r. 261–246) of Syria, provides a broad *terminus post quem* for the deposit of the material in the well.[12] Two or perhaps three nearby houses (the House of the Mosaics and its neighbors) were destroyed by fire in the first part of the 3rd century, an event that the excavators tentatively ascribe to action during the Chremonidean War (267–262/1),[13] and the war may also be implicated in the deposit of the coin hoard. The bones in the well appear to have been in the same layer. Above the level of the hoard, the well contained a uniform deposit of debris that is consistent with a date of deposit in the first half of the 3rd century. It is possible that the hoard bears witness to anticipation of the conflict, while the dumped debris reflects cleanup operations soon after the attack.

According to accounts published shortly after excavation, the well included the bones of one infant along with the remains of five or six dogs. Isabelle Chenal-Velarde now reports, however, that the number of infants is 19, with a minimum of 26 dogs.[14] All were found at the bottom of the well, in association with the coin hoard. The infants range from 31 gestational weeks to neonatal; the dogs present a mixture of ages.[15] The age range of the infants closely parallels that of the infants in the Agora Bone Well. Liston has been given permission to study the infant skeletons and has examined them briefly.[16] They offer convincing parallels to the Agora infants, including evidence for endocranial pathologies that may have contributed to the early deaths of these babies. Although a full study of the case has yet to be published, it is possible that military action contributed to this extraordinary deposit. Whether or not the children died as a result of the attack, either a prolonged siege or disruption of normal activities in the wake of the attack might have occasioned a breakdown of usual burial practices. If this well was dry, it could have been a reasonable solution to the problem of the disposal of infant dead during the siege; alternatively, if it had been fouled by the invaders, it could have served the same purpose in the wake of the attack. Chenal-Velarde suggests that the dogs are not part of cleanup debris, but rather bear witness to some sort of symbolic act, although animals left dead in the wake of the attack might have been discarded here as well. What is not clear, however, is why only late-term fetuses and neonates were deposited here, since in the case of an attack or

11. Ducrey and Schmid 1997; Schmid 2000.

12. Schmid 2000, pp. 370–371 (Antiochos I); Houghton and Lorber 2002, vol. I, p. 182, no. 511.3 (Antiochos II). We thank Guy Ackermann for alerting us to this difference of opinion.

13. *Eretria* VIII, p. 177. For the siege of the city in 268 and its capitulation the following year, see Knoepfler 1993, pp. 339–341; 1995, p. 144.

14. Chenal-Velarde 2006, pp. 25–28.

15. Three fetal/neonatal puppies, seven less than six months old, one between six and 12 months, and 13 adult dogs.

16. We are grateful to Stephan G. Schmid of the Institut für Archäologie, Humboldt University of Berlin, for his kind permission to examine the human remains from this well.

siege, they would not have been the only individuals to die. If the infants in the well are the result of a breakdown of normal societal practices, the age range should be much broader. The association of complete dogs with the remains of neonates also provides a close parallel to the Agora deposit. The smaller numbers are a certain indication that the deposit accumulated over a very short period of time, but until a final study is published it is difficult to associate the deposit with an attack definitively, and it may reflect instead a normal practice in the city of disposing of infants who died in the perinatal period.

The more recent discovery of a Roman well in the gymnasium at Eretria provides evidence that this pattern of infant disposal was more widespread than previously recognized. Excavation was completed in 2017, and the contents of the well have not yet been fully studied.[17] The well contained a dense deposit of human remains of all ages, including a minimum of eight adults, four juveniles, and 23 infant and fetal skeletons found in the first season. At least that many additional infant skeletons are represented in the material from the second season of excavation, which has not yet been studied. Like the majority of the infants from the Agora Bone Well, these range in age from the fetal period, as young as 18 weeks *in utero,* to no older than one to two weeks post–full term. The older juveniles are no younger than three years, so there is a gap in ages between the infant group and the older children. The skeletons of the adults and older children appear to have been deposited in the well as disarticulated bones, not intact bodies. The inventory of the infant and fetal skeletons, however, strongly suggests that they entered the well as intact bodies. While the cranial bones are not well preserved, there are at least two cases of cleft palate, a birth defect also seen in the Agora Bone Well. Finally, while the animal bones from the well have not yet been examined, it is clear that they include a large number of dog remains. The age distribution of the infants, the pathologies, and the presence of large numbers of dogs in the two wells in Eretria offer the closest parallels to the deposit in the Agora.

Messene

Another site with striking similarities to the Agora case was discovered by Petros Themelis in his excavations at Messene.[18] In a Hellenistic well in a public area, near the council hall and the temple of the deified queen Messenia, were found the skeletons of a minimum of 262 infants as well as considerable faunal material, primarily dog bones. Many fragments of large vessels, including locally made amphoras, were notable among the artifacts in the well. According to Chryssi Bourbou, the anthropologist entrusted with the study of human bone from the well, the age of the infants clusters closely around the time of birth, within a range of 26–42 weeks, with some post-term (more than 42 weeks) infants as well. Bourbou and Themelis concluded that their deaths were the result of the complications of pregnancy. The correspondence between the Messene and Agora wells seems to be close in the large numbers of individuals, the uniformity of their ages, and their association with large vessels and dogs. In view of the fact that amphoras are very commonly used as containers in infant burials, however, Bourbou and Themelis concluded that these infants were deposited

17. We are grateful to Karl Reber, director of the Swiss School of Archaeology in Greece, for the invitation to study the human skeletons from this well and to discuss them here ahead of formal publication. For preliminary notices of the excavation, see Ackermann, Tettamanti, Pradervand, and Reber 2016, p. 9; 2017, pp. 133–134; Ackermann, Tettamanti, Pop, and Reber 2017, pp. 7–8.

18. Bourbou and Themelis 2010, pp. 112–120. We are grateful to Chryssi Bourbou for sharing information about this deposit in advance of publication.

secondarily in the well at Messene, having previously been buried elsewhere in ceramic vessels. They also suggested, however, that once the site had been established as a recipient of infant dead, mothers and midwives may also have used the well for the primary disposal of remains.[19] The dog bones still await study, but the authors leave open the possibility that the animals played a ritual role.

Ashkelon

Excavations in the large town of Ashkelon, on the southern coast of present-day Israel, revealed another concentration of infant bones.[20] The remains of over 100 individuals were recovered from the gutter of a large sewer, where they lay mixed with assorted rubbish (animal bones, potsherds, and coins). The sewer ran under a bathhouse that had been built in the 3rd century A.D. and went out of use during the 5th century,[21] after which the area lay abandoned until the construction of a large apsidal building that sealed in the bath and the sewer. No detailed account of the stratigraphy of the building has been published, but those who have written about the deposit assume that the bones accumulated during the time when the bath was active. Based on bone lengths, dentition, and the absence of neonatal lines in the teeth, the children were identified as neonates, no more than one or two days old. Although the bones were commingled, their good state of preservation and the fact that all parts of the skeleton were accounted for suggested that the babies entered the sewer whole and very shortly after their deaths.

Because of the apparently casual manner of their discard, and, more significantly, the great uniformity of their ages, clustered in the first two days of life, the anthropologists who examined the bones concluded that the children were victims of infanticide.[22] Had the children died of natural causes (in an epidemic, for instance) or as a result of violence, they reasoned, a range of ages would have been represented. Possible support for this conclusion was found in a further examination of the tooth buds, some of which were stained dark brown and had a high content of iron oxide, which they interpreted as a symptom of death by asphyxiation.[23] Pursuing this research further, they were able to extract DNA from some of the bones, which in 19 cases could be amplified and analyzed. This study showed, surprisingly, a marked majority of males in this sample (14 as opposed to five females). Since it is generally assumed that the peoples of the ancient Mediterranean, like so many others, preferred male to female offspring, this is the opposite of what one would have expected in a population of ancient infanticides.[24] The researchers speculated that the bathhouse may have served as a brothel in which the mothers of the unwanted babies plied their trade; as prostitutes, they might have preferred to rear girls (as future members of the profession) rather than boys.

The Ashkelon deposit resembles the Agora Bone Well in the large number of neonatal individuals, but it is hard to draw comparisons without a better understanding of the period during which the Ashkelon deposit accumulated. The bathhouse, and presumably its sewer, were apparently in use for about 200 years; if this is the period during which the infants were deposited, then the Ashkelon case differs significantly from the Agora

19. Bourbou and Themelis 2010, pp. 115–117.
20. Stager 1991a, pp. 49–51; Smith and Kahila 1992; Faerman et al. 1998; Stager et al. 2008, pp. 293–297.
21. There is some uncertainty about the date. In their most recent report, the excavators date the construction to the 3rd century and the abandonment to the 5th century (Stager et al. 2008, pp. 293, 297). Earlier reports place the building between the 4th and 6th centuries (Smith and Kahila 1992, p. 669; Faerman et al. 1998, p. 862).
22. Smith and Kahila 1992, pp. 669, 673–674.
23. Smith and Kahila 1992, p. 673.
24. Faerman et al. 1998.

one, with its far shorter period of deposition. It is possible, however, that at Ashkelon too the span was shorter. The presence of over 100 infant bodies, even if they did not all go into the sewer at the same time, would have created a significant blockage in a major drain that served the bathhouse. The resulting odor would potentially have been overwhelming, even in a culture more accustomed to biological smells than our own. Both of these considerations cast doubt on the assumption that the bodies were deposited while the bath was in use. The final publication of the bathhouse notes that after repeated attempts to fix leaks in the bath, it was abandoned in the 5th century and its bathing pool filled with amphoras; the hypocaust system and other drains became choked with debris at this time as well.[25] It is unclear why the infant skeletons are assigned to the period of use of the sewer, while the debris in the other drains and the bath itself is identified as post-use. It seems more likely that the infants were deposited in the period between the abandonment of the bath in the 5th century and the construction of the apsidal building over it sometime later.[26] At Ashkelon, then, the accumulation of bodies could have taken place over more than a century or it could have happened more quickly, but neither scenario necessarily supports the interpretation of infanticide as the cause of these deaths.

The interpretation of the Ashkelon infants as victims of infanticide rests on the number of infants present in the sewer, the fact that the age at death clusters around the age of neonatal infants, and the assertion that natural deaths would have a flatter age distribution.[27] Other than the suggestion that dark staining of the teeth was evidence of strangulation,[28] no paleopathological evaluation of the skeletons has been reported.

There are a number of reasons to challenge the interpretation of infanticide as the cause of the infant deaths at Ashkelon. The distribution of humerus lengths, used to estimate age in the two collections, demonstrates that the ages at death of the infants follow very similar patterns at both Ashkelon and the Agora. Using regression equations to estimate age from humerus length, we can compare the age distributions of the infants in the two collections.[29] While the Agora sample is much larger, it is clear from the frequency distribution that the pattern of age at death is quite similar (Fig. 94). The absence of the neonatal line in the Ashkelon infants indicates that all were stillbirths or died at less than two days of age. It does not, however, indicate that they died after a normal full-term live birth. The analysis of the Ashkelon remains fails to consider the high probability of death by natural causes in the immediate perinatal period, and the presence of a large percentage of preterm-size infants who would be more likely to die within hours or days of birth, if they were born alive. The distribution of age at death in the Ashkelon sewer does not differ from the expected pattern of natural perinatal death in preterm and full-term infant births.[30]

The interpretation of staining in the teeth of the Ashkelon infants as evidence of suffocation or strangulation is also suspect. While "pink teeth" are associated with strangulation in recent forensic contexts, there is no evidence that this results in discoloration of the teeth in long-dead infants. The staining found at Ashkelon, which is common in most infant dental

25. Stager et al. 2008, p. 297.
26. As Scott has also suggested (Scott 1999, p. 68; 2001, p. 12).
27. Smith and Kahila 1992, p. 669: "We reasoned that if all infants were neonates we could assume that they were the victims of infanticide. We dismissed the possibility that they were stillborn because of the large number of individuals represented. On the other hand, if they were of different ages, then we could assume that they either died from natural causes, or were massacred."
28. Smith and Kahila 1992, p. 673.
29. Smith and Kahila (1992, p. 670, fig. 2) give frequencies of humerus lengths from the site, providing the data to compare age estimates using regression equations (Scheuer, Musgrave, and Evans 1980).
30. Konigsberg and Liston 2013.

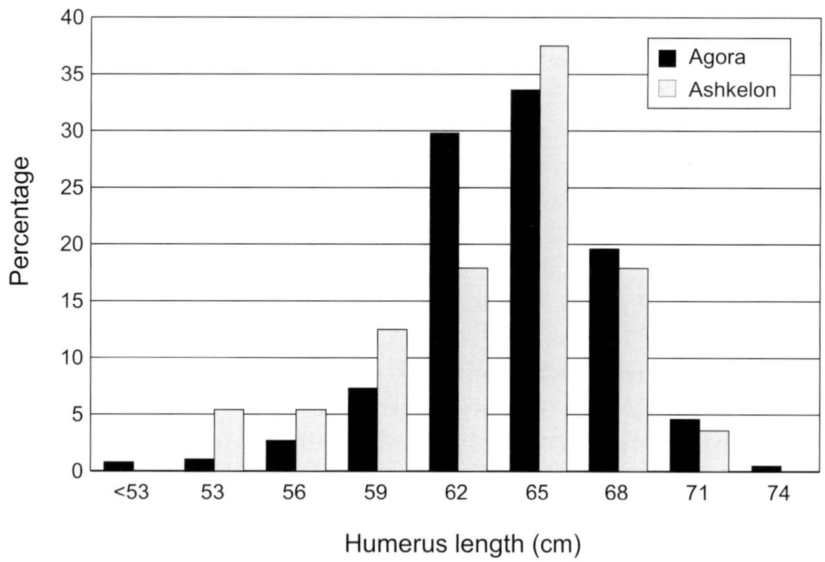

Figure 94. Humerus length distributions for the infants in the Agora Bone Well and in the Ashkelon sewer. Ashkelon data after Smith and Kahila 1992, p. 670

remains recovered from burial contexts, has been shown at other sites to be the result of diagenetic processes, including fungal infiltration and uptake of iron and other minerals from the surrounding soil.[31]

As a result, we feel that the Ashkelon deposit of infants in an abandoned sewer may very closely mirror the deposit of infants in an abandoned well in the Athenian Agora, but we hesitate to accept the Ashkelon deposit as evidence of infanticide.

Infant Burials in Settlements

Archaeology the world over provides many instances of infant burial within settlements, often under the floors of houses. It is often assumed that this is simply another instance of differential treatment of infant and adult dead, and for the ancient Mediterranean there is a text that supports this interpretation. Fulgentius, in a treatise on obscure words probably written in the late 5th century A.D., recalls this ancient practice, explaining that "in earlier times the ancients used the term *suggrundarium* for the burial of an infant who had not yet lived 40 days" (*Expositio sermonum antiquorum* 7: *Priore tempore suggrundaria antiqui dicebant sepulchra infantum qui necdum quadraginta dies implessent*). The term suggests burial under the eaves of the house.[32] In some cases, however, unusual concentrations of intramural neonatal graves have been interpreted as sacrifices or infanticides rather than normal interment. Whatever the interpretation, the concentration of the remains of newborns within a settlement invites comparison with the Agora deposit.

A complete survey of this material is beyond the scope of this work, but a few examples can illustrate the various interpretations that have been applied to such finds. Neonatal burials have been found in several Late Roman villa sites. In a brief paragraph, the excavator of the Yewden Villa at Hambleden in southern England (occupied ca. A.D. 50–410)

31. Dye, Lucy, and Pollard 1995, pp. 344–346; Lewis 2007, p. 24.

32. See the derivation in *OLD*, s.v. *suggrunda*.

describes how the northern half of the excavation was "positively littered with babies."[33] He unearthed 97 skeletons there, mostly of neonates but a few "rather older." The bodies were often contracted, the knees pulled up above the head in what sounds like fetal position. No evidence of markers was found, and one burial sometimes encroached upon another, suggesting to the excavator that "the interments took place secretly, after dark." Although the excavator offers no further explanation, the implication is that these were illicit births, concealed by their mothers probably because of illegitimacy, and secretly buried here; presumably, then, their deaths were not natural.[34]

Bringing modern anthropological techniques to bear on this phenomenon, Simon Mays analyzed the skeletal data from six Romano-British sites (two cemeteries, two villas, and two settlements) and, for comparison, the medieval churchyard at Wharram Percy.[35] He found that statistics for the Roman sites were fairly homogeneous, with a marked peak of births at full term, while the medieval cemetery showed a flatter distribution of age at death. Comparing these data with 20th-century statistics for the distribution of gestational age for stillbirths, live births dying within seven days, and all live births, he found that the Romano-British data matched the latter—all live births—most closely. Because infanticide usually occurs within a day or two of birth, Mays reasoned that the data for infanticides should mirror the modern data for all live births, and he therefore concluded that infanticides made up a sufficiently large number of the Romano-British deaths to be visible in the statistics at these sites. The flatter age-at-death distribution among infants in the Christian churchyard at Wharram Percy presumably resulted from the exclusion of the unbaptized, including victims of infanticide, who would have contributed to the absent peak. While the flatter age-at-death distribution of the Wharram Percy burials has been challenged,[36] Mays's argument is much like that advanced at Ashkelon: a concentration of true neonates is likely to be made up in large part of infanticides.

Mays's work has elicited a strong reaction. Rebecca Gowland and Andrew Chamberlain examined the data for the skeletons of 396 infants from 19 Romano-British sites, including the same six sites that formed the basis of Mays's study.[37] Applying a different statistical technique to

33. Cocks 1921, p. 150; Scott 1999, pp. 110–113. Watts (1989, p. 373) gives a date of late 3rd century A.D. for the burials.

34. See also Frere 1987, pp. 303–304, where these burials are taken to be the "unwanted female offspring of a slave-run establishment." Mays and Eyers (2011), in a recent analysis of the skeletal material, agree that the children were primarily infanticides, though Hassan et al. (2014) have demonstrated through DNA analysis that there was no preference for females. The following are some similar sites where infanticide has been invoked as a possible explanation of multiple infant burials: Owslebury (Collis 1977, pp. 29, 34); Springhead (Penn 1967, p. 269; he ultimately rejects this explanation in favor of epidemic); and Sallèles d'Aude and Poundbury (Molleson 2003, pp. 119–121; for Sallèles d'Aude, see also n. 40, below).

35. Mays 1993; Mays and Eyers (2011) add a third villa to the list, with data from 35 of the Yewden Villa infants, recently rediscovered in their original packing cases.

36. In a reanalysis of the data using Bayesian statistics, Lewis and Gowland found that the mortality curve of the infants at Wharram Percy was not flat, but peaked at a gestational age of 38–42 weeks, and thus more closely resembled "normal" infant mortality for the time period (Lewis and Gowland 2007, pp. 125–127, fig. 8). In response, Mays and Eyers have produced further analyses in support of the flat distribution (Mays and Eyers 2011, pp. 1936–1937, figs. 3–6). See also Bonsall 2013.

37. Gowland and Chamberlain 2002. For Mays's response, see Mays 2003.

the aging of the infants, they found a spread of age at death significantly wider than that calculated by Mays, and closely approximating natural perinatal mortality. While Gowland and Chamberlain do not discount the probability that infanticide was practiced in Roman Britain, to them the skeletal evidence indicates that it did not occur so frequently as to be reflected in the statistics of age distribution of the deceased.

Eleanor Scott, who has made a study of infant burials at Romano-British villas, has come to much the same conclusion.[38] For her, large numbers of perinatal infant burials are more likely to be the result of natural infant mortality in the premodern world than of the regular practice of infanticide, and she interprets the villa sites as infant cemeteries rather than the venues of illicit burials. She sees the emergence of this burial rite in the Late Roman period as a revival of ancient practices from the Celtic past, a revitalization movement responding to developments within Romano-British society. Mays's argument for infanticide, in her opinion, is more a reflection of a "Romano-Victorian" worldview than a realistic interpretation of either the social mores of the time or the dangers that faced newborn infants in the Roman period.[39]

Similar concentrations of newborns have been found under the floors of farmhouses and workshops elsewhere, and a similar diversity of explanations explored. A few examples of the many instances will suffice. The skeletons of 22 or 23 children were found within a late-5th- to early-4th-century B.C. settlement at Gailhan, in southern France, and, as at the British sites, the great majority (18–19) were perinatal.[40] In their presentation of this material, Bernard Dedet and his colleagues consider but immediately dismiss the possibility of sacrifice and, while admitting that the age of the children may suggest infanticide, conclude that the deaths were instead natural. As evidence for this conclusion, they invoke the location of the burials within houses and the proportion of burials to domestic units, which seems in accord with expected neonatal mortality. Furthermore, infant burials within settlements are a frequent feature of prehistoric sites in the region, suggesting that this is an indigenous custom, although one not practiced in every village. They also cite the absence of newborns from contemporaneous cemeteries, concluding that burial within the house was simply the normal practice for the very young at this particular time and place.

The skeletons of 14 children ranging in age from 36 gestational weeks to two months after birth were found in and around a farmhouse at Neftenbach, near Zurich.[41] They had been buried during two phases of the site: two in the third quarter of the 1st century A.D., the others in the 2nd century. Although there were only slight traces of grave gifts or special treatment of the bodies, Elisabeth Langenegger has no doubt that this represents the normal burial practice for the very young, and sees it as confirmation of a comment made by Pliny (*HN* 7.72) that those who died before the appearance of their teeth should not be cremated.

All of these sites resemble the Agora Bone Well in their unusual concentration of the remains of infants within a settlement and in the fact that the majority of the individuals died around the time of birth, and they illustrate again the differing conclusions that can be drawn from such material.

38. Scott 1991; 1999, pp. 110–115.

39. Scott 1999, p. 110.

40. Dedet, Duday, and Tillier 1991, with a summary of similar material elsewhere in Languedoc and Provence. For a similar though later site at Sallèles d'Aude (a pottery works of the 1st–2nd century A.D.), meticulously excavated and analyzed by some of the same scholars, see Duday, Laubenheimer, and Tillier 1995, with more comparative material on pp. 111–112; here too they conclude that the deaths were natural.

41. Langenegger 1996, with references to similar sites in the region.

Infant Cemeteries

Infant cemeteries, per se, are unexceptional; many are documented in the Greek world and they bear witness to nothing more than compliance with the widespread human tendency to isolate the very young in special burial places. There are three cemeteries, however, that bear comparison with the Agora well.

Lugnano in Teverina

At Poggio Gramignano, near the town of Lugnano in Teverina on the upper reaches of the Tiber, an infant cemetery was excavated within a disused Roman villa.[42] Forty-seven infants—the largest such concentration so far reported from Roman Italy—were found spread throughout five rooms of the villa, which had fallen into ruins by the time these burials were made. Ages clustered at full term to two months old, with a few fetal and older individuals; only one child was older than six months. Burial of many (though not all) of the younger children was very casual; isolated in two of the rooms, they had simply been tossed away with other debris. Other children, and usually older ones, received more care (for example, burial within ceramic vessels or under tiles). All indications are that the burials took place within a very short period of time—a few days or a month, perhaps—around the middle of the 5th century A.D.

What sets this cemetery apart, in the eyes of the excavators, is substantial evidence of unusual ritual practices. Parts of 12 puppies less than six months old and the skeleton of a dog approximately one year of age were found in the area restricted to neonates (though not within the burials themselves). Some of the animals had been cut in pieces, and the excavators interpret these animals as remains of propitiatory sacrifices. The skeleton of a toad and the talon of a raven (both animals attested as efficacious in witchcraft), as well as a cooking pot placed upside down, a bone doll, and stones placed on the hands of the oldest child, can also be read as measures of aversion.[43] They conclude that the children were the victims of a malaria epidemic, the rituals enacted in an attempt to avert the plague.[44] It is easy enough to invoke plague when any unusual concentration of human remains is discovered.[45] The Lugnano team, however, was subsequently able to support this hypothesis through DNA analysis, which identified traces of *Plasmodium falciparum,* the agent of a virulent form of the disease, in some of the bones.[46] The Lugnano cemetery, then, provides a documented instance of multiple deaths as a result of epidemic and is therefore an important comparandum in assessing the meaning of the Agora deposit.

Although 16 of the Lugnano babies were full term (36–40 gestational weeks), more were judged to be in the first two months of life. The uniformity of the deposit at the Agora thus appears to be much greater, with all but a very few of the infants dying in the late fetal or perinatal period. The cemetery is similar to the Agora well, however, in the association of infants and dogs—although the severing of the dogs into pieces is not paralleled at Athens, and other than the dogs and the female herm, the Agora deposit preserves very little evidence of ritual activity, and nothing to parallel the toad and the raven of Lugnano. The bones of other species

42. Soren and Soren 1999, pp. 486–530.

43. Soren and Soren 1999, pp. 517–519.

44. Soren and Soren 1999, pp. 520–523.

45. E.g., Penn 1967; he invokes the plague under Marcus Aurelius to explain the graves of 18 children at Springhead.

46. Sallares and Gomzi 2001, pp. 202–211; Sallares et al. 2003; Soren 2003.

from the Agora appear to be typical butchering or consumption debris or simple bone tools presumably discarded after use.

The Tophet of Carthage

A second example highlights the difficulties of interpretation even in cases where considerable amounts of written testimony may be brought to bear on the question. The Tophet of Carthage has been a focus of archaeological exploration since the early 20th century,[47] and thousands of infant burials have been found there. The individuals had been cremated and placed within urns, their graves often associated with a marker in the form of a stele or a cippus. Numerous Greek, Roman, and biblical texts refer with horror to the Carthaginian practice of child sacrifice;[48] on this basis, the Tophet has long been regarded as the resting place of sacrificed infants and children.[49] Anthropological analysis by Jeffrey Schwartz of the skeletal material from some of the more recent excavations has revealed, as expected, that all of the deceased were children; a few were older than four years, but most were younger than six months.[50] One-quarter of the urns contained the remains of two different individuals, usually separated by only a few months of age; animal bones were also present, in isolated urns or mixed with human remains. It has also emerged, however, that at least 54% of the deceased, and possibly as many as 81%, are late-third-trimester fetuses; as such, they are improbable victims of sacrifice and are much more likely to have died naturally as a result of premature birth. All in all, Schwartz reckons that 90% of the sample he examined can best be seen as stillbirths, spontaneous abortions, or neonates who died of natural causes. For Schwartz, then, the Tophet is an infant cemetery plain and simple, not the repository of sacrificed infants. Although he is not alone in this position,[51] his work is of particular relevance to the present case in that it is based on the interpretation of skeletal remains rather than other archaeological or literary evidence. In any event, the Carthaginian case illustrates how, even when written accounts seem to mandate a verdict of unnatural death, it is possible to interpret the evidence in a different light.

Astypalia

The largest ancient infant cemetery so far discovered is located at Kylindra, on the Greek island of Astypalia, in the Dodecanese. Over 2,700 infant burials, most dating to the 6th and 5th centuries B.C., have been identified thus far in the ongoing excavations.[52] The infants were buried

47. Brown 1991; Bénichou-Safar 2004. For the history of the excavations, see Brown 1991, pp. 39–57; Bénichou-Safar 2004, pp. 7–25.

48. For a summary of the literary and epigraphical evidence, see Brown 1991, pp. 21–35.

49. Stager 1982; Brown 1991, pp. 56–57, 148–149, 167–170.

50. Schwartz 1993, pp. 52–57.

51. In a fascinating essay in intellectual history, Brien Garnand (2002, pp. 4–15) recounts how, since 1987, many scholars of Phoenician archaeology have repudiated the infant sacrifice model. Nor were they the first. Schaeffer (in Virolleaud 1956, p. 67; Schaeffer 1962, pp. 77–83) had led the way with brief notes to similar effect, followed by Weinfeld (1972, p. 134), who, while conceding that the Carthaginians may have performed such sacrifices, dismissed them as occasional responses to crisis rather than institutionalized cult. See Bénichou-Safar 2004, pp. 159–163, 171, for a summary of the arguments in support of this view, with bibliography.

52. Clement, Hillson, and Michalaki-Kollia, 2009; Hillson 2009.

in ceramic jars, often amphoras that were used to bring products to the island, but occasionally also domestic vessels. No detailed data have been published, but preliminary studies indicate that most of the infants died in the perinatal period, near full-term births, although some are preterm and a few are post-term infants who survived for some time after birth. The total age range is approximately 24 weeks *in utero* to three years. Most vessels contained a single infant, but a few had more than one, although the second and occasional third skeletons were usually represented by only a few elements and may be intrusive from other, disturbed burials. However, approximately 1.9% of the vessels have two complete skeletons and may represent twins who did not survive. This percentage is similar to the prevalence of natural twins in modern-day Europe, that is, those conceived without assistive technologies. Most of the infants were buried with their heads toward the mouth of the vessel, but approximately 10% were placed with their feet toward the mouth. The excavators speculate that these may represent breech births, and that the position and number of the infants in vessels was meant to simulate the conditions of birth. Surprisingly, no evidence for pathologies or congenital anomalies has been detected, but the current research focuses almost exclusively on dental remains and growth and development studies.

The origin of the infants remains unclear, but the numbers are too vast to be accounted for on this small island during the period of the cemetery's use. Maria Michalaki-Kollia, the project director, suggests the site may be associated with the worship of goddesses of childbirth, such as Artemis Lochia and Eileithyia, but no definitive interpretations are available as yet.[53]

THE INFANTS: THREE HYPOTHESES

The above discussion illustrates the different ways in which large collections of infant dead have been interpreted in the archaeological literature. One of four explanations is invariably suggested—sacrifice, plague, infanticide, or normal infant mortality—and, as we have seen, it is often not easy to choose among them. One of the problems that bedevils the analysis of unusual burial contexts is the search for a single cause. The reality of human culture or biology is rarely so simple, however, and the causes will almost always be varied and more nuanced than a single explanation, particularly one that is shocking or exciting, such as large-scale infanticide. To understand complex human behaviors, we must recognize that there may be multiple motivations and causes, and seek to tease these out by a careful examination of the evidence.

Among the likely explanations of the Agora Bone Well deposit, symbolic sacrifice, invoked as a motivation by Shear at the time of excavation,[54] can safely be dismissed; although rumors of human sacrifice in out-of-the-way places persisted, this was clearly not a normal part of Greek religious practice in the time and place with which we are concerned.[55] This leaves three possibilities: the infants died as a result of an epidemic or famine; they are the victims of infanticide; or the well provides evidence for one of the ways in which the bodies of newborns who died of a variety of causes

53. Clement, Hillson, and Michalaki-Kollia 2009, p. 21.

54. Shear 1939, p. 239.

55. For human sacrifice among the Greeks, see Brown 1991, pp. 159–162; Hughes 1991.

were disposed of in Hellenistic Athens. In the following pages we examine the likelihood of each of these possibilities, keeping in mind that they are not mutually exclusive.

Famine and Epidemic

In his discussion of the babies in 1945, Angel suggested "starvation or plague" as the agency of their deaths.[56] The first of these two explanations was no doubt encouraged by Angel's understanding that the deposit accumulated during the Sullan siege. We now know, however, that this was not the case; the accompanying pottery dates the deposit nearly a century earlier. The interactions of famine, epidemic, and infant mortality are complex, but in general, poor maternal nutrition is correlated with higher perinatal mortality, and the epidemics that often accompany famine contribute to further perinatal and postnatal mortality.[57] There is evidence, however, that in otherwise well-nourished populations experiencing conditions of food shortage, infants, fed on breast milk, are much less at risk than the rest of the population.[58]

The period after 167 is generally thought to have been a prosperous one for Athens, with the city's economy stimulated by the control of Delos and Lemnos, granted to her by Rome in that year.[59] There is no mention of plague or epidemic in the historical record during those years.[60] Athens may, however, have weathered many difficulties that are not attested in the surviving testimonia, so this explanation should not be dismissed out of hand. In their analysis of the baby skeletons at Ashkelon, Patricia Smith and Gila Kahila rejected epidemic as a cause of death on the basis of the fact that all of the babies in their deposit died at the same age, shortly after birth.[61] If we examine the data from the Lugnano cemetery, the single case in which epidemic seems to have been proven as a cause, we do indeed find more variety in the ages of the deceased, which range from fetal to two or three years, with older children in the majority. By contrast, at Kylindra on Astypalia—a vast infant cemetery likely to reflect ordinary rather than extraordinary conditions—while the ages of the infants range from the mid-fetal period to early childhood, most died in the late fetal to neonatal period. In the Agora Bone Well, the age range is similar, with most of the infants falling into the late fetal period up to normal full-term birth. Only four of the infants survived more than one month after full-term birth.

56. Angel 1945, p. 311.

57. Scott, Duncan, and Duncan 1995, pp. 250–251.

58. Livi-Bacci 1991, pp. 73, 75.

59. Habicht 1997, p. 220.

60. Pausanias, writing three centuries later, ascribes an Athenian raid on Oropos in the 150s to "extreme poverty" in the wake of the Macedonian war (7.11.4: πενίας γὰρ ἐς τὸ ἔσχατον Ἀθηναῖοι τηνικαῦτα ἧκον ἅτε ὑπὸ Μακεδόνων πολέμῳ πιεσθέντες μάλιστα Ἑλλήνων), but modern commentators see it rather in the context of wider political developments and Athens's long-standing claim to this border territory (Habicht 1997, pp. 264–269). A hint of possible difficulties a decade earlier comes from the epigraphical record. John Morgan (pers. comm.) has identified serious calendrical irregularities in the spring of the year of the archon Achaios, whom he dates in 166/5. According to Livy (Julius Obsequens, *De prodigiis* 13), Italy suffered from plague and famine *(pestilentia fameque)* in that same year. Morgan points out that one possible cause of the irregularities in the calendar is drought, which might have delayed the harvest and hence the festivals for a month or so. Drought could also, if sufficiently widespread, have precipitated the difficulties in Italy. He concedes, however, that the calendrical irregularities could also have been the result of internal political events.

61. Smith and Kahila 1992, p. 674.

To argue that an epidemic was responsible for this deposit, we would have to postulate either that the illness in question targeted neonates exclusively, or—except for the four older infants, the 11-year-old, and the adult—all victims more than a few days old were buried elsewhere. Neither of these two possibilities can be conclusively ruled out, but we think that they are unlikely.

Many diseases that particularly target newborns and that may account for high infant mortality can be observed in premodern populations and in developing countries.[62] We might imagine, then, an increase in one of these diseases. A dramatic example of such a case is recorded for St. Kilda, a remote and today uninhabited island in the Outer Hebrides, where a remarkably high incidence of *tetanus infantum* killed the majority of babies born between 1830 and 1861.[63] The islanders called the illness "the sickness of eight days," since it usually killed children before they had reached that age. Why it was so widespread on this particular island is unknown, although unsanitary conditions and folk customs surrounding birth (possibly anointing the umbilical cord with fulmar oil) may have been involved.[64] In ancient births, Soranus (*Gyn.* 2.7.11) records the use of various tools for cutting the cord, none of which can have been very sterile: glass, a reed, a potsherd, or a crust of bread. But even if some of the Agora infants may have died of this malady, there is no way to confirm this from an analysis of their physical remains. It is entirely possible that the deposit did not accumulate steadily, and instead there were periods of increased mortality due to disease, but the lack of detailed stratigraphic information about the bone deposit obscures this if they indeed occurred. The clear paleopathological evidence for a range of causes or contributing factors in the infant deaths indicates that, even if epidemic disease had some impact, it is not the only reason these infants died.

Perhaps, however, older victims of our hypothetical epidemic were buried elsewhere, and only those who died before they had crossed a certain threshold were buried so unceremoniously. As we shall see below, Athenian children were accepted into society through the agency of the Amphidromia, a ceremony that took place between the fifth and the tenth day of life, and funeral arrangements for children who died before the ceremony might well have been more casual than the rites for older children. The Amphidromia, then, could have filtered out anyone over the age of 10 days, leaving us with only the youngest victims of a plague along with a few older individuals who were hastily interred here during the crisis. Although this scenario, too, is possible, there are some arguments against it. It is questionable whether the distinction between a pre- and post-Amphidromia demise would be rigorously observed during an epidemic; it seems more likely that

62. Charlier 2003; Sallares et al. 2003, p. 120.

63. Steel 1975, pp. 150–155; a mortality rate of 80% was reported by one source (we thank James Russell for bringing the case of St. Kilda to our attention). In more recent times, neonatal tetanus has accounted for at least 60% of neonatal mortality in Pakistan; other areas with percentages over 50% are Bangladesh, Bhutan, Indonesia, and the Ivory Coast (S. O. Foster 1984, p. 120).

64. See S. O. Foster 1984, pp. 119–122, for factors increasing the risk of this disease. Foster reports that many cultures term this the seventh- or eighth-day disease; death occurs within the first month.

some slightly older infants would have been placed in the well in such a crisis. Evidence from a mass burial of victims of the 5th-century plague in Athens indicates that infants of unspecified age were buried together with adults and older children,[65] and two mass graves from Thebes probably associated with the Justinianic plague contain preterm and neonatal infants as well.[66] It is also questionable whether noncitizen dead, whether free or slave, to which group many of the infants arguably belong, would have been governed by Athenian customs. Lastly, pathologies and trauma in the cases of the four older individuals where enough is preserved for evaluation suggest causes of death that have nothing to do with epidemic.

Infanticide

Ethnographic studies show that infanticide—or more properly, neonaticide, the killing of a child on the day of its birth[67]—occurs in most, if not all societies.[68] Incidence in the United States has been estimated at hundreds if not thousands of neonaticides per year, despite draconian laws against it,[69] and selective killing of female infants has resulted in catastrophically skewed sex ratios in some modern countries.[70] It has also been conjectured that human beings of the remote past practiced neonaticide,[71] and some authors have argued that it is an adaptive behavior that promotes survival of the group in some conditions. Infants are most at risk for infanticide when they have visible birth defects, are born too soon after an older sibling, are illegitimate, are of the "wrong" sex, or if the society is experiencing severe stresses, including famine, disease, or conflict.[72] No one doubts that neonaticide took place in ancient Greece, although there is considerable debate about the extent to which it was practiced at any one period.[73] Many fictional and quasi-historical narratives revolve around the elimination of an unwanted child through exposure, and the recognition of the foundling was a staple of New Comedy and romance.[74] The existence of the motif in literature, of course, is only indirect evidence that exposure (and the neonaticide that would often result) took place in the real world; but there is other documentary evidence as well, discussed below. None of the sources for the period with which we are concerned admit to the outright killing of an infant; rather the baby simply "is not reared," or is "set out" (ἐκτίθημι, ἀποτίθημι) or, more harshly, "thrown out" (ἐκβάλλω),[75] abandoned in

65. Papagrigorakis et al. 2006, p. 206.

66. Unpublished data collected by Liston.

67. The term was coined by psychiatrist P. J. Resnick (1970) in a study stressing the difference between this and the killing of older children.

68. Williamson 1978.

69. Hundreds and possibly thousands of cases: Resnick 1970, p. 1419; between 150 and 300: Meyer and Oberman 2001, p. 46.

70. *Economist*, "Gendercide."

71. See Dickemann 1975 for a review of the historical and ethnographic literature on this topic.

72. Dickemann 1975, pp. 129–131; Hausfater 1984; Lummaa et al. 1998, pp. 196–197.

73. There is not surprisingly a large bibliography on the subject. Earlier scholars, following the authoritative opinion of Glotz (DarSag II.1, pp. 930–939, s.v. *expositio*), saw exposure as widespread. Subsequently, several scholars argued that, although it was a common practice in the Hellenistic period, exposure was the exception in Classical times (Van Hook 1920; Bolkestein 1922; Gomme 1933, pp. 79–82; Viljoen 1959; Eyben 1980–1981). The debate continues; for a recent summary, mostly for the Roman period, see Evans Grubbs 2013.

74. For a review of the literary material in the Roman period, see Boswell 1988, pp. 95–137.

75. For the terminology, see Golden 1981, pp. 330–331; Patterson 1985, pp. 104–105; Huys 1989.

some place where another person may (and in fiction, always does) rescue and rear it. There is no way of knowing whether these locutions are merely euphemisms or whether abandonment was the primary means of ridding oneself of a child that one did not wish to rear.[76] The use of exposure rather than other means would have depressed the number of neonaticides, since some babies would have survived.[77]

It is likely that many parents would have been unwilling to attempt to rear a child with a serious visible deformity.[78] Several ancient texts bear on this problem. In Plato's *Theaetetus* (160e–161a), Socrates, midwifing the birth of an argument, insists that it should be scrutinized, as a child would be at the ceremony of the Amphidromia, to determine if it is "worth rearing"; if not, its fate would be to be "put out" (ἀποτιθέναι).

> Τοῦτο μὲν δή, ὡς ἔοικεν, μόλις ποτὲ ἐγεννήσαμεν, ὅτι δή ποτε τυγχάνει ὄν. μετὰ δὲ τὸν τόκον τὰ ἀμφιδρόμια αὐτοῦ ὡς ἀληθῶς ἐν κύκλῳ περιθρεκτέον τῷ λόγῳ, σκοπουμένους μὴ λάθῃ ἡμᾶς οὐκ ἄξιον ὂν τροφῆς τὸ γιγνόμενον, ἀλλὰ ἀνεμιαῖόν τε καὶ ψεῦδος. ἢ σὺ οἴει πάντως δεῖν τό γε σὸν τρέφειν καὶ μὴ ἀποτιθέναι, ἢ καὶ ἀνέξῃ ἐλεγχόμενον ὁρῶν, καὶ οὐ σφόδρα χαλεπανεῖς ἐάν τις σοῦ ὡς πρωτοτόκου αὐτὸ ὑφαιρῇ;
>
> Well, we have at last managed to bring this forth, whatever it turns out to be; and now that it is born, we must in very truth perform the rite of running round with it in a circle—the circle of our argument—and see whether it may not turn out to be after all not worth rearing, but only a wind-egg, an imposture. But perhaps you think that any offspring of yours ought to be cared for and not put away; or will you bear to see it examined and not get angry if it is taken away from you, though it is your first-born?[79]

This text indicates that in Plato's day a newborn child was examined shortly after its birth and, on the basis of that examination, a decision was taken whether to raise it or not. The decision would have lain with the father, and the specific criteria he consulted are unknown.[80] Much later, Soranus (*Gyn.* 2.6.10) wrote a checklist for midwives as a guide to recognizing "the newborn that is worth rearing" (πῶς γνωρίζεται τὸ πρὸς ἀνατροφὴν ἐπιτήδειον). Positive signs were the health of the mother, the proper length of gestation, a vigorous cry, and a judgment that the child "is perfect in all its parts, members, and senses." Soranus's criteria closely resemble those of the Apgar score that is used today to evaluate newborns,[81] and it is perhaps not fanciful to imagine that these criteria also had a long prehistory before

76. Most sources referring to other means (drowning, strangulation) date to the Roman period (they are collected by Eyben 1980–1981, p. 15, n. 36). Terence (*Haut.* 632–643) preserves the view that other means of disposal are kinder than exposure, but it is impossible to know whether this refers to Greek or Roman opinion, or both. A Delphic inscription of 73 B.C., if correctly read, grants a manumitted woman the shocking right to kill an unwanted child by strangulation (Couve and Bourguet 1893, pp. 383–384, no. 80).

77. There is anecdotal evidence for their rescue, and legislation and legal debate about the status of foundlings make it clear that, in the Roman period, at least, a sufficient number of exposed infants were reared to make their status a legal concern (Boswell 1988, pp. 123–126).

78. Garland 1995, pp. 13–16. For the extent to which parents may have raised such children, see Schmidt 1983–1984; Edwards 1996.

79. Trans. H. N. Fowler, Cambridge, Mass., 1952.

80. Dasen 1993, pp. 205–206.

81. Galanakis 1998.

Soranus committed them to paper. Responsible medical opinion, then, held that a child that did not meet these criteria was unlikely to survive; responsible parents ought not to attempt rearing it (though no doubt many did).[82]

We can assume, and there is considerable indirect evidence to support the assumption, that illegitimate babies were often exposed.[83] These might include illegitimate or adulterous births to citizen and metic women, but also the children of courtesans (whether slave or free) and the offspring of slaves impregnated by their masters, or in fact any unwanted slave offspring, however parented.

In a global perspective, however, it is economic factors that most frequently provide the motive for infanticide,[84] and this was probably true of exposure in ancient Greece. W. K. Lacey, in his study of the Classical family, stresses the importance of the *oikos* in this connection; for the good of all its members, this family unit needed to be managed and maintained with care and forethought. Lacey concludes that "when children were more numerous than two, the economic resources of the family must have been an important factor in deciding whether or not to rear additional children."[85] Texts provide support for the principle. In a much-cited passage, Polybios (36.17) pinpoints the cause of the low birthrate and consequent depopulation that he observed in his own time (about the time of the Agora Bone Well): the unwillingness of people to marry or, once married, to raise large families. The motive is unambiguously economic; they want to maintain a comfortable lifestyle and wish to leave any offspring well provided for:[86]

> τῶν γὰρ ἀνθρώπων εἰς ἀλαζονείαν καὶ φιλοχρημοσύνην, ἔτι δὲ ῥᾳθυμίαν ἐκτετραμμένων καὶ μὴ βουλομένων μήτε γαμεῖν μήτ,' ἐὰν γήμωσι, τὰ γινόμενα τέκνα τρέφειν, ἀλλὰ μόλις ἓν τῶν πλείστων ἢ δύο χάριν τοῦ πλουσίους τούτους καταλιπεῖν καὶ σπαταλῶντας θρέψαι, ταχέως ἔλαθε τὸ κακὸν αὐξηθέν.

> For as men had fallen into such a state of pretentiousness, avarice, and indolence that they did not wish to marry, or if they married to rear the children born to them, or at most as a rule but one or two of them, so as to leave these in affluence and bring them up to waste their substance, the evil rapidly and insensibly grew.[87]

82. Other texts commonly cited in discussions of this issue are Pl. *Resp.* 459d–e, 460c, 461c; Arist. *Pol.* 7.1335b.20; Plut. *Vit. Lyc.* 16. Both Plato and Aristotle express the notion that deformed children and, in Plato's case, children of lesser parents and parents beyond the approved childbearing age should not be reared in the ideal state; this, however, says nothing about whether or not such children actually were reared in Athens. Plutarch describes eugenic neonaticide in Sparta in (from Plutarch's perspective) the distant past; his text is of limited value for assessing the situation in Hellenistic Athens.

83. In the parabasis of the *Clouds* (530–532), Aristophanes uses the metaphor of exposure (and subsequent rescue by another) to describe the production of a play of his that was written at an early age under the name of another. There are many examples in literature; a frequently cited Athenian example is Euripides' *Ion.* We need not belabor the point that these narratives are fictions; the real situation must have arisen often enough. See Patterson 1985, pp. 115–116.

84. Writing of the practice in general, Williamson (1978, p. 73) comments, "The great majority of infanticides have been performed to keep the size of families and, indirectly, societies adjusted to their environmental and economic conditions." Bolkestein (1922, p. 239, n. 1) presents figures linking a dramatic increase in abandoned children in 19th-century Amsterdam directly to economic depression.

85. Lacey 1968, p. 165.

86. Much earlier, Plato advised limiting the size of the family in accord with its resources (*Resp.* 2.372b–c).

87. Trans. W. R. Paton, Cambridge, Mass., 1927.

Polybios clearly has in mind people of some means, but other ancient texts also assert poverty as a reason for not rearing children.[88]

A final motive to be considered in our review of exposure is gender. In societies where infanticide is practiced, it is female infants who are most commonly its victims, and it is estimated that, in parts of the modern world, female "gendercide" had resulted by 1990 in the deaths of over 100,000,000 infant girls though sex-selective abortion, neonaticide, and differential neglect. The process has only accelerated since then.[89] There is no doubt that Greek society was rampantly patriarchal and that women held an inferior position in that society; the question is whether this resulted in the exposure of a larger number of female infants, as the ethnographic data would lead us to believe. Again, a handful of texts seem to provide a hint. In a comedy produced in the first half of the 3rd century B.C., Poseidippos wrote,

> υἱὸν τρέφει πᾶς κἂν πένης τις ὢν τύχῃ,
> θυγατέρα δ'ἐκτίθησι κἂν ᾖ πλούσιος.
>
> Everyone rears a son even if he's poor,
> But he exposes a daughter even if he's rich.[90]

As lines taken out of context from a comedy, this sentiment is difficult to assess; it is, however, repeated at frequent intervals. In the following century, in Terence's *Heauton timoroumenos* (626–627), a wife says to her husband,

> *Meministin me gravidam et mihi te maxumo opere edicere,*
> *Si puellam parerem, nolle tolli?*
>
> Do you remember I was pregnant and you gave strict
> instructions that,
> If it was a girl, you didn't want it to be raised?[91]

Later, life imitated art in Hellenized Egypt, in the famous letter that the soldier Hilarion wrote to his wife Alis a year before the birth of Christ: "If . . . you give birth, if it's male, leave it be, if it's female, throw it out" (ἐὰν πολλοπολλων τέκῃς, ἐὰν ἦν ἄρσενον ἄφες, ἐὰν ἦν θήλεα ἔκβαλε).[92]

Since the texts, few and fragmentary as they are, cannot settle the issue, scholars have turned to demographic evidence and arguments to throw light on the problem. On the one hand, Donald Engels argued that a high rate of female infanticide (20% of female births) was impossible, for it would quickly have led to a staggering reduction of the population.[93] His

88. Menander, *Epitrepontes* 254–255; *Perikeiromene* 810–812; and, much later, Plut. *Mor.* 497e. For further discussion, see Patterson 1985, pp. 116–119.

89. *Economist,* "Gendercide," p. 11. See also Brulé 1992 for detailed discussion of some well-documented instances. See Scott 2001 for arguments against the universality of the practice.

90. *Hermaphroditos,* fr. 12 (*PCG* VII, pp. 567–568; trans. Robert Lamberton).

91. Trans. J. Barsby, Cambridge, Mass., 2001.

92. *POxy.* IV 744 (trans. Robert Lamberton). The text is not without problems, and the word πολλαπολλων has never been satisfactorily explained. Stephanie West (1998) has suggested that the expected child may be that of a female relative, not Hilarion's wife. Be that as it may, the passage still supports the existence of female preferential exposure/infanticide. Vatin (1970, p. 234, n. 1), however, is not convinced that the passage refers to a human birth. For subsequent instances of the same sentiment, see Ov. *Met.* 9.675–679; Apul. *Met.* 10.23, eerily repeated many centuries later in Medieval Icelandic saga (Wicker 1998, p. 205).

93. Engels 1980, pp. 118–119.

demographic argument was quickly and decisively refuted by both Mark Golden and Richard Harris,[94] who maintain that a high rate of infanticide (10%) could not be ruled out. Golden argues in favor of preferential female exposure on other grounds as well,[95] concluding that "it is likely (though not beyond reasonable doubt) that the exposure of newborns, especially newborn girls, was widespread and even common in the ancient world."[96] Epigraphical evidence has also been brought to bear on the problem, first by W. W. Tarn and more recently by Sarah Pomeroy; they conclude that men outnumbered women in the ancient Greek world and that this imbalance was the result of female infanticide.[97] The most complete data, however, involve the families of Cretan mercenaries who settled in Miletos in the latter part of the 3rd century—not a typical sample, and far removed from Athens.[98]

A final question is whether exposure increased dramatically in the Hellenistic period, as several scholars have maintained.[99] They offer as evidence the passage of Polybios quoted above and epigraphical evidence pointing to a low number of children and of female children in particular in the population. As causes, they underline the impoverishment of the Greek cities in the Hellenistic period. Their testimony has been influential, and even those who maintain that levels of exposure were low in the Classical period are inclined to concede that the practice was widespread later on.[100] Others, however, reject this conclusion[101] or remain agnostic on the issue.[102] As Golden has commented, "There is simply no series of data which permits any reasonably reliable conclusion on the levels of exposure during the classical or the Hellenistic periods, let alone on variations between them."[103]

Two questions need to be asked in assessing neonaticide as the primary agent of our deposit. Is it feasible that this many children would have suffered this fate within the time the deposit accumulated? And what indications in the archaeological record would provide support for the hypothesis?

94. Golden 1981; Harris 1982. See also Brulé 1992. We might also note that societies that have killed almost 100% of their female offspring have survived for centuries; see Dickemann 1979.

95. Golden 1981, pp. 321–330. He maintains that if all female babies had been raised in Athens, the result would have been a "marriage squeeze," that is, a surplus of women of marriageable age. Since there is no evidence of such a situation, Golden concludes that the female population must have been artificially reduced. For opinions to the contrary, see Sallares 1991, pp. 157–158, with references to additional bibliography.

96. Golden 1988, p. 158.

97. Tarn 1930, pp. 92–94; Pomeroy 1983. For arguments to the contrary, see Patterson 1985, pp. 119–121; she concludes, "Until we have convincing positive evidence that in fact female infanticide was prevalent, we should not assume it was."

98. Sallares (1991, pp. 153–154) discounts this as demographic evidence because of the small sample size.

99. Tarn (1930, pp. 92–93) claims that "for the late third and the second centuries the inscriptions are conclusive" and "infanticide on a considerable scale, particularly of girls, is not in doubt." Rostovtzeff (1941, pp. 623–624) asserts that "abortion, exposure of children, and the like" had reached "disastrous proportions," and speaks of "race suicide." As causes he adduces the insecurity of the times (warfare, revolution, piracy) and impoverishment of the Greek cities (pp. 625–628). Vatin (1970, pp. 230–235) sees clear evidence of reduced population and a shortage of women in the 3rd and 2nd centuries that, in his view, could only have been caused by female preferential infanticide. Sallares (1991, pp. 136, 158–160) maintains that infanticide was negligible in the Classical period but was adopted in Hellenistic times as a response to overpopulation in the 4th century: "By adopting infanticide Hellenistic Greeks were tackling rationally a problem which their classical ancestors had failed to get to grips with."

100. Bolkestein 1922, pp. 238–239; Viljoen 1959, p. 58; Eyben 1980–1981, p. 14.

101. Patterson 1985, p. 104, n. 3; Brulé 1992, p. 64.

102. Golden 1997, pp. 177–179.

103. Golden 1997, p. 178.

To the first question we can answer a tentative yes. If, as we have estimated, the deposit in the Agora Bone Well accumulated over a period of 15 years, an average of just under 31 infants must have entered the well each year to make up the final total of 459. Taking Harris's hypothetical figures (a birthrate of 40 births per 1,000 adults, and an infanticide rate of 10%),[104] we can calculate that a population of 7,650 would have been required to produce this number of infanticides.[105] This figure is within the parameters for the population of this part of Athens in the 2nd century (see below for estimates of the population and of the catchment area of the well). If, however, the well was filled over a period of five years or less (which it could have been), infanticide as a single cause would have to be ruled out; the population of this part of Athens is unlikely to have been large enough to have experienced the requisite number of births.

In answer to the second question, if the infants in the deposit are victims of infanticide, we should expect that they all be the same age, and probably no more than a day old. We might further expect some evidence of deformity, and a high incidence of females might also be predicted. If the children were exposed rather than killed outright, as our sources lead us to believe was the normal practice, their bodies may have been subject to disturbance by animals, and consequently marks of gnawing might be expected. Some sources suggest that children were not merely laid on the ground, but were placed within a pot or a fragment of a pot.[106] Whoever collected the remains would presumably have picked up the pot too and discarded it together with its occupant; pottery appropriate to this task, then, might be found in the well.

The contents of the well, however, do not conform to this picture. While the vast majority of the infants are late fetal and perinatal in age, the size distribution suggests that many did survive for at least a few days, or up to a week. By modeling age at death, it has been shown that the median age at death of the Agora infants is about 287 days after conception, if 280 days is a normal full-term birth. This age-at-death distribution closely resembles that of the Native American Arikara tribe of North America, a group not known ethnohistorically to have practiced infanticide. We have identified fewer than 10 instances of deformity among the infants in the deposit, though here we should point out that most of the conditions listed by Soranus as grounds for not rearing a child would not be manifested on the bones. Furthermore, deformities visible at birth would probably have occurred quite rarely.[107] The sex ratio, as tentatively evaluated using the

104. Harris 1982, p. 115.

105. If the infanticide rate is 10%, 306 births are required to produce 30.6 bodies for our well. If there are 40 births per 1,000 adults annually, a population of 306/40 × 1,000 = 7,650 adults would produce 306 births in a single year.

106. In the *Frogs* (1190), Aristophanes writes of Oedipus, "they put him out in a pot" (ἐξέθεσαν ἐν ὀστράκῳ). Scholiasts comment (here and elsewhere) that babies were exposed in chytrai. Aristophanes also describes in his *Thesmophoriazousai* (505) how a suppositious child was carried into the house in a chytra (obviously something very different from exposure). The notion that this was the common container for an exposed infant is probably based on the scholiasts' misunderstanding of the words ἐγχυτρίζω and ἐγχυτρίστρια (see Bolkestein 1922). In Athens, at any rate, chytrai were only rarely used as containers for the infant dead who received burial in cemeteries; other shapes, particularly amphoras, were preferred.

107. Hassan (1981, p. 155) reports that "the incidence of malformation identifiable at birth for several populations is about 1%."

morphology of the ilium, is not statistically significantly different from 1:1, suggesting that there was probably no systematic bias against either sex in the infant deaths represented here. It is also important to note that most of the evidence for female preferential infanticide refers to citizen populations, not metics or slaves—the groups to which a substantial proportion of the infants in this study are likely to have belonged, and for whom other and completely unknown factors were probably operating.[108] As for exposure, no traces of weathering or other taphonomic processes have been found on the bones. Together with the presence of adapocere (grave wax) formation on some of the bones, this strongly suggests that the infant corpses were not left exposed to the environment for any length of time, but instead went into the well as intact bodies. The large fragments of pottery found in the well may have contained infant bodies, but whether these infants were exposed or died of natural causes we cannot say. In the end, there is no compelling reason to conclude that the majority of these infants were killed or allowed to die, although the simple fact that infanticide is attested for Greek society, coupled with the presence of a small number of infants with visible birth defects, suggests that some were victims of infanticide.

Natural Mortality

The simplest and least dramatic explanation for the presence of the babies in the well is that most are children who died of natural causes in the first few days of life. Infant mortality (the death of a child in its first year) must have been high in antiquity. Although it is true, as one skeptical commentator maintains, that "there is no useable evidence for childhood mortality from Classical antiquity,"[109] scholars who have addressed this question estimate infant mortality at between 20% and 40%.[110] Whatever the figure, the statistics for more recent populations suggest that a high proportion of those infant deaths will have taken place very shortly after birth. Figures collected for England and Wales for 1984 indicate that 57.5% of the children who died before the age of one died in the first month of life, and 46.5% in the first week.[111] In a group of German village populations of the 18th and 19th century, neonatal deaths (deaths in the first month) accounted for 40% of infant mortality.[112] Massimo Livi-Bacci opines that in the days before

108. For example, recent investigation of a mass grave at Pydna, probably containing the bodies of slaves, has revealed an equal number of males and females, in contrast to the overrepresentation of males in contemporary Thessalian cemeteries (Triantaphyllou and Bessios 2005).

109. Scheidel 2001, p. 7.

110. Frier 1982, p. 247, and Bagnall and Frier 1994, p. 34 (33%, Roman Egypt); Hopkins 1983, p. 225 (28% in the Roman period); Garnsey and Saller 1987, p. 138 (25% or higher in the Roman Empire); Golden 1988, p. 155, and 1990, p. 83 (30%–40% in antiquity); Sallares 1991, p. 135 (25%–30% estimated at Olynthos; see *Olynthus* XI, p. 166); Parkin 1992, p. 93 (30% in the early Roman Empire); Scott 1999, p. 115 (25%, Roman Britain). Rega 1997 gives an estimate of 15%–30% for prehistory in general. A few authors place the number higher: Durand 2003, p. 97 (43%–52% for both antiquity and preindustrial societies); Becker 2007, p. 282, and 2011, p. 24 (50% for nonindustrial societies). Infant mortality rates extracted from records of preindustrial Europe vary widely; Woods (1993, pp. 199, 202, 212, tables 1, 2, 5) records rates ranging from 94/1000 (9.4%) to 399/1000 (39.9%).

111. Parkin 1992, p. 180, n. 12.

112. Knodel 1988, p. 48, table 3.2; among the villages, the figure ranged from a low of 34% to a high of 63%, the latter in a village where infants were generally not breast-fed.

immunization, "a good half of infant deaths occurred in the first month of life."[113] These figures do not include stillbirths, which modern statistics suggest may account for 2% or more of total births.[114]

That ancient Athenian infant deaths also clustered in the days immediately following birth is suggested by Aristotle's observation that most babies die before their seventh day (*Hist. an.* 9[7].588a.8: τὰ πλεῖστα δ' ἀναιρεῖται πρὸ τῆς ἑβδόμης).[115] Standards and practices of infant care will have had an enormous impact on mortality. If ancient Athenian mothers followed some of the advice that has been preserved in surviving texts on infant care, the effect on mortality could have been substantial. It seems to have been widely believed that colostrum, a form of milk containing antibodies produced by the mother in the first days after birth, was bad for a child. Soranus (*Gyn.* 2.11.17–18), for instance, advises against feeding a newborn anything at all during the first two days of life, and then, after administering hydromel (a mixture of honey and water), to have the baby fed by a wet nurse; the mother's own milk is to be avoided for at least three days, ideally for 20. This practice would not only run the risk of introducing bacteria from the honey into the infant's system, but would also deprive the newborn of the immunity conferred by the colostrum.[116] Breast milk from a wet nurse brought in from outside the household would not have included colostrum, nor would her own antibodies necessarily have afforded protection from the pathogens in the infant's immediate environment. Soranus's suggested alternative diet of honey is particularly dangerous for infants, as unpasteurized honey is a reservoir for spores of *Clostridium botulinum*, the cause of botulism. The symptoms of infant botulism include lethargy, difficulty feeding, weak crying, and eventually paralysis of the limbs and respiratory muscles.[117] It would have been almost inevitably fatal in antiquity. Not all physicians concurred with Soranus's advice, however, and what midwives suggested, and what mothers did, we do not know.[118]

In examining the hypothesis of natural mortality as the primary agent of our deposit, we need to consider whether the population that used this well for the disposal of newborns was sufficient to produce 459 natural neonatal deaths within the 15-year maximum during which the deposit accumulated. The only serious attempt to estimate the size of the population within the walls of the city on the basis of empirical evidence was made by

113. Livi-Bacci 1991, p. 77; this estimate is based on data from the 18th century.

114. Stillbirths accounted for 2% of a total of 819,234 births among white American children (statistics quoted by Mays 1993, p. 885, fig. 1). A 2003 survey of 27 studies indicated stillbirth rates of 0.15% to 2.2% in developed countries; in other regions, with one exception (10% in rural Rwanda), the highest was 2.59% (West Africa) (Caracostea 2003). Stillbirths accounted for 5.7% of total births at the Harare Maternity Hospital in Zimbabwe in 1997–1998, a recent increase from 3.4% (Feresu et al. 2005).

115. Presumably he means most of those who die in infancy, not most of those who have been born.

116. Mistrust of colostrum is documented ethnographically as a factor in infant mortality and morbidity from infectious diseases: Green, Jurg, and Djedje 1994, p. 15; Whittemore and Beverley 1996, pp. 51, 55. See also Knodel (1988, pp. 47–48), who attributes elevated infant mortality in Bavarian villages of the 19th century to the fact that mothers there did not generally breast-feed their infants; and Fildes (1986), who credits the adoption of immediate breast-feeding with the decline in neonatal mortality in England and Wales beginning in the late 17th century.

117. Tanzi and Gabay 2002, p. 1479.

118. In this same passage (*Gyn.* 2.11.18), Soranus cites Damastes and Apollonios Biblas (both probably writing in the 2nd century B.C.; see Parker 1999, p. 518) among those who recommend immediate breast-feeding, and Aristotle remarks that the mother's milk becomes useful at the same time the child becomes viable (*Hist. an.* 9[7].585a.29–31; see also 9[7].587a.31–32).

Travlos in 1960.[119] Writing of the period just after the construction of the Themistoklean wall in 478, he calculated the area of the city as 215 ha; of this, he reckoned that 30 ha were devoted to public spaces and buildings and 65 ha to hills and unoccupied land,[120] leaving 120 ha free for private houses and roads. To judge from the few that have been excavated, the average footprint of an Athenian house, with its accompanying roads, is about 200 m^2; the total number of Athenian houses would therefore have been ca. 6,000. Estimating an average of six people per house, Travlos arrived at a figure of 36,000 for the total population of the city—a density of 167/ha for the city as a whole, or 300/ha within the residential areas.[121]

More recent studies offer slight adjustments, but the final result is not very different. The work of Thomas Gallant tends to suggest a smaller household size than Travlos's estimate of six members; according to his calculations, an ancient household would have fluctuated between two and five members over a 24-year cycle.[122] Assuming that every stage of Gallant's eight-triennia model of household wax and wane was equally represented in the city at any one time, the average household would have encompassed 4.375 family members. This reduction is offset, however, by the insights of Richard Alston, who draws on data from Roman and Byzantine Egypt, where he observes that more than one household frequently shared a single dwelling.[123] If this was the case in Athens, using Alston's ratio of 1.41 to 1 for houseful to household, the average Athenian house would have sheltered 6.17 people, exclusive of slaves. Alston also notes that at any one time, as many as 10% of the houses in a settlement are likely to have been empty. Applying these further adjustments, there would have been 5,400 occupied dwellings and thus a little over 33,000 free persons living in Athens just after 480; there were also slaves, but we have no idea of how many.

Many things must have changed between the 5th century and the 2nd.[124] The extent of the walls remained the same, but formerly empty

119. Travlos 1960, p. 71. Most studies have focused instead on the number of Athenian citizens, on the population of Attica as a whole, or on the urban nucleus of Athens, Phaleron, and Piraeus (e.g., Gomme 1933, pp. 26, 37–47, table 1; Hansen 1985; 1988, pp. 7–12; Habicht 1997, p. 58). For a discussion of the difficulties encountered in making such estimates, see Zorn 1994. He outlines three methods: area estimates (based on assumed density of persons per area or on the minimum sheltered living space required for each person), dwelling-based estimates (Travlos's method), and estimates based on natural resources. The natural resources of Attica were shared by city and country dwellers, so an inventory of these cannot help us. We cannot, on the basis of the foundations of the approximately 20 houses that have been excavated, get close to estimating the amount of sheltered living space available in the city, especially since we do not know how many stories those houses had.

120. Both Thucydides and Xenophon speak of parts of the city that were not built upon (Thuc. 2.17: τά τε ἐρῆμα τῆς πόλεως; Xen. *Poroi* 2.6: πολλὰ οἰκιῶν ἔρημά ἐστιν ἐντὸς τῶν τειχῶν). Taking this into account, Travlos reconstructs houses only up to within about 150 m of the city wall (see his plan in Fig. 95).

121. Reviewing these figures in the light of more recent work on urban demography, Osborne (1985, p. 99) finds them "rather high," but nonetheless estimates a population of 35,000–40,000 in 431 B.C.

122. Gallant 1991, pp. 27–30.

123. Alston's study of Egyptian households of the Roman period suggests that urban households numbered between 4.02 and 4.11 individuals, while "housefuls" (all the inhabitants of a house) ranged from 5.66 to 5.78 individuals; thus the ratio of houseful to household is 1.41 to 1 (Alston 2002, pp. 69–72).

124. An overall decline in population is often claimed for Hellenistic Greece as a whole. Corvisier and Suder (2000, pp. 112–116) summarize the evidence, concluding that there was no dramatic decrease in population in the Hellenistic period, though perhaps a slow decline. Ferguson (1911, p. 374) believed that population increased in the period 166–86 and (p. 317) estimated the population of Attica at 100,000–150,000. Sallares (1991, p. 107) believes the decline in Athens was less marked than elsewhere. We do not know whether the number of individuals within the city grew, declined, or remained stable in the Hellenistic period.

spaces might have been built over, and as much as 140 ha might have been occupied by residences. If so, there could have been as many as 6,300 occupied houses and a free population of nearly 39,000, giving a density of 181/ha for the city area as a whole and a bit over 278/ha for the residential areas. Although the population might have been much lower, it probably was not higher.[125] Urban density is unlikely to have been less than 100/ha (21,500); even if the Hellenistic population of Attica was in decline, the city continued to offer opportunities and would have continued to attract residents. Even this lower population figure could have generated a sufficient number of deceased infants for the deposit in the well through natural mortality over only a few years.

It is unlikely, however, that the well served the whole population within the walls. One would not have wanted to travel any further than necessary to dispose of a deceased newborn (or an adult, for that matter), and crossing exposed public space would have been something to be avoided. We therefore conjecture that the population that used the well would have included only those living in the northern and western parts of the walled city. A circle with a radius of 400 m with the well at its center includes an area of 50.24 ha, of which about 33.5 ha were possibly or probably occupied by dwellings (Fig. 95).[126] Using the minimum and maximum estimates of population density calculated above, we would guess that these neighborhoods housed between 5,024 and 9,313 people.[127] Applying a birthrate of 40/1000 and a probable rate of infant mortality of 20% to 40% to these population parameters, and assuming that half of those infants died in the first week of life, we can calculate that between 20 and 75 neonates died yearly within the hypothetical catchment area of the well, and that it would take between 6 and 23 years to produce the total of 459 that were found in the well. The figures on which these estimates are based are imprecise in the extreme, but this exercise suggests that the wider vicinity of the well could have experienced the requisite number of natural infant deaths within the period the well was active as a burial place.

Although we cannot know the size of the population with any certainty, we can make some educated guesses about its character. A large percentage of the city-dwellers were not Athenian citizens but a mixture of metics, slaves, and visiting foreigners. A. W. Gomme believed that, by the end of

125. In a review of evidence for cities of the Roman Empire, Russell (1958, p. 68) found that a population density of over 200/ha was rare and restricted to large cities. Cities of medium size (among which Athens might be classed) would be more likely to have a concentration of 100–150/ha.

126. Much of the area within the circle is unexcavated; we base our estimate of the portion available for residential use on the reconstruction of Travlos (1960, p. 71, fig. 20), assuming that formerly unoccupied areas had been built over by the 2nd century. Four hundred meters is, of course, an arbitrary figure, but it reaches the city wall and avoids in most cases the necessity of crossing public space.

127. Applying the general population density figures for the city as a whole, a high population estimate of 39,000 (181/ha) would place 9,093 people within the 50.24 ha of our circle; a low extreme of 21,500 (100/ha) would place 5,024 people there. Much of the area within our circle was public land, and hence unoccupied. We get similar figures, however, if we base our estimates instead on the ca. 33.5 ha likely to have been available for residences and the higher density estimated for residential areas. The high population estimate of ca. 39,000 gives a residential population density of ca. 278/ha, and so 9,313 within an area of 33.5 ha; the low estimate of ca. 21,500 gives a residential population density of ca. 154/ha, or 5,159 within our area.

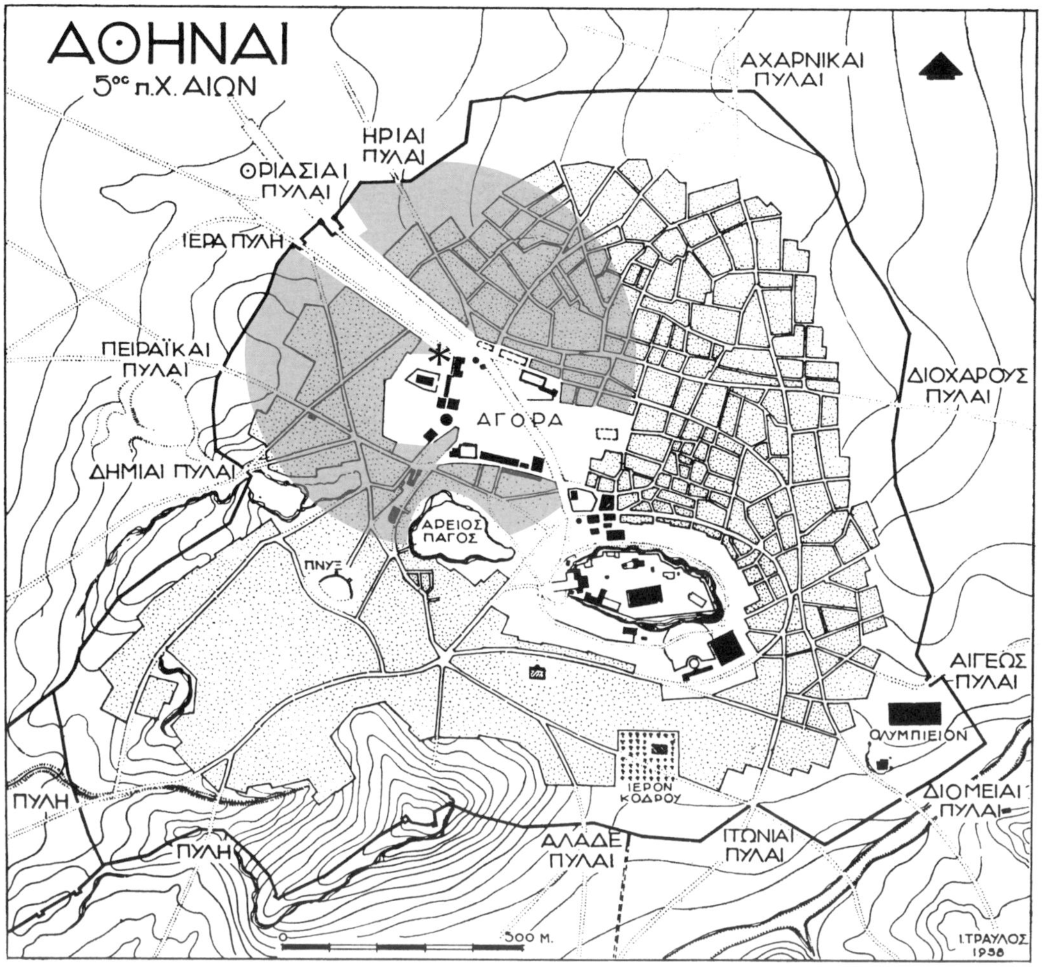

Figure 95. Hypothetical area served by the Agora Bone Well, a circle with a 400-meter radius centered on the well (marked by an asterisk). Travlos 1960, p. 51, fig. 20, with additions by S. I. Rotroff

the 4th century, half of the citizenry had come to live in the urban area constituted by the city, Piraeus, and the surrounding demes.[128] A more recent review of the evidence argues that this may overstate the case, but confirms that population steadily gravitated to the city;[129] we might imagine that perhaps 20% of the citizens lived within the walls. But the city was the favored place of residence for metics and other landless people; fully 50% of the metics whose place of residence is known lived in one of the five demes within the walls of Athens.[130] If we apply these percentages to the conjectured proportions that citizens and metics contributed to the

128. Gomme 1933, p. 47. The five demes within the walls (Koile, Kollytos, Kydathenaion, Melite, and Skambonidai) account for only 27–28 (ca. 5%) of the bouletic representatives. Although this might represent the percentage of citizens resident in the city at the time of Kleisthenes, it is generally agreed that later a much larger portion of the citizens lived there. The urban area, in Gomme's calculation, included not only the demes within the city walls but also Phaleron, Piraeus, and Alopeke. For the city alone, we would have to reduce his figure, perhaps by a third or a half.

129. Rosivach 1993.

130. Whitehead 1986, p. 63.

population as a whole, we would find that between 38% and 45% of the free population was non-Athenian.[131] To these we would have to add an unknown number of slaves, which could bring the number of noncitizen inhabitants to half the total population or more. It is likely, then, that half of the babies in the well were the children of non-Athenians, whether free or slave, and we should be wary of applying the mores of Athenian society (such as we know them) to the activities of these noncitizens. The evidence for low birth weight further suggests that many of these infants were from the lowest economic strata of the city: slaves and the very poor.

Why, however, if these babies died natural deaths, did they end up in the Agora Bone Well rather than in one of the many cemeteries of Athens, which included metics and slaves as well as citizens? We have seen above that, in many cultures, infants receive funerary rites different from those accorded to adults. This was also the case in the ancient Greek world, where infants and small children were often buried in their own cemeteries away from adult tombs.[132] Sanne Houby-Nielsen has traced the mortuary treatment of children at Athens from the Bronze Age to Hellenistic times.[133] She reports that differential burial practices can first be distinguished in the Submycenaean and Protogeometric periods and are well established by the end of the 8th century. In the 5th century, cemeteries with concentrations of infants and small children in excess of 50% are found in the Kerameikos and outside the Diochares Gate. In the 4th century, however, these concentrations disappear, and there is only one Hellenistic cemetery where more than 10% of the burials are of children: a plot outside the Acharnian Gate.[134] Houby-Nielsen sees this as the result of a change in female attitudes, as women no longer focused on an identity as a "dutiful, child-bearing mother" but indulged in more selfish interests of luxury and body care. Be this as it may, the inhabitants of the city were now only rarely burying their children in extramural cemeteries—at least, in any of the extramural cemeteries that have been excavated so far.[135]

131. There is no documentary evidence for the size of the Attic population in the Hellenistic period. The figures closest in date are those reported from the census conducted by Demetrios of Phaleron in the late 4th century (Ath. 6.272c). Estimates of the population of Attica have been concocted on this basis, with a wide range of results. Some estimate about 150,000 individuals, including 60,000–80,000 citizens, no more than 20,000 metics, and 20,000–50,000 slaves (Osborne 1987, p. 46; see also Sallares 1991, p. 60). Others envision a total population of between 200,000 and 250,000 individuals, with 100,000–140,000 citizens, 33,000–46,000 metics, and 66,000–93,000 slaves (Ferguson 1911, p. 54; Hansen 1988, pp. 7–12). More important than the numbers for our purpose is the suggested proportion of metics to citizens—1:3 or 1:4. If 50% of the metics and 20% of the citizens lived within the walls, the ratio of metics to citizens among the city-dwellers would be closer to 5:6 or 5:8.

132. See Sabetai 2000, with bibliography in p. 494, n. 1.

133. Houby-Nielsen 2000.

134. Houby-Nielsen 2000, pp. 158–160, figs. 12.4–12.6.

135. Ian Morris (1992, pp. 78–80) interprets a similar dearth of children's burials from ca. 925 to 725 as evidence that in those centuries Athenians disposed of dead children in ways that left few recoverable remains. If so, Hellenistic Athenians were reverting to an earlier custom.

What, then, were they doing with the corpses of these small children? A glance at Houby-Nielsen's figure 12.6, a plot of Hellenistic burials in and around the city, shows a significant increase in graves situated within the walls: 18 burial sites *intra muros,* in contrast to three in each of the two centuries of the Classical period.[136] These are adult burials, but this Hellenistic shift towards intramural burial is not irrelevant to the Agora Bone Well, which itself constitutes an intramural burial site.

This shift still does not explain why almost all of the infants are newborns. It was observed above that many cultures do not consider a child fully human until some threshold has been passed, and that children who have not passed that threshold tend to be buried in a more casual manner. As it happens, there is evidence of rituals that served just this purpose at Athens, at least for its citizen inhabitants. At the Amphidromia,[137] on the fifth, seventh, or tenth day after the birth, a group of people (midwives? relatives? the father?) either ran around the family hearth[138] with the child or ran around the child, who had been placed on the ground. The passage from Plato's *Theaetetus* quoted above (p. 120) indicates that one purpose of the ceremony was to decide whether or not the child was viable; we might imagine, then, that there was an inspection by responsible persons in order to determine the answer to this question. Of course, having survived to the age of the Amphidromia, the infant would already have demonstrated its probable viability; the ceremony took place after the greatest danger of mortality had passed and was probably timed to account for this. Presents and a feast with a traditional menu (squid, octopus, cheese, cabbage, lamb, and small birds, along with abundant wine) were involved, though presumably only if the decision about the child's rearing was positive.[139] The sources also mention the Dekate, the tenth day after the birth, some conflating it with the Amphidromia; most agree that it was at this point that the baby was named.[140] With this, the child had been accepted into the family and hence into society; he or she was now a person. Although this was a ceremony of Athenians, and thus applicable only to an unknown and possibly small percentage of the babies in the well, it is likely that other Greeks did something similar; for instance, the Cyrenaican poet Kallimachos, who spent much of his career in Alexandria, wrote a poem for the seventh-day

136. Houby-Nielsen 2000, pp. 158–160: compare her fig. 12.6 (Hellenistic) with figs. 12.4 and 12.5 (5th and 4th centuries). She also claims (p. 153) that cremation was used more frequently for children in the Hellenistic period, although the instances she cites are all of Classical date. While infant (and other) burials occurred in the area around the Agora in the 6th century, especially in well-defined precincts that were probably family cemeteries (Young 1939; 1951b, pp. 72–110; see also *Agora* XII, pp. 384, 395, deposits A 20:10[?], M 18:6), no certain examples of later infant graves have been found there. For possible instances, see *Agora* XII, pp. 389, 394, 396, deposits F 12:8, L 20:2, O 19:3, all of the 5th century. There are no such Hellenistic graves. The pyres that Young (1951b, pp. 110–130) interpreted as infant cremations of the 4th and 3rd centuries have now been shown to represent the remains of animal sacrifice (Rotroff 2013). The bones in other deposits originally identified as infant graves have proven upon expert examination to be animal rather than human (see *Agora* XXXIII, pp. 356, 361, deposits F 16:7, H 17:1).

137. Hamilton 1984 collects and discusses the testimonia. See also Paradiso 1988; Garland 1990, pp. 93–95.

138. The stipulation of a hearth is troubling, since very few fixed hearths have been found in Athenian houses.

139. Ath. 2.65c–d (Euboulos, fr. 148, *PCG* V, p. 272); 9.370c–d (Ephippos, fr. 3, *PCG* V, p. 133).

140. The orators in particular mention the celebration of the Dekate as proof of legitimacy (Dem. 39.20, 22–24, 40.28; Isae. 3.30).

ceremony of the infant daughter of a friend (*Ia.* 12). The prevalence of such ceremonies documented by ethnographic study of living societies encourages us to believe that non-Athenian and even non-Greek inhabitants of the city also followed customs of this same sort. It is likely that little effort would have been expended on the disposal of the bodies of children who died before they celebrated these rituals,[141] and we have demonstrated that it is these who make up the majority of the individuals in the Agora Bone Well.

THE OLDER INDIVIDUALS

Six of the deceased individuals in the well stand apart from the rest by virtue of their greater age: four infants well beyond the neonatal stage, a child 8–10 years old, and an adult. Different reasons and social attitudes must lie behind their presence in the well. Studies by John Papadopoulos and Lisa Little, building on the work of Talia Shay, have investigated the identification of deviant individuals or social outcasts in the mortuary record.[142] Deviance resists definition, as it is a concept constructed differently by different societies, but, on the basis of anthropological research, Shay outlines various conditions that contribute to the classification of a person as "different." These include both behavior during life (e.g., committing a crime, suffering from an illness, being a twin or a sorcerer) and the circumstances of a person's death (e.g., suicide, drowning, lightning strike, death in battle). The "otherness" of such individuals is likely to be reflected in the way in which their bodies are treated after death. As examples, Papadopoulos has collected instances of burial in wells, a survey in which he includes the Agora Bone Well.[143]

We would also do well to recall again the all-important place of the *oikos* in Greek society. The degree to which one might be treated as "deviant" in death might well depend upon whether or not one belonged to such a unit; families would probably provide ritually proper burial to their members even if those members were not deemed acceptable by society at large. Consider the example of Antigone, who risks everything to give the last rites to her brother, declared an enemy of the state. In real life, we know that the bodies of executed criminals were at least sometimes given to their families for burial (Socrates is a frequently cited example here). Thus another reason why a person might not receive proper burial is that he or she, for whatever reason, was not a member of a functioning *oikos*. Athens must have had its share of friendless strangers, beggars, and homeless persons. Their deaths were a considerable enough problem that provision was made

141. Plutarch (*Mor.* 612a) writes some centuries after our period that it was not customary to bring libations or to celebrate the usual funerary rites for those who died in infancy. The context is a letter of consolation to his wife on the death of their two-year-old daughter; the text implies that she will receive burial, but that it will be carried out as expeditiously as possible and strictly without public display. Cicero (*Tusc.* 1.39.93) says something similar (closer to the time of the well, but from another culture), namely, that if a child dies in the cradle, one takes no notice. For discussion of parents' emotional response to the deaths of their children, see Golden 1988.

142. Shay 1985; Little and Papadopoulos 1998; Papadopoulos 2000.

143. The Agora Bone Well is the only instance of historical date; the other five cases date in the Bronze or Early Iron Age (Papadopoulos 2000, pp. 104–111). More recently, another Early Iron Age instance has been unearthed at the Agora (well J 3:9, excavated in 2002).

for the disposal of their bodies. The *Athenaion Politeia* (50) stipulates that the Astynomos shall collect the bodies of those who died in the streets (the actual work was done by the public slaves under his supervision). The text does not say what was to be done with the corpses, but a law cited by Demosthenes (43.58) governing unclaimed corpses found in the demes instructs the Demarch to "contract for the taking up and burial of the body, and for the purification of the deme on the same day at the lowest possible cost" (ἐὰν δὲ τοῦ δημάρχου ἐπαγγείλαντος μὴ ἀναιρῶνται οἱ προσήκοντες, ὁ μὲν δήμαρχος ἀπομισθωσάτω ἀνελεῖν καὶ καταθάψαι καὶ καθῆραι τὸν δῆμον αὐθημερόν, ὅπως ἂν δύναται ὀλιγίστου).[144] Burial of some sort, then, would be the normal procedure, but it is not impossible that from time to time the public slaves might remember a convenient well not too far away.

The pathology of the skeletons provides some hints about the status of the older individuals in the well. The adult suffered from hemochromatosis, a debilitating and potentially disfiguring disease. It would have left him severely crippled and unable to perform most physical tasks, and can also cause discoloration of the skin, which is why it is sometimes referred to as the "bronze disease." The child probably suffered from brucellosis, a likewise debilitating disease, characterized by 24-hour fever cycles and, in this case, extensive destruction of the vertebrae and inflammation of the endocranial membranes. Neither of these people is likely to have been able to participate in any normal activities by the time they died, and both were probably a significant burden to their families or associates; they could have been considered "deviant" and thus received this minimal form of burial.

The oldest of the infants was a victim of child abuse, the earliest case of Battered Child Syndrome documented thus far. Another of the older infants suffered from hydrocephalus and would have been abnormal, if not frightening, in appearance. Someone must have cared for the child, however, which suggests that he or she was not without support in the community. In that case, why was there no formal burial? Perhaps the child was a slave whose master would have been happy to see him or her recover but did not wish to undertake the expenses of burial (however small), or perhaps the family was indigent and without resources.

The Agora provides other instances of skeletons in wells, all of which have been or are now being studied,[145] and it is clear that many of these individuals could be considered deviant in either their lives or the manner of their deaths. Some, including a young man of the 5th century, were clearly murdered. Others died violently in the Herulian sack in A.D. 267. The evidence for violent death also includes a Mycenaean skull of an individual who was beheaded. In the Geometric period, at least two adults with severely debilitating injuries were formally buried on top of debris in wells.[146] In the 18 instances when the skeletons of adults who had been placed in wells were saved, the individuals had all died violently or suffered from debilitating disease or injury before death. In other cases, unfortunately, the skeletal remains were not kept. For example, the skull and bones of an adult were found in the 3rd-century fill of the Bronze Head Well (H 6:4), located just behind the Stoa of Zeus, some 30 m south of the Agora Bone Well. Only the skull was saved, however, and it is silent on the cause

144. Trans. A. T. Murray, Cambridge, Mass., 1939.

145. Liston is currently conducting a study of all of the extant human remains found in wells in the Agora; the following examples derive from this research.

146. Little and Papadopoulos 1998; Liston 2017, pp. 542–543, 558–560.

or manner of death and the health of the individual in life.[147] In only two instances can the skeletal remains found in wells be demonstrated to come from an early grave that was disturbed by the well diggers.

THE DOGS

A final puzzle that requires resolution is the presence of the dogs. Are they simply urban refuse, or is there a deeper message to be read in their association with the infants?

The disposal of dead strays is a common urban problem; ancient Athens must have had many masterless dogs, and when they died their bodies had to be dealt with. Recalling the tasks of the public slaves under the direction of the Astynomoi (*Ath. Pol.* 50), we might imagine that they also removed dead animals from Athenian streets, and the well would have been a convenient place to discard them. Fortunately, this is a hypothesis that can easily be tested. If the dogs were collected in this manner, the age profile of the collection should be the same as that of natural die-off, with a heavy concentration of puppies and aged adults. Such was the case, for example, in the huge 5th-century dog cemetery excavated at Ashkelon, where 60%–70% of the animals were puppies.[148] By contrast, however, 65%–70% of the dogs in the Agora Bone Well were adults, a strong indication that these animals do not represent a cross-section of deceased Athenian strays, but rather were chosen for a particular reason. It might be that the small bodies of puppies would have been tossed onto ordinary trash heaps rather than transported to the well. It is significant, however, that whole skeletons of other animals of the sort that, when dead, would have been a nuisance on the street (such as donkeys or mules) have not been found in the well, though here the relative size of animal and well diameter might be a factor.

The dogs, then, are likely to have something to do with the circumstances of the well. Dogs are not infrequently associated with graves and seem in some cases to have played a part in the rituals accompanying burial. At the funeral of Patroklos, Achilles slit the throats of nine of the hero's dogs and threw them on the pyre (*Il.* 23.173–174). Whether these were sacrifices or grave gifts, meant to accompany the hero in the next life, may be debated,[149] but the passage establishes the association of dogs and human burial at the beginning of the Greek literary tradition. The archaeological literature provides numerous examples of dogs buried with or near

147. Shear 1933, pp. 453–454. The well (7.10 m deep and about 1.0 m in diameter), which has a period-of-use fill at the bottom, was filled near the end of the 3rd century with a mixture of gray clay, rocks, roof tiles, and broken pottery (for the date, see *Agora* XXXIII, p. 360). The bones were found in this debris at a depth of 6.0 m, and the excavation summary makes it clear that more than just the skull was discovered: "a well-preserved adult skull along with many of the body bones of an adult" (notebook A 5, p. 829).

148. Stager 1991b, pp. 25–26; he comments that this accords well with the mortality profile of present-day urban dog populations. See also Wapnish and Hesse 1993.

149. See Mylonas 1948, p. 59; Vermeule 1979, pp. 58–61; Day 1984, p. 27.

humans, among which those in Athens are particularly relevant here.[150] A few unburned dog bones accompanied the Middle Geometric cremation of a woman buried on the slopes of the Areopagus; in her publication of the grave, Evelyn Smithson suggested that the animal might have been a sacrifice of purification, perhaps for a woman who died in childbirth.[151] The remains of two dogs, interpreted as a chthonic offering, were found in the fill of an 8th-century grave at the Kerameikos.[152] A dog burial lies directly above the grave of a 40-year-old woman in precinct VII of the Eckterrasse at the Kerameikos; right beside the woman's grave is the amphora interment of a newborn child, prompting the suggestion that the woman died in childbirth.[153] The date is around the middle of the 4th century. Another, contemporaneous dog burial was found not far away, in the same precinct, but not closely associated with a preserved grave.[154] Several dog burials were found in and around precinct XIII, the large burial plot of the Messenians also in the Eckterrasse. A pit containing three dog skeletons lay directly over the grave of a 45-year-old woman, probably dating in the early 3rd century.[155] A single dog was buried near the entrance to the precinct at about the same time,[156] and another (undated) was found just outside the precinct.[157] Two more dog burials in the Kerameikos were uncovered in the Südhügel, east of the Eckterrasse. One belongs to the 3rd-century grave of Thallis,[158] the other to a nearby grave of about the same date.[159]

Clearly dogs were a regular feature of the graveyard, where they were also represented on grave monuments in the role of guardians or pets.[160] From the instances cited above, however, it appears that the animals are frequently associated with female graves, and sometimes with infants and possibly with women who died in childbirth. A close tie between dogs and infant death is further suggested by the discovery at Messene of a group of 25 infant burials, beside some of which small dogs had also been buried.[161] The excavator suggested that the dogs were there as companions for the children. In other instances, however, the dog clearly does not play the

150. For other instances, see Day 1984, pp. 22–24, with 18 examples, mostly of the Bronze Age and Early Iron Age; Soren and Soren 1999, pp. 479–481, 627–630, with eight examples, mostly from Britain and dating to the Roman Imperial period. For instance, several complete dog skeletons were found in an infant cemetery at Owslebury (Collis 1977, p. 26), and canine and infant skeletons were buried together in shafts in what appears to have been a shrine at Ridgeons Gardens in Cambridge (Goodburn et al. 1976, pp. 340–341; Pullinger 1978, pp. 58–59).

151. Smithson 1974, pp. 334, 362.

152. *Kerameikos* V.i, pp. 269–270, no. 94.

153. *Kerameikos* XIV, p. 61, no. 63, fig. 33 (where the grave is labeled 29), pl. 46:2 (Eck 25).

154. *Kerameikos* XIV, p. 60, no. 61, fig. 33 (Eck 41).

155. *Kerameikos* XIV, p. 125, no. 153, fig. 48, pl. 15:7 (Me 46). The associated grave is no. 152 (Me 51).

156. *Kerameikos* XIV, p. 125, no. 154, fig. 48 (Me 48).

157. *Kerameikos* IX, p. 157, no. 346, plan 3 (SW 110).

158. *Kerameikos* IX, pp. 18, 158, no. 355 (HW 140), there dated to the end of the 4th century; the accompanying unguentaria (pl. 67:4), however, appear to date to the first half of the 3rd century. Interestingly, an amphora lay directly over the pit for the grave (p. 163, no. 382 [HW 139]); although no bones were preserved, it is likely to have been the burial of a child.

159. *Kerameikos* IX, pp. 18, 160, no. 365 (HW 141); the skeleton of the dog lay under a tile and over the eastern end of grave 362 (HW 145): see plan 2. The unguentaria in the grave suggest a 3rd-century date (pl. 68:1).

160. Ohly 1965, col. 323, figs. 23, 28, pl. I; Vermeule 1968, p. 97, pl. 38:5; Koch 1984, pp. 68–70.

161. Themelis 1999, p. 97, fig. 7, pls. 63:γ, 66:α; 2000, pp. 98–99, fig. 7, pls. 61:β, 62:α; Bourbou and Themelis 2010, p. 111, figs. 1–3. The date is 2nd to 1st century. The recurrence of dog burials at Messene and in the burial precinct of Messenian metics at the Kerameikos is intriguing and warrants further investigation.

role of a pet. As described above, some of the dogs found in the cemetery at Lugnano had been dismembered, probably as part of rituals of aversion that accompanied the burial of the children.[162] The role of the dogs in the Agora Bone Well may have been similar.

It was a belief deeply ingrained in Greek religion that contact with either birth or death brought on pollution.[163] Theophrastos's superstitious man equally avoids graves, corpses, and women in childbirth for fear of pollution (*Char.* 16.9).[164] The combination of both birth and death might engender a particularly serious case of impurity,[165] and those who placed the infants in the well therefore had a special need for purification. Martin Nilsson lists the piglet, followed by the dog, as the most common purificatory offering.[166] Recalling that the well contained bones from seven young pigs, we may view these as possible sacrificial victims, and the dogs are also strong candidates for this role. According to Nilsson, dogs were sacrificed exclusively in rites of purification—though we need to keep in mind that the bones of the dogs in the well preserve no evidence of sacrificial killing. Many ancient texts mention the special ability of the dog to absorb malign influences. Illnesses, for instance, could be transferred from patient to animal by applying a puppy to the affected part of the sufferer (Plin. *HN* 30.16.42; 30.64); the animal, having absorbed the malady, either dies of its own accord or is killed, and then buried. Plutarch (*Quaest. Rom.* 68 [*Mor.* 280b]) reports that even in his own day some people dealt with pollution by rubbing the infected person with a puppy in a rite called *periskylakismos.* It is perhaps to this rite that Theophrastos refers when his superstitious man calls for purification by means of a puppy (*Char.* 16.13).[167] This last citation is of special importance, since it establishes a link between dogs and purification in Hellenistic Athens.

The dogs need not, then, have been sacrifices, but simply the vessels of impurity, discarded here after they had absorbed the pollution engendered by the birth and death documented by the infant bones. But if they were sacrifices, there are only a limited number of divinities that could have received them.[168] What is particularly interesting in the context of the Agora Bone Well is the use of the dog for sacrifices to goddesses of childbirth. Plutarch (*Quaest. Rom.* 52 [*Mor.* 277a–b]), investigating the Roman custom of sacrificing a bitch to the goddess Genita Mana,[169] explains it

162. See above, p. 114, and n. 150.

163. Nilsson 1941, pp. 85–88; Parker 1983, pp. 32–73.

164. "He refuses to step on a gravestone, view a corpse or visit a woman who has given birth, and says it's the best policy for him not to incur pollution" (καὶ οὔτε ἐπιβῆναι μνήματι οὔτ' ἐπὶ νεκρὸν οὔτ' ἐπι λεχὼ ἐλθεῖν ἐθελῆσαι, ἀλλὰ τὸ μὴ μιαίνεσθαι συμφέρον αὑτῷ φῆσαι εἶναι); trans. J. Rusten, Cambridge, Mass., 2002.

165. It is noteworthy that the period of pollution following a miscarriage cited in sacred laws is generally longer than that after either a birth or a death (Parker 1983, p. 355).

166. Nilsson 1941, p. 95.

167. "He goes away, takes a shower, summons priestesses and orders a deluxe purification by sea onion or puppy" (ἀπελθὼν κατὰ κεφαλῆς λούσασθαι καὶ ἱερείας καλέσας σκίλλῃ ἢ σκύλακι κελεῦσαι αὑτὸν περικαθᾶραι); trans. J. Rusten, Cambridge, Mass., 2002, adapted.

168. Sources are collected and summarized by Zaganiaris (1975). See also Masson 1950 on a Hittite rite of purification where an army marches between the sundered bodies of various victims, including a dog; the rite has parallels in the Greek world (Curt. 10.9.11–12; Livy 40.6; Plut. *Quaest. Rom.* 111 [*Mor.* 290c]). Greenewalt (1978, p. 41, n. 4) has collected the known recipients of dog sacrifice in the context of his study of ritual puppy dinners at 6th-century Sardis: he lists Ares/Enyalios, Eilioneia/Eileithyia, Hekate and other chthonic figures, the hero Linos at Argos, Pan/Faunus at the Lupercalia, Diana Trivia, Genita Mana, and Robigo.

169. Pliny (*HN* 29.14.58) also mentions the sacrifice of a puppy to Genita Mana.

by the connection of the goddess with birth. He goes on to comment that the Argives sacrifice a bitch to the birth goddess Eilioneia because of the apparent ease with which dogs give birth. He cites Socrates as the source of this information, so we may assume that the custom was an old one. A passage of Hesychios (s.v. Γενετυλλίς), unfortunately corrupt, hints at a similar custom. The lexicographer derives the name Genetyllis from γένησις, adding that she is a foreign goddess and her cult is celebrated by women. A garbled phrase in the passage has been emended to read that she receives dog sacrifices because of a similarity to Hekate, but both the words "Hekate" and "dogs" are conjectures.[170] Pausanias (1.1.5) informs us that Genetyllis was worshipped along with Aphrodite in a sanctuary at Cape Kolias. That the cult is at least as old as the 5th century is confirmed by references in the plays of Aristophanes (*Clouds* 52; *Lysistrata* 2; *Thesmophoriazusai* 130); they also confirm that the cult was one of women. A scholion on *Thesmophoriazusai* 130 associates Genetyllis with Aphrodite and echoes Hesychios's derivation of the name; it further associates the Genetyllides with Artemis and calls them the τοκετῶν ἔφοροι, a phrase often translated as "divine midwives."[171] No source other than the suspect Hesychios, however, mentions dog sacrifice. In view of the identity of the herm, Eileithyeia (another birth goddess, and one who also occurs in plural form) may also be suggested as a recipient, but again we have no positive evidence of canine (or other) sacrifices to her at Athens.

The goddess with whom dogs are perhaps most intimately associated is Hekate; packs of hounds accompany her, dogs bay at her approach, and dogs were sacrificed to her so frequently that the animal was known as the Ἑκάτης ἄγαλμα.[172] In addition, not only did Hekate have a long history as a goddess of birth, she was also intimately connected with death; her special province seems to have been the point at which a soul either entered or left a body.[173] She was also particularly associated with the *aoroi* (ἄωροι),[174] those who died before their time—a description that can aptly be applied to most of the individuals in the well.

The dogs in the well, then, may have served to draw off the pollution incurred by the recent birth and death of these infants, either by direct application to the polluted person or by sacrifice. They may also have served as a protection against the possible malign influence of the untimely dead. Greek sources have little to say about the way in which newborn dead were regarded. Death in early infancy was ascribed to various bogey-women, childless creatures who preyed on the newborn,[175] but what happened to

170. The text reads: . . . ἐοικυῖα τῇ ἑορτῇ, διὸ καὶ ταύτῃ κείνας προετίθησαν. Schmitt (1858) prints the conjecture of Vossius and Scaliger: . . . ἐοικυῖα τῇ Ἑκάτῃ, διὸ καὶ ταύτῃ κύνας προετίθησαν; the more recent edition of Latte (1953) gives . . . ἐοικυῖα τῇ Ἀρτεμίδι, διὸ καὶ ταύτῃ ἐκαίνας [births] προσετίθησαν.

171. Farnell 1896, vol. 2, p. 519. Ps.-Lucian (*Amores* 42) classifies the Genetyllides among divinities vaguely associated with love affairs, worshipped by women and disapproved of by men. Hadzisteliou-Price (1978, p. 127) further characterizes Genetyllis as the "goddess of one's birth hour."

172. For Hekate in general, see Kraus 1960; Johnston 1990. For her association with dogs and dog sacrifice, see Zaganiaris 1975, pp. 323–324; Eur. fr. 968 (Nauck); Theoc. *Id.* 2.12–14, and the scholion on these lines; Plut. *Quaest. Rom.* 68, 111 [*Mor.* 280b–c, 290d]; Paus. 3.14.9; Hsch. s.v. Ἑκάτης ἄγαλμα.

173. Rohde 1925, pp. 297, 322 (n. 91); Kraus 1960, pp. 25–26; Johnston 1990, pp. 144–145.

174. Rohde 1925, pp. 593–595, appendix VII.

175. Gello, Lamia, and Mormo; see Johnston 1995 for their stories and the various spells and charms that were supposed to protect children against them.

the infants after death, and whether or not they were likely to return to harass the living, is uncertain.[176] But if they were thought to do so, Hekate, as the leader of the *aoroi*, could protect against those influences—another reason, perhaps, to offer her a dog in these circumstances.

CONCLUSIONS

It is not a straightforward matter to choose among the possible reasons behind the deposit in the Agora Bone Well, and to insist on a single cause for this complex assemblage would, in the end, ignore the complexities of biology and culture. The most efficient explanation for the deposition of the infants, however, is that this was the way in which the newborn dead were normally interred in 2nd-century Athens. Natural infant mortality could account for the numbers, but some infanticides are doubtless present as well. In the frequent instances in which a newborn died, someone—probably the midwife—took the body to a secret place that she knew, and we have by chance found one of those places. Midwives would also have had to dispose of the placenta and other afterbirth tissues following every birth, whether the infant lived or not—soft tissues that have not survived but may also have found their way into the well. Access to a convenient place of disposal would have been an essential part of a midwife's professional practice, and the Agora Bone Well offered many advantages. It was conveniently located near the center of town, but in an out-of-the-way and deserted corner. It also lay just up the hill from the sanctuary of Demos and the Graces, which may have lent the well a sacred character and gone some distance toward ameliorating the apparent casualness of this means of dealing with the corpse.

Those who needed such facilities must always have been on the lookout for likely places. They began to use the Agora Bone Well soon after it became available through the abandonment of the surrounding neighborhood. Once it was established as an unofficial burial place, the well occasionally received the remains of older individuals, all of them in some way compromised. It is more difficult to explain why it went out of use. Most likely, someone objected to these activities and deliberately filled the well, weighting down the burials with a heavy deposit of stones—just as someone placed stones on the hands of one of the buried Lugnano children, or, indeed, as we fix our own burial places with heavy tombstones, anchoring the dead firmly in their graves. Or perhaps another place more suitable was found. Only a tiny fraction of the residential area of ancient Athens has been excavated;

176. The things that the reborn Er said about those who died in early infancy are dismissed by Socrates as not worth recalling (*Resp.* 10.615c: τῶν δὲ εὐθὺς γενομένων καὶ ὀλίγον χρόνον βιούντων πέρι ἄλλα ἔλεγεν οὐκ ἄξια μνήμης). Much later, Plutarch reports that Timarchos, when consulting the oracle of Trophonios, hears the wailing of innumerable babies coming from the abyss (*De gen.* 22 [*Mor.* 590f]: μυρίων δὲ κλαυθμὸν βρέφων), and Virgil's Aeneas encounters dead newborns just inside the entrance of Hades (*Aen.* 6.426–429). Roman texts suggest that the infant dead were sometimes regarded as threatening; see Baills 2003, pp. 86–87.

if our conjecture is correct, other similar deposits still lie undiscovered beneath the modern city.

The discovery of two wells in Eretria with faunal and human remains closely similar to those in the Agora Bone Well confirms that this practice was not unique to Athens or to the second century B.C. Preliminary examination of the human remains there has revealed that the infants, though less numerous, reflect an age distribution similar to that of the infants in the Agora deposit and that they suffered from some of the same pathologies and developmental defects. It is clear that the Agora well simply documents a more extreme example of a common practice that persisted over a long period of time.

While the disposal of the infants in the well may strike us today as unfeeling and callous, there are indications that it was not practiced heedlessly. The numerous ceramic vessels large enough to serve as "coffins" are analogous to those used in the more formal burial of infants. Unguentaria and the feeding vessel recall the grave gifts of the cemetery, and other, less durable gifts may also have accompanied the infants. The dogs suggest ritual practice with parallels in the cemetery, and the herm of Eileithyia acknowledges divine oversight of the birth process. Ancient literature and art introduce us to only the very richest of Athenians, and it is easy to forget that life for many more was always precarious. Many of the free poor must have lived at close to subsistence levels, often one catastrophe away from serious deprivation, and they were not in a position to invest significant resources in the burial of infants who entered the life of the family so briefly. The deaths of infant slaves will have elicited even less ceremony. The Agora Bone Well may have offered a pragmatic solution to the all-too-common phenomenon of perinatal infant death, but its use does not necessarily suggest the absence of grief among the mothers and other members of the families who suffered these losses. This remarkable collection opens a window onto a very private aspect of ancient experience, offering a vivid and intimate view of a distressing but inevitable part of Hellenistic Athenian lives. It also provides a remarkably detailed picture of the sufferings of four older individuals, who can stand as proxies for the many ancient Athenians who succumbed to serious ailments and harsh mistreatment.

It is usually cause for regret when an excavation remains unpublished long after the completion of fieldwork. In the case of the Agora Bone Well, however, the delay has been beneficial. At the time the well was excavated, only a single, overworked bioarchaeologist was active in Greece, zooarchaeology had yet to become an established specialty, and the chronological framework that dates the well had not yet been developed. Furthermore, the intense degree of interdisciplinary collaboration necessary for the study of such a deposit was not commonly encountered in Classical archaeology as it was practiced in the 1930s.

Changes in the field since that time have made the present study possible, and the project has emerged as a remarkable exercise in the long-term cooperation of experts in disparate fields. Separate studies and analyses of the human remains, faunal assemblage, ceramics, and sculpture are unlikely to have taken us far towards an understanding of the phenomena that led to the formation of this deposit. What was required was the integration of these analyses in order to reinforce, clarify, and correct our individual conclusions, and ultimately to develop a coherent interpretation of this complex assemblage. That interpretation may, of course, miss the mark entirely, but it is the fruit of long discussions, a give-and-take among collaborators, as the work of each raised new questions for the others to consider.

The undertaking has not been without its challenges. All of the participants were concurrently involved in other projects and had heavy demands on their time. We were rarely free to work on the material at the same time, and some parts of the study would race ahead while others sat on a back burner. Unlike most excavations, the Agora functions year-round as a research center, and our visits to the excavation often did not coincide. Face-to-face meetings were a rarity, and disagreements of interpretation more often than not had to be worked out long-distance and intermittently. We feel, however, that the results published here compensate for those inconveniences, and demonstrate the virtues of such an interdisciplinary approach.

Catalogue

INTRODUCTION

Catalogue entries include the following information.

Agora inventory number.
Reference to illustration.
Previous publication, if any.
The depth at which the object was found, if known. The Agora records describe most of the objects as coming "from the filling from the surface to 20.00 m" (notebook ΛΛ 9, p. 1763), i.e., the entire excavated depth of the well. Because the records also specify that there was little pottery above a depth of 13 m, approximately where the bone deposit began, we assume that most of this material was found in association with the bones.
Dimensions: H. (height) or p.H. (preserved height); L. (length) or p.L. (preserved length); W. (width); Diam. (diameter); Th. (thickness); max. p.dim. (maximum preserved dimension); Wt. (weight). All linear measurements are in meters.
State of preservation, described in detail because of its bearing on the question of whether the object was a chance discard or relevant to the bone deposit.
Description. Except for objects that have not been published elsewhere, this is brief. Unless otherwise noted, fine ware is of the typical Attic fabric, as described in *Agora* XXIX, pp. 10–11. Unguentarium fabric is gray with an occasional red core, as described in *Agora* XXXIII, pp. 140–141. With a few exceptions (noted in the entries), household fabric is Attic Pink temper ware (see *Agora* XXXIII, pp. 23–28) and cooking pots are of Schist cooking fabric (see *Agora* XXXIII, pp. 40–43). Fabric color, where mentioned, is described with reference to the *Munsell Soil Color Charts*.
Comparanda are included for some objects that have not previously been published.

Dates are offered mainly for stamped amphora handles, for which there is considerable external evidence.

Details about uninventoried objects are given after the catalogue entries for each object type. For the sake of completeness, a few objects specifically identified as coming from the upper part of the well (above the bone deposit) or from its mouth are included at the end of the catalogue.

FINE-WARE VESSELS

Vessels for Food

Bowl with Outturned Rim, Classical Type

1 (P 13678) Fig. 51

Agora XXIX, p. 333, no. 900, fig. 60; Rotroff 2014, p. 525, no. 8, pl. 170:a. H. 0.045; Diam. 0.130. Mended from five frr.; four frr. of wall restored; four large chips missing from foot. No wear on resting surface. Scraped groove at junction of foot and wall. Four tiny palmettes within rouletting on floor. Shiny black gloss. Graffiti on underside: two Xs.

2 (P 13488) Figs. 51, 52, 91

Rotroff 2014, p. 525, no. 9, pl. 170:a. Found at 16.00. H. 0.040; Diam. 0.120. Intact except for four small chips in rim. No wear on resting surface. Scraped groove at junction of foot and wall. Four lightly stamped palmettes within rouletting on floor. Black glaze. Graffito on underside: H.

3 (P 13672) Fig. 53

Diam. of foot 0.096. Single fr. preserves foot and a bit of lower wall. Worn resting surface. Scraped groove at junction of foot and wall. Four palmettes within rouletting on floor. Shiny black gloss, stacking circle.

Uninventoried: frr. of three.

Bowl with Outturned Rim, Hellenistic Type

4 (P 13676) Fig. 51

Agora XXIX, p. 337, no. 949, pl. 73; Rotroff 2014, p. 525, no. 10, pl. 170:a. H. 0.085; est. Diam. 0.270. Mended from eight frr.; less than half of foot and more than half of rim and wall missing (partly restored). Resting surface slightly worn. Dull black gloss.

5 (P 13677) Figs. 51, 91

Agora XXIX, p. 336, no. 945, fig. 61; Rotroff 2014, p. 525, no. 11, pl. 170:a. H. 0.060; Diam. 0.169. Mended from four frr.; two rim frr. missing (restored); large chip missing from foot. Dull black gloss, red on part of outside and foot.

6 (P 13679) Fig. 51

Agora XXIX, p. 336, no. 939, fig. 61, pl. 73; Rotroff 2014, p. 525, no. 12, pl. 170:a. H. 0.035; Diam. 0.095. Single fr.; half of wall and rim missing. Battered; worn resting surface. Red gloss, mostly missing.

Uninventoried: 20, with 19 small bowls (three more than half preserved, five less than half preserved, frr. of 11) and frr. of one medium-sized bowl.

Echinus Bowl

7 (P 13680) Fig. 51

Agora XXIX, p. 343, no. 1033, fig. 64, pl. 77; Rotroff 2014, p. 525, no. 13, pl. 170:a. H. 0.038; est. Diam. 0.095. Three-fourths of rim and upper wall missing. Worn resting surface. Dull thin gray-black gloss.

8 (P 13500) Figs. 51, 91

Agora XXIX, p. 421, no. 1745, fig. 103, pl. 137; Rotroff 2014, p. 525, no. 14, pl. 170:a. Found at 17.85–18.45. H. 0.036; Diam. 0.080. Intact. Worn circles on floor, possibly from mixing or crushing something in the bowl, though possibly just gloss flaking along wheel marks. Reddish yellow fabric (5YR 6/8) with voids, small red and larger white inclusions; dull red gloss inside and upper exterior. Probably not Attic.

Uninventoried: frr. of four, one of them semiglazed.

Echinus Bowl, Grooved Wall

9 (P 13671) Fig. 51

Agora XXIX, p. 344, no. 1036, fig. 64, pl. 77; Rotroff 2014, p. 525, no. 15, pl. 170:a. H. 0.056; rest. Diam. 0.254. Mended from two pieces; slightly less than half of wall and rim and one-third of foot preserved; most of floor missing. Worn resting surface; some scratches on floor. Shiny black gloss.

Uninventoried: frr. of two.

Bowl, Beveled Rim

Uninventoried: one small rim fr.; cf. *Agora* XXIX, p. 344, no. 1037, fig. 64, pl. 78.

Deep Bowl, Projecting Rim

10 (P 13674) Fig. 51

Agora XXIX, p. 349, no. 1103, fig. 67, pl. 80; Rotroff 2014, p. 525, no. 18, pl. 170:a. H. 0.142; Diam. 0.290. Shattered (mended from ca. 27 frr.); over half of rim and some wall frr. missing (restored); foot heavily chipped. Considerable wear on resting surface. Hole pierced through rim, probably for hanging. Shiny black glaze.

Uninventoried: frr. of one or two.

Rolled-Rim Plate

11 (P 13670) Fig. 51

Agora XXIX, p. 312, no. 676, fig. 48; Rotroff 2014, p. 525, no. 16, pl. 170:a. H. 0.037; rest. Diam. 0.252. Mended from four frr.; two-thirds of rim and wall and half of foot missing (restored); almost all of floor present. Worn resting surface. Dull black gloss, very worn with much missing.

Uninventoried: eight (three less than half preserved, frr. of five, including one-fourth of the floor of a stamped plate probably dating to the 3rd century).

Rilled-Rim Plate

12 (P 13501) Fig. 91

Found at 17.85–18.45. H. 0.034; Diam. 0.133. Intact except for two chips from rim. Scratches below rim on outside; traces of bronze adhering to rim. Dull red gloss inside only.

13 (P 13673) Figs. 51, 91

Agora XXIX, pp. 323–324, no. 806, fig. 55, pl. 68; Rotroff 2014, p. 525, no. 17, pl. 170:a. H. 0.030; Diam. 0.129. Mended from four frr.; one small piece missing (restored). Worn resting surface. Traces of thin red gloss inside only.

Uninventoried: five (one more than half preserved, two less than half preserved, frr. of two).

Fishplate

Uninventoried: frr. of three large and two small. For the shape, see *Agora* XXIX, pp. 146–149.

Saucer

Uninventoried: rim frr. of nine. For the shape, see *Agora* XXIX, pp. 149–150.

Vessels for Drink

Moldmade Bowl

14 (P 13687) Fig. 54

Agora XXII, p. 48, no. 31, pls. 6, 94; Rotroff 2014, p. 525, no. 1, pl. 167. H. 0.082; Diam. 0.142. Mended from 19 frr.; almost all of rim and some parts of wall missing (restored). Almost no wear on resting surface. Medallion: double four-petal rosette. Wall: imbricate fronds. Rim: egg and dart, double spirals, alternating rosettes and leaves(?). Mostly dark red gloss, brown/black on upper wall. Workshop A, but not at the beginning of the tradition: the mold was not new, as details are visible but not crisp.

15 (P 13684) Fig. 55

Agora XXII, p. 61, no. 144, pl. 27; Rotroff 2014, p. 525, no. 3, pl. 167. H. 0.087; Diam. 0.155. Mended from 20 frr.; several pieces of wall and rim restored. Considerable wear on resting surface. Medallion: gorgoneion surrounded by rosettes. Calyx: fronds and ferns with flying Erotes between tips. Wall: pairs of flying Nikai flanking frontal Nike. Rim: double spirals, leaves. Dull black gloss. Class 1.

16 (P 13686) Fig. 56

Agora XXII, p. 53, no. 73, pls. 13, 94; Rotroff 2014, p. 525, no. 2, pl. 167. H. 0.094; Diam. 0.165. Most of rim and two-thirds of wall missing (restored). Very worn resting surface. Medallion: gorgoneion, barely legible. Calyx: imbricate ferns. Wall: large fronds. Rim: double spirals. There are traces of a large leaf stamp on the pimple at the middle of the floor. Black gloss. Class 2.

17 (P 13683) Fig. 57

Agora XXII, p. 57, no. 109, pls. 19, 94; Rotroff 2014, p. 525, no. 5, pl. 367. H. 0.089; Diam. 0.143. Mended from ca. 25 frr.; one-fourth of rim and frr. of wall missing (restored). Very little wear on resting surface. Medallion: double six-petal rosette. Calyx: imbricate ferns. Wall: pairs of rampant goats flanking kraters alternating with pairs of flying Erotes carrying masks. Rim: egg and dart, double spiral, flowers springing from tendrils. Gloss largely red, except on part of rim on outside. M Monogram Class. Mold fairly fresh.

18 (P 13685) Fig. 58

Agora XXII, p. 73, no. 236, pls. 45, 85; Rotroff 2014, p. 525, no. 4, pl. 167. H. 0.082; rest. Diam. 0.140. Mended from 11 frr.; half of rim and about one-fourth of wall missing (restored). No wear on resting surface. Medallion: eight-petal rosette.

Calyx: small ferns. Wall: riders, kantharos, amazon, Eros on goat, and foot soldier. Rim: guilloche, double spirals crowned by leaves. Dull red gloss, black near rim.

Uninventoried: ca. 113 nonjoining segments (mostly single frr.) from a minimum of 30 bowls (one pine cone, five imbricate, two floral, twelve figured, ten unknown).

Two-Handled Cup

19 (P 13681) Fig. 51

Agora XXIX, p. 284, no. 400, fig. 23, pl. 38; Rotroff 2014, p. 525, no. 6, pl. 170:a. H. 0.067; Diam. 0.178. Mended from seven frr.; handle and one-third of rim missing (restored). Worn resting surface. Thick brown to black glaze.

Uninventoried: rim frr. of one or two.

Hemispherical West Slope Cup

20 (P 13682) Fig. 59

Agora XXIX, p. 281, no. 372, pl. 36. Max. p.dim. 0.136. Mended from four frr.; one-third of lower wall preserved. Grooves on exterior. Black to red glaze. Medallion: asterisk with zigzag streamers between rays. Wall: wheat garland with long incised beards (cf. *Agora* XXIX, pp. 305–306, no. 603, pl. 58). A remarkably large example: greatest preserved diameter is 0.145 about halfway up wall.

Uninventoried: frr. of one.

Other Cups

Uninventoried: frr. of five West Slope kantharoi (cf. *Agora* XXIX, pp. 262–270, nos. 188–216, 232–270, figs. 14–18, pls. 17–20, 22–25) and possibly of one black-gloss Hellenistic kantharos (cf. *Agora* XXIX, pp. 272–273, nos. 283–301, fig. 19, pls. 28–30).

Closed Vessels for Wine Service

Uninventoried: frr. of two West Slope amphoras with garlands on necks (cf. *Agora* XXIX, p. 287, no. 419, fig. 26, pl. 41 [shape and decoration], pp. 304, 326, nos. 587, 832, pls. 55, 70 [garland only]), a rim fr. of a trefoil oinochoe, the mouth of an olpe (cf. *Agora* XXIX, p. 296, nos. 502, 503, fig. 37, pl. 49).

Other Shapes

Lug-Handled Krater

21 (P 13675) Fig. 51

Agora XXIX, p. 304, no. 592, fig. 42, pl. 56; Rotroff 2014, p. 525, no. 7, pl. 170:a. P.H. 0.120; Diam. 0.310. Mended from ten frr.; half of rim, one third of wall, and one handle preserved (partly restored). Very battered. Shiny black gloss, mostly missing.

Uninventoried: single frr. of two more.

Round-Mouth Jug

22 (P 13688) Figs. 60, 91

Agora XXIX, p. 299, no. 531, fig. 39, pl. 51; Rotroff 2014, p. 525, no. 19, pl. 170:a. H. 0.176; Diam. 0.150. Mended from six frr.; half of mouth and small pieces of body missing (restored). Worn resting surface. Dull brown gloss.

Uninventoried: frr. of one medium-sized juglet (cf. *Agora* XXIX, p. 299, nos. 533–535, fig. 39, pl. 51).

Lekythos

23 (P 13689) Fig. 60

Agora XXIX, p. 350, no. 1117, fig. 69, pl. 81; Rotroff 2014, p. 525, no. 20, pl. 170:a. H. 0.154; Diam. 0.112. Mended from ca. eight frr.; over half of belly and half of mouth missing (restored); foot chipped. Worn resting surface. Shiny black gloss, missing on one side.

Canteen

24 (P 13690) Fig. 61

Agora XXIX, p. 359, no. 1206, pls. 89, 147; Liston and Rotroff 2013b, p. 76; Rotroff 2014, p. 525, no. 22, pls. 168:a. H. 0.323; Diam. 0.271. Shattered (mended from ca. 35 frr.); both handles, many pieces of belly, and chips of rim missing (restored). Stamped [Δ]ΩΡΟΘΕΟΥ at the center of the concave side. Metallic black gloss.

25 (P 25554) Fig. 60

Agora XXIX, p. 359, no. 1205, fig. 74, pl. 89; Rotroff 2014, p. 525, no. 23, pl. 170:a. Est. diam. of body 0.270. Neck, mouth, and nine frr. of body preserved. Body probably round. Corner of rectangular stamp preserved. Shiny black gloss.

Feeder

26 (P 13498) Figs. 60, 62, 91

Agora XXIX, p. 358, no. 1195, fig. 73, pl. 87; Liston and Rotroff 2013a, pp. 65–66, fig. 3.2; 2013b, p. 74; Rotroff 2014, p. 525, no. 21, pl. 170:a. Found at 16.85–17.85. H. 0.061; Diam. 0.075. Handle restored; chip missing from foot and a few small chips around mouth; otherwise unbroken. End of nozzle slightly chipped and gloss around end abraded in places. Worn resting surface. Dull black gloss.

Panathenaic Amphora

27 (P 25553) Fig. 63

Edwards 1957, p. 339, no. 9, pl. 77. P.H. 0.068. Small fr. preserving part of helmet, with trace of white of Athena's face at lower right.

Pyxis

Uninventoried: one type B pyxis body fr.

Lamps

28 (L 3584) Fig. 64

Rotroff 2014, p. 525, no. 24, pl. 168:b. Diam. 0.088. Lower half and tip of nozzle missing. Type 45C, handleless version; large, with crisp detail. Shiny black gloss. Cf. *Agora* IV, p. 147, no. 584, pl. 47 (from deposit E 14:1, deposited ca. 200), and L 4749 (small fr. from deposit Q 8–9, deposited ca. 170).

29 (L 3580) Figs. 64, 91

Agora IV, p. 103, no. 440, pls. 15, 42; Rotroff 2014, p. 525, no. 25, pl. 168:b. H. 0.032; Diam. 0.068. Intact except for one chip from end of nozzle. Some burning around nozzle. Type 33A. Dull black gloss, mostly missing. For date of type, see *Agora* XXIX, p. 501.

Uninventoried: frr. of six Classical, with one type 22C, one Classical nozzle (perhaps type 23), one uncertain Classical type, and three type 25, and four Hellenistic, with three wheelmade (perhaps type 33 or 34) and one type 43D.

Classical Votives

Uninventoried: a miniature black-gloss oinochoe(?), an unglazed two-handled cup (cf. *Agora* XXIX, p. 380, no. 1409, pl. 108), and fr. of a cooking-ware lopadion (cf. *Agora* XXIX, p. 387, no. 1483, fig. 87, pl. 112).

Early Fine Ware

Uninventoried: frr. of 13 Classical and earlier vessels, with one Iron Age(?), one Corinthian skyphos handle, one Corinthian skyphos foot, six red-figure, one plate rim, one lidded pelike rim, one stamped base, and one black-gloss wall fr.

PLAIN-WARE VESSELS

Unguentaria

Category 3

30 (P 32492) Figs. 65, 66

Rotroff 2014, p. 525, no. 26, pl. 170:b. P.H. 0.056; Diam. 0.030. Half of lower body preserved; foot chipped all around.

Category 4

31 (P 13499) Figs. 65, 66, 90

Agora XXXIII, p. 292, no. 441, fig. 63, pl. 53; Rotroff 2014, p. 525, no. 27, pl. 170:b. Found at 17.85–18.45. H. 0.173; Diam. 0.059. Rim and foot chipped.

Category 5

32 (P 13490) Figs. 65, 90

Agora XXXIII, p. 294, no. 463, fig. 64; Liston and Rotroff 2013b, p. 76; Rotroff 2014, p. 526, no. 28, pls. 168:c, 170:b. Found at 16.00–16.85. H. 0.115; Diam. 0.025. Intact.

33 (P 13491) Figs. 65, 90

Agora XXXIII, p. 293, no. 460, fig. 64; Liston and Rotroff 2013b, p. 76; Rotroff 2014, p. 526, no. 29, pls. 168:c, 170:b. Found at 16.00–16.85. H. 0.115; Diam. 0.027. Small chip of rim and several of foot missing.

34 (P 13492) Figs. 65, 90

Agora XXXIII, p. 293, no. 461, fig. 64; Liston and Rotroff 2013b, p. 76; Rotroff 2014, p. 526, no. 30, pls. 168:c, 170:b. Found at 16.00–16.85. H. 0.104; Diam. 0.022. Intact.

35 (P 13493) Fig. 90

Agora XXXIII, p. 293, under no. 461; Liston and Rotroff 2013b, p. 76; Rotroff 2014, p. 526, no. 31, pl. 168:c. Found at 16.00–16.85. H. 0.104; Diam. 0.022. Intact.

36 (P 13494) Figs. 65, 90

Agora XXXIII, p. 293, no. 459, fig. 64; Rotroff 2014, p. 526, no. 32, pls. 168:c, 170:b. Found at 13.00. H. 0.129; Diam. 0.035. Rim slightly chipped, foot chipped.

37 (P 13495) Fig. 90

Agora XXXIII, p. 294, under no. 462; Rotroff 2014, p. 526, no. 33, pl. 168:c. Found at 13.00. H. 0.110; Diam. 0.028. Intact.

38 (P 13691) Figs. 65, 90

Agora XXXIII, pp. 293–294, no. 462, fig. 64; Rotroff 2014, p. 526, no. 34, pls. 168:c, 170:b. H. 0.111; Diam. 0.028. Rim slightly chipped, one chip missing from foot.

39 (P 32491) Fig. 65

Rotroff 2014, p. 526, no. 35, pls. 168:c, 170:b. P.H. 0.152; Diam. 0.057. Neck and mouth missing.

Uninventoried: nine (two complete, two more than half preserved, frr. of five).

Household Ware, Open Shapes

Lekane, Form 1

40 (P 13502) Fig. 67

Agora XXXIII, p. 271, no. 243, fig. 40, pl. 34; Rotroff 2014, p. 526, no. 37, pl. 171. Found at 17.85–18.45. H. 0.116; Diam. 0.305. Rim chipped. Ring foot. Dull orange gloss inside.

41 (P 13697) Fig. 93

Agora XXXIII, p. 271, under no. 243; Liston and Rotroff 2013a, p. 66, fig. 3.3; 2013b, p. 76; Rotroff 2014, p. 526, no. 38, pl. 169:a. H. 0.126; Diam. 0.322. Mended from 14 frr.; a few frr. of rim and wall missing (restored). Ring foot. Thin brown wash inside.

42 (P 13698) Fig. 67

Agora XXXIII, p. 271, no. 248, fig. 41, pl. 34. H. 0.134; Diam. 0.323. Mended from ten frr.; center of floor, parts of wall, over half of rim, and parts of both handles missing (restored). Evidence of burning inside. Disc foot. Thin red wash inside.

Uninventoried: frr. of four.

Lekane, Form 3

43 (P 13699) Fig. 67

Agora XXXIII, p. 272, no. 257, fig. 43, pl. 36; Rotroff 2014, p. 526, no. 39, pl. 171. H. 0.281; rest. Diam. 0.357. Mended from 11 frr.; over half preserved: center of floor, part of foot, over half of rim and upper wall, and one handle missing (restored). Dull reddish brown gloss inside, on rim, and on handle.

Uninventoried: frr. of two.

Lekane, Form 4

44 (P 13703) Fig. 67

Agora XXXIII, p. 274, no. 270, fig. 46, pl. 38. No depth recorded, but bronze staining suggests it was probably found at 16.00–16.85. H. 0.162; Diam. 0.413. Mended from seven frr.; one handle missing and parts of rim, wall, and bottom missing but restored. Raised base.

45 (P 13704) Figs. 67, 93

Agora XXXIII, p. 274, no. 271, fig. 47, pl. 38; Liston and Rotroff 2013a, p. 66, fig. 3.3; 2013b, p. 76; Rotroff 2014, p. 526, no. 36, pls. 169:a, 171. H. 0.161; Diam. 0.434. Mended from 13 frr.; small parts of wall and rim missing (restored). Flat bottom.

Uninventoried: frr. of 20 (11 less than half preserved, frr. of nine). Four have a ring base, four have a raised base, and three have a flat bottom. One is lacking the thumbprint on the handle.

Deep Bowl

46 (P 13503) Figs. 67, 93

Agora XXXIII, p. 275, no. 287, fig. 50; Rotroff 2014, p. 526, no. 40, pl. 171. Found at 17.85–18.45. H. 0.203; Diam. 0.316. One-third of rim missing; otherwise intact. Raised base. Hellenistic water jug fabric; imported.

47 (P 13700) Fig. 68

Agora XXXIII, p. 275, under no. 287. H. 0.163; Diam. 0.255. Mended from 10 frr.; frr. of rim, wall, and bottom missing (restored). Raised base. Pale fabric with red inclusions; faint traces of gloss inside.

Shallow Bowl, Large

48 (P 13693) Fig. 69

Agora XXXIII, p. 277, under no. 300; Rotroff 2014, p. 526, no. 42, pl. 169:b. No depth recorded, but traces of bronze on walls indicates probably found at 16.00–16.85. H. 0.125; Diam. 0.322. Mended from nine frr.; small parts of rim and wall missing (restored). Ring foot. Thin red wash inside.

49 (P 13692) Fig. 67

Agora XXXIII, p. 277, no. 300, fig. 51, pl. 41; Rotroff 2014, p. 526, no. 41, pl. 171. H. 0.157; Diam. 0.380. Mended from 14 frr.; center of floor, part of foot, and about one-third of rim and body missing (partly restored). Thin brown gloss inside.

Uninventoried: one, less than half preserved.

Shallow Bowl, Small

50 (P 13694) Fig. 67

Agora XXXIII, p. 277, no. 303, fig. 52, pl. 41; Rotroff 2014, p. 526, no. 43, pl. 171. H. 0.064; Diam. 0.206. Mended from seven frr.; small pieces of wall missing (restored).

51 (P 13695) Fig. 69

Agora XXXIII, p. 277, under no. 303; Rotroff 2014, p. 526, no. 45, pl. 169:b. H. 0.061; Diam. 0.203. Mended from four frr.; small piece of rim and wall missing (restored).

52 (P 13696) Fig. 67

Agora XXXIII, p. 277, no. 304, fig. 52, pl. 41; Rotroff 2014, p. 526, no. 44, pl. 171. H. 0.051; Diam. 0.195. Mended from seven frr.; one-fourth of rim missing (restored).

Uninventoried: three (two more than half preserved, one less than half preserved).

Krater

53 (P 13701) Fig. 70

Agora XXXIII, p. 269, no. 222, fig. 38, pl. 31; Rotroff 2014, p. 526, no. 47, pl. 171. H. 0.278; Diam. 0.275. Mended from 14 frr. One handle and one-fourth of rim and wall missing (restored); foot chipped. Decoration in dull orange gloss.

54 (P 13702) Figs. 70, 93

Agora XXXIII, pp. 268–269, no. 221, fig. 37, pl. 31; Rotroff 2014, p. 526, no. 46, pl. 171. H. 0.301; Diam. 0.310. Mended from 42 frr.; center of floor, large parts of body, one-fourth of rim, and one handle missing (restored).

Uninventoried: four (two less than half preserved, frr. of two).

Mortar

55 (P 13705) Fig. 70

Agora XXXIII, p. 265, no. 188, fig. 31, pl. 25; Rotroff 2014, p. 526, no. 48, pl. 171. H. to rim 0.100; est. Diam. 0.363. Mended from three frr.; most of rim and spout missing (restored). Wear on floor. Raised base.

Uninventoried: two (one more than half preserved, one less than half preserved).

Beehive

56 (P 35218) Fig. 71

P.H. 0.205; Diam. of base 0.220. Mended from nine frr.; bottom and two-thirds of lower body preserved. Mended in antiquity: part of one lead clamp in situ, holes for others in wall. Floor and two-thirds of wall scored. Gritty light red fabric (5YR 6/8) with many small inclusions. Parts of three loose clamps in the well may come from this hive.

Other Household-Ware Open Vessels

Uninventoried: rim of pithos or vat; foot of vat or amphora stand; large knob of lid.

Household Ware, Closed Shapes

Jug, Form 2

57 (P 13712) Fig. 70

Agora XXXIII, p. 249, no. 42, fig. 8, pl. 8; Rotroff 2014, p. 526, no. 49, pl. 171. H. 0.447; Diam. 0.259. Mended from 38 frr.; large parts of body and small piece of rim missing (restored).

Amphora, Form 2

58 (P 35220) Fig. 72

Rotroff 2014, p. 526, no. 50, pl. 171. P.H. of fr. a 0.138; est. Diam. of rim 0.060. Two joining frr. preserving less than half of neck and mouth, one handle, and part of shoulder and upper body, and six more nonjoining sections of belly (not illustrated). Flaring rim with square profile; short, narrow neck with drip ring at point of upper handle attachment. Strap handle. Angular shoulder. Cf. *Agora* XXXIII, p. 257, nos. 120, 121 (both imported), 122 (local), fig. 19, pl. 18.

Lagynos

59 (P 35219) Fig. 73

Diam. of foot 0.099, est. Diam. of body 0.280. Three nonjoining sections mended from 19 frr.; foot, about one-third of lower body, parts of shoulder, and lower handle attachment preserved. Patches of residue inside, perhaps resin. Fine fabric with small flecks of silver mica, mottled to reddish yellow outside (ca. 7.5YR 6/6), darker inside (ca. 10R 5/4).

Uninventoried: 1 fr.

Other Household-Ware Closed Vessels

Uninventoried: frr. of two jugs, form 4; frr. of two storage bins, form 1.

Cooking Ware

Chytra, Form 1

60 (P 13489) Fig. 92

Agora XXXIII, p. 304, under no. 567; Rotroff 2014, p. 526, no. 51, pl. 169:c. Found at 16.00–16.85. H. 0.105; Diam. 0.122. Intact; apparent sooting on wall approximately opposite handle and on part of underside.

61 (P 13496) Figs. 74, 92

Agora XXXIII, p. 304, no. 567, fig. 72, pl. 61; Rotroff 2014, p. 526, no. 52, pls. 169:c, 172. Found at 16.85–17.85. H. 0.100; Diam. 0.115. Rim chipped; slight sooting approximately opposite handle and on part of underside.

62 (P 13497) Fig. 92

Agora XXXIII, p. 304, under no. 567; Rotroff 2014, p. 526, no. 53, pl. 169:c. Found at 16.85–17.85. H. 0.107; Diam. 0.110. Rim chipped, small holes in wall; slight sooting on underside.

63 (P 13706) Figs. 74, 75

Agora XXXIII, p. 304, no. 568, fig. 72, pl. 61; Rotroff 2014, p. 526, no. 54, pls. 169:c, 172. H. 0.120; Diam. 0.119. Mended from four frr.; most of rim and much of wall missing (restored); no sooting. Soft light red fabric (ca. 2.5YR 6/8) with many inclusions, probably local.

Uninventoried: four (one less than half preserved, frr. of three) of the same form and size as **60–62**.

Chytra, Form 4

64 (P 13707) Fig. 74

Agora XXXIII, p. 307, no. 594, fig. 74, pl. 63; Rotroff 2014, p. 526, no. 56, pl. 172. H. 0.315; Diam. 0.332. Mended from ca. 60 frr.; small pieces of wall and rim missing (restored); lower two-thirds of interior darkened (possibly residue, not sooting); exterior irregularly darkened, with undarkened stacking circle on underside. Gritty ochre cooking fabric; imported.

Uninventoried: one, less than half preserved, identical but with heavy deposit (possibly lead putty?) on floor.

Chytra, Form 10

65 (P 13708) Fig. 74

Agora XXXIII, p. 310, no. 629, fig. 81, pl. 67; Rotroff 2014, p. 526, no. 55, pl. 172. H. 0.255; Diam. 0.261. Mended from 41 frr.; large pieces of wall and most of rim missing (restored); heavy sooting on floor, underside, and part of one side.

Lopas, Form 3

66 (P 13710) Fig. 74

Agora XXXIII, p. 313, no. 657, fig. 83, pl. 69; Rotroff 2014, p. 526, no. 57, pl. 172. H. 0.104; Diam. 0.140. Mended from six frr.; most of floor, part of wall, and half of rim missing (restored); sooting.

Lopas, Form 4

67 (P 13709) Fig. 74

Agora XXXIII, p. 314, no. 665, fig. 84, pl. 69; Rotroff 2014, p. 526, no. 58, pl. 172. H. to rim 0.087; Diam. 0.315. Body mended from 24 frr.; most of bottom, parts of wall and rim, and part of one handle missing (restored); four frr. of lid preserved; underside of body heavily sooted. Lopas 5 cooking fabric; imported.

Other Cooking-Ware Vessels

Uninventoried: frr. of two lids, one pan.

Brazier

68 (P 13711) Fig. 76

Agora XXXIII, p. 323, no. 752, pl. 75; Rotroff 2014, p. 526, no. 59, pl. 169:d. P.H. 0.110. Pot support from brazier, with moldmade head; part of attached rim preserved; tip of beard worn, interior sooted. Male with pointed cap: Agora type I.2c. Quartz cooking fabric; imported. Cf. Rahmani 1984, p. 225, no. 5, pl. 29:E (Akko).

69 (P 34970) Fig. 77

Rotroff 2014, p. 526, no. 60, pl. 169:e. P.H. 0.240. Single large fr. Stand of brazier, flaring out to bottom, with part of one ventilation hole preserved at break; large upturned, ribbed handle attached to wall above and below with thumbprint. Yellowish fabric with shell temper; probably Benghazi Local Fabric 1 (Riley 1979, pp. 94–95). For other braziers imported from Berenike, see *Agora* XXXIII, p. 333, no. 814.

Transport Amphoras

The readings of the stamped handles are those of Virginia Grace and her staff, as preserved in the Virginia R. Grace Papers at the Archives of the American School and as entered on the inventory cards.

Koan

70 (SS 8214) Fig. 78

Grace 1949, pp. 186, 188, pls. 19:8, 20:10; 1971, p. 85, n. 86 (with revised reading); 1979, fig. 56, second from left; Whitbread 1995, p. 82, pl. 4:15. H. 0.785; Diam. 0.450. Mended from ca. 50 frr.; large frr. of wall and rim missing (restored). Short peg toe; broad shoulder, rolled rim; double handles. Stamp on one handle.

club
[Ἀ]σκλη(–)
(retr.)

Finkielsztejn (2004, p. 157, figs. 2:4, 3:a, b) illustrates an amphora with a similar stamped handle from Marissa that dates to the first half of the 2nd century and bears the abbreviation Ἀσκληπι(–).

First quarter of the 2nd century?

Uninventoried: frr. of at least four.

Knidian

71 (SS 8217)

Upper part of handle with attachment. Small incuse stamp (hook with crosspiece: fishhook?). Early Knidian (ca. 240–220).

72 (SS 8216) Fig. 79

P.H. 0.360. Mended from three frr.; neck, one handle, and upper part of the other preserved. Stamps on both handles: eponym Sokrates, fabricant Philokrates (KT 1252).

a	*b*
[Ἐπὶ Σωκρ]ά̣(τευς)	Ἐπὶ Σωκρά(τευς)
φρο̣υ̣ρ̣ά̣ρ̣χ̣ο̣υ̣	φρο̣υ̣ρ̣ά̣ρ̣[χ]ο̣υ̣
Φ̣ιλο̣κ̣ρ̣ά̣τ̣ε̣υ̣ς̣	Φ̣ιλοκ̣[ρά]τ̣ε̣υ̣ς̣
(retr.)	(retr.)

Cf. Jöhrens 1999, pp. 113–114, no. 312 (same KT), with commentary. Early in Period IV A (after 188 or a decade later).

73 (SS 8196)

Agora XXII, p. 100; *Agora* XXXIII, p. 358. Found at 13.00. Upper part of handle with attachment. Stamp: eponym Euphragoras I, fabricant Aristandros, oar device (KT 197).

Ἐπι Ε[ὐφ]ρ̣[αγό]ρ̣α̣
Ἀριστ[άνδρ]ου
Κνίδι(ον)
oar

Cf. Jöhrens 1999, p. 151, no. 458 (same KT). For fabricants associated with Euphragoras, see Jefremow 1995, pp. 125–131, table X, and Jöhrens 1999, p. 151, under no. 457. A stamp of the same KT was found in the nearby cistern F 5:1 (SS 7717). The eponym was formerly dated late in period IV B, around the mid-2nd century (Grace and Savvatianou-Petropoulakou 1970, p. 335, under E 102), but is now placed early in period IV A (Empereur and Garlan 1987, p. 90), after 188 or a decade later.

74 (SS 8215) Fig. 79

P.H. 0.370. Mended from six frr.; most of rim and neck and two handles preserved (partly restored). Stamped on one handle only: eponym Aristarchos, fabricant Skirtos, boukranion device (KT 1174).

Ἐπὶ Ἀ̣ριστάρχο
Σκ̣ί̣[ρτ]ου *bou-* υ
Κνί̣[δι]ον *kran*
(retr.)

Cf. Jöhrens 1999, p. 142, no. 430 (same KT); see also p. 121, under no. 343. Period IV A, not early (after ca. 180 or a decade later).

75 (SS 8197)

Found at 13.00. Upper part of handle with attachment. Stamp: eponym Asklepiodoros, fabricant Astragalos, boukranion device (KT 327).

Ἐπὶ Ἀσκληπι̣ο̣δ[ώ]
ρου Ἀσ̣ *bou-* τ̣ρ̣α̣
γ̣ά̣λ̣ο̣υ̣ Κ *kran* νίδι[ον]

For Asklepiodoros, see Jöhrens 1999, p. 126, under no. 363 (not the same KT). For the fabricant Astragalos named on this handle, see Jöhrens 1999, pp. 103–104, nos. 272, 273, as well as p. 275, no. AS 24 (associated with the eponym Poliouches, late period III). Period IV A, not early (after ca. 180 or a decade later).

Uninventoried: frr. of at least six more.

Other Types

Uninventoried: frr. of one Mendaean (late 5th or early 4th century), one Erythraean (3rd century), three Thasian (one early 3rd century, two late 3rd–early 2nd century), one Chian (late 3rd–early 2nd century), one Corinthian/northern Peloponnesian (early 2nd century), one Rhodian, two Greco-Italic (one from Campania), and four unidentified. We owe identifications and dates to Mark Lawall.

OTHER OBJECTS MADE OF CLAY

Molds and Figurine

76 (T 1895) Fig. 80

Max. p.dim. 0.070. Single fr. with one original edge preserved. Mold for center and left part of chest of heavily draped figure, taken from a figurine; rough area above folds marks position of neck.

77 (T 1896) Fig. 81

P. W. 0.048. Single fr. Mold with squared end, possibly for nozzle of lamp. String mark shows it was a double mold.

Uninventoried: possible head of figurine, very worn.

Loomweight

78 (MC 520) Fig. 82

H. 0.082; Diam. 0.054. Intact. Biconical loom weight; suspension hole pierced at a slight angle, two holes pierced in bottom for firing.

Uninventoried: nine biconical (three intact, six chipped), one pyramidal (more than half preserved).

Roof Tile

79 (A 938) Fig. 83

Stevens 1950, pp. 179–180, fig. 3, pl. 82:2. L. 0.985; W. 0.500. Much of one side and middle restored. Laconian pan tile. Red to black gloss on upper face.

Uninventoried: four frr. of Laconian tiles, seven of Corinthian tiles, one of a possible opaion tile.

HERM

80 (S 1086) Fig. 84

Shear 1939, pp. 238–239, fig. 37; Travlos 1949, p. 391, n. 19; 1971, pp. 79, 82, fig. 105; Langlotz 1954, p. 28, n. 41; Thompson 1963, p. 145, under no. 301 (noncommittal); *Agora* XI, pp. 167–169, no. 218, pl. 58 (Artemis); *LIMC* II, 1984, pp. 11–12, no. 20, s.v. Aphrodite (A. Delivorrias); p. 630, no. 76, pl. 447, s.v. Artemis (L. Kahil); Osanna 1988–1989, p. 81; Kunze 1992, p. 40; Pirenne-Delforge 1994, pp. 19–20; Rosenzweig 2004, p. 125, n. 14 (not Aphrodite); Weber 2006, pp. 180–183, pl. 23:2; Lippolis 2009, pp. 264–265; Schoch 2009, pp. 72–73; Stewart 2012, p. 272, n. 13 (Artemis, Eileithyia, or Hekate); 2017, pp. 118–123, fig. 26 (Eileithyia, with fuller description). Those not otherwise noted follow Shear (1939) in identifying the herm as a replica of Pheidias's Aphrodite Ourania or as a support for such a replica. Found at 18.45. P.H. 0.330; W. 0.080. Bottom of shaft broken away; tip of nose, chin, shoulders, and edges of herm chipped. Armless; back of head unfinished; rear of herm continues upwards for 0.053 as back pillar for the head, its top chipped and battered. Crown of head roughly pointed and chiseled. Gray-white marble, either Pentelic or Hymettian.

The goddess wears a long, symmetrical, undergirt "Argive" peplos with a U-shaped neckline and an overfold, modeled only on the front of the shaft. The modeling is impressionistic. The mouth is short and the lips upturned at the corners in a slight smile; the eyes are wide, but only the left one has clearly defined eyelids; the ears are not modeled. The hair is styled in the "hair roll" manner introduced in the 5th century. The locks are fairly straight in typical 2nd-century fashion. Ca. 200–150 B.C.

CHAPE

81 (BI 457) Fig. 86

Shear 1939, pp. 239–240, fig. 38; Thompson 1971, fig. 55. Found at 16.85. H. 0.059; W. 0.135; Th. 0.021; Wt. 149.73 gr. Intact except for chips, especially on lower projection, where chape was attached to rest of scabbard. Straight upper edge with projecting button at center. Sides slope outward slightly. Lower edges slope up toward center. Projecting flange at bottom. In each of the four lower corners, an identical anthemion within a teardrop-shaped field; originally inlaid in gold (of which traces remain), which was attached with six small nails. Elephant ivory. Letters picked into the top surface: if Greek, one is unquestionably N, the other perhaps Γ, Ξ, or X.

BRONZE

Straight Edging

82 (B 907) Fig. 87

Found at 16.00–16.85. P.L. of one side 0.095, of the other 0.065; W. of plain face 0.021, of scalloped face 0.018. Broken at both ends and badly corroded. Bronze edge reinforcement for an inner, right-angled corner. At the outer edge of the horizontal(?) face, a scallop pattern: broad curved protrusions alternating with small triangular teeth. In the vertical face, near the angle, two rivet holes, only one of which goes all the way through. Near the break, another with rivet in place.

Uninventoried: two similar frr.

83 (B 2245) Fig. 88

Found at 16.00–16.85. P.L. 0.138; W. of sides 0.015, 0.020. Broken at both ends. Two lengths of straight bronze edging with a right-angled bend, corroded together. A scalloped edge is preserved on one side of the longest bar. Wrapped around it at a 45-degree angle are the remains of woven organic material, in strips ca. 0.025 wide but splitting into narrower widths. Possibly rail for a bed or chair and its webbing.

Uninventoried: 50 frr. of straight edging from three different series, with slightly varying widths and heights and different distances between the teeth (total p.L. ca. 2.80). In addition, 21 slightly lighter frr., where the angle between the two sides is oblique (total p.L. ca. 1.75).

Curved Edging

84 (B 908) Fig. 87

Found at 16.00–16.85. P.L. 0.165; W. of scalloped face 0.015, of plain face 0.022 (before cleaning); est. Diam. 0.580, if this is an arc of a circle. Broken at both ends. Reinforcement for curved edge, with one face plain, the other concave with scallop decoration (pattern as **82**). Rivets in the plain face for attachment. The piece was cleaned in 1955 but could not be located as of 1958 and may not have survived treatment.

Uninventoried: five similar frr. in two series, with different widths and distances between the teeth, not all of them arcs of a circle (total p.L. ca. 0.750).

85 (B 909) Fig. 87

Found at 16.00–16.85. P.L. 0.220; W. of scalloped face 0.012, of plain face 0.017; est. Diam. 0.580, if this is an arc of a circle. Broken at both ends. Reinforcement for curved edge, possibly with a scallop pattern on the convex face. Three rivets in plain face, with spacings of 0.065 and 0.063.

Uninventoried: five similar frr. in three(?) series (total p.L. ca. 0.650). There are also two or three frr. with edging for a curved element, but with the scallop pattern on the straight rather than the curved surface (total p.L. 0.185).

Bead-and-Reel Ornament

86 (B 906) Fig. 89

Found at 16.00–16.85. P.L. 0.101; Diam. of bead 0.009; ornament spacing 0.011. Broken at both ends and badly corroded. Bead and reel, flattened on one side where it was attached.

Uninventoried: 12 frr. of similar ornament (total p.L. ca. 0.550); two frr. from another series, one of them curved (total p.L. ca. 0.100).

Twisted Rod

87 (B 905) Fig. 89

Found at 16.00–16.85. P.L. 0.157; Th. 0.0055–0.0060. Broken at both ends and badly corroded. Rod approximately square in section, with S-twist. Cf. Andonova 2013, pp. 239, 245, fig. N 2:4 (iron hearth rake).

Uninventoried: 18 frr. with S-twist, one with Z-twist, of varying thicknesses (total p.L. ca. 1.62 [S-twist], 0.10 [Z-twist]).

Other Bronze

Uninventoried: solid knob or finial with molded profile, vertically pierced (H. 0.063); three frr. of plain heavy rods (total p.L. ca. 0.870); six frr. of thinner rods (total p.L. ca. 0.097).

OBJECTS FROM THE UPPER FILL

88 (P 10848)

Found at 10.50–11.05. Diam. of foot 0.057. Single fr.; two-thirds of foot preserved. Broad-based bowl with reserved resting surface. Shiny black glaze. Graffito on resting surface: ΔA. Cf. *Agora* XII, p. 299, no. 887, fig. 9; *Agora* XXIX, p. 345, nos. 1051–1053, fig. 65, pl. 78.

89 (SS 7794)

Found at 2.15–4.10. P.H. 0.165. Upper part of vertical of handle with beginning of arch.

Κλει(–)

Cf. *Salamine de Chypre* III, p. 18, no. 15. Early Rhodian (before ca. 270).

OBJECTS FROM THE MOUTH OF THE WELL

A 794, a marble triglyph; L 3585 and P 13713–P 13718, a Byzantine lamp and pottery; SS 7793, a Knidian amphora handle, period V (146–108 [KT 432]).

REFERENCES

Ackermann, G., R. Tettamanti, L. Pop, and K. Reber. 2017. "Le gymnase d'Érétrie," *École suisse d'archéologie en Grèce/Schweizerische archäologische Schule in Griechenland: Rapport annuel/Jahresbericht* 2017, pp. 6–9.

Ackermann, G., R. Tettamanti, A.-L. Pradervand, and K. Reber. 2016. "Le gymnase d'Érétrie," *École suisse d'archéologie en Grèce/Schweizerische archäologische Schule in Griechenland: Rapport annuel/Jahresbericht 2016,* pp. 6–9.

———. 2017. "Le gymnase d'Érétrie," *AntK* 60, pp. 126–134.

Adriani, A. 1940. "Fouilles et découvertes," *Annuaire du Musée gréco-romain [Alexandrie]* 1935–1939, pp. 15–163.

Agora = *The Athenian Agora: Results of Excavations Conducted by the American School of Classical Studies at Athens,* Princeton

IV = R. H. Howland, *Greek Lamps and Their Survivals,* 1958.

V = H. S. Robinson, *Pottery of the Roman Period: Chronology,* 1959.

X = M. Lang and M. Crosby, *Weights, Measures, and Tokens,* 1964.

XI = E. B. Harrison, *Archaic and Archaistic Sculpture,* 1965.

XII = B. A. Sparkes and L. Talcott, *Black and Plain Pottery of the 6th, 5th, and 4th Centuries* B.C., 1970.

XIV = H. A. Thompson and R. E. Wycherley, *The Agora of Athens: The History, Shape, and Uses of an Ancient City Center,* 1972.

XVIII = D. J. Geagan, *Inscriptions: The Dedicatory Monuments,* 2011.

XIX = G. V. Lalonde, M. K. Langdon, and M. B. Walbank, *Inscriptions: Horoi, Poletai Records, Leases of Public Lands,* 1991.

XXII = S. I. Rotroff, *Hellenistic Pottery: Athenian and Imported Moldmade Bowls,* 1982.

XXVI = J. H. Kroll, *The Greek Coins,* 1993.

XXIX = S. I. Rotroff, *Hellenistic Pottery: Athenian and Imported Wheelmade Table Ware and Related Material,* 1997.

XXXIII = S. I. Rotroff, *Hellenistic Pottery: The Plain Wares,* 2006.

Alston, R. 2002. *The City in Roman and Byzantine Egypt,* New York.

Andersen, J., J. Watt, J. Olson, and J. Van Aerde. 2006. "Perinatal Brachial Plexus Palsy," *Paediatrics and Child Health* 11, pp. 93–100.

Andonova, A. 2013. "Topography and Classification of Metal Tools from Pistiros (Preliminary Report)," in *Pistiros* V: *Excavations and Studies,* ed. J. Bouzek, L. Domaradzka, A. Gotzev, and Z. H. Archibald, Prague, pp. 238–249.

Andreiomenou, A. K. 1972. "Ἔρευναι καὶ τυχαῖα εὑρήματα ἐν τῇ πόλει καὶ τῇ ἐπαρχίᾳ Χαλκίδος," *ArchDelt* 27, Α΄, pp. 170–184.

Andrianou, D. 2009. *The Furniture and Furnishings of Ancient Greek Houses and Tombs,* Cambridge.

Andronikos, M. 1984. *Vergina: The Royal Tombs and the Ancient City,* trans. L. Turner, Athens.

Angel, J. L. 1945. "Skeletal Material from Attica," *Hesperia* 14, pp. 279–363.

———. 1971. *The People of Lerna: Analysis of a Prehistoric Aegean Population,* Princeton.

Aufderheide, A. C., and C. Rodríguez-Martín. 1998. *The Cambridge Encyclopedia of Human Paleopathology,* Cambridge.

Bagnall, R. S., and B. W. Frier. 1994. *The Demography of Roman Egypt* (Cambridge Studies in Population, Economy, and Society in Past Time 23), Cambridge.

Baills, N. 2003. "Statut et place de l'enfant dans la société romaine," in Gourevitch, Moirin, and Rouquet 2003, pp. 83–89.

Bari, W., R. I. Chowdhury, M. A. Islam, N. Chakraborty, and H. A. H. Akhter. 2002. "The Differentials and Determinants of Perinatal Mortality in Rural Bangladesh," *European Journal of Contraception and Reproductive Health Care* 7, pp. 216–222.

Barnes, E. 1994. *Developmental Defects of the Axial Skeleton in Paleopathology,* Niowot, Colo.

Barnett, R. D. 1982. *Ancient Ivories in the Middle East and Adjacent Countries* (Qedem 14), Jerusalem.

Bass, W. M. 1995. *Human Osteology: A Laboratory and Field Manual* (Special Publications of the Missouri Archaeological Society 2), 4th ed., Columbia, Mo.

Becker, M. H.-J., F. Lassner, J. Bahm, G. Ingianni, and N. Pallua. 2002. "The Cervical Rib: A Predisposing Factor for Obstetric Brachial Plexus Lesions," *Journal of Bone and Joint Surgery* 84, pp. 740–743.

Becker, M. J. 2007. "Childhood Among the Etruscans: Mortuary Programs at Tarquinia as Indicators of the Transition to Adult Status," in *Constructions of Childhood in Ancient Greece and Italy* (*Hesperia* Suppl. 41), ed. A. Cohen and J. B. Rutter, Princeton, pp. 281–292.

———. 2011. "Etruscan Infants: Children's Cemeteries at Tarquinia, Italy, as Indicators of an Age of Transition," in *(Re)Thinking the Little Ancestor: New Perspectives on the Archaeology of Infancy and Childhood* (*BAR-IS* 2271), ed. M. Lally and A. Moore, Oxford, pp. 24–36.

Beers, M. H., and R. Berkow. 1999. *The Merck Manual of Diagnosis and Therapy,* 17th ed., Whitehouse Station, NJ.

Benco, N. L., A. Ettahiri, and M. Loyet. 2002. "Worked Bone Tools: Linking Metal Artisans and Animal Processors in Medieval Islamic Morocco," *Antiquity* 76, pp. 447–457.

Bénichou-Safar, H. 2004. *Le tophet de Salammbô à Carthage: Essai de reconstitution* (*CÉFR* 342), Rome.

Binford, L. R. 1981. *Bones: Ancient Men and Modern Myths,* New York.

Bocquet-Appel, J.-P., and C. Masset. 1982. "Farewell to Paleodemography," *Journal of Human Evolution* 11, pp. 321–333.

Bol, P. C. 1972. *Die Skulpturen des Schiffsfundes von Antikythera* (*AM-BH* 2), Berlin.

Bolkestein, H. 1922. "The Exposure of Children at Athens and the ἐγχυτρίστριαι," *CP* 17, pp. 222–239.

Bonar, B. E. 1937. "Problems of the Newborn," *Journal of Pediatrics* 11, pp. 572–595.

Bonsall, L. 2013. "Infanticide in Roman Britain: A Critical Review of the Osteological Evidence," *Childhood in the Past* 6, pp. 73–88.

Börker, C., and J. Burow. 1998. *Die hellenistischen Amphorenstempel aus Pergamon* (Pergamenische Forschungen 11), Berlin.

Boswell, J. 1988. *The Kindness of Strangers: The Abandonment of Children in Western Europe from Late Antiquity to the Renaissance,* New York.

Bourbou, C., and P. Themelis. 2010. "Child Burials at Ancient Messene," in *L'enfant et la mort dans l'Antiquité* I: *Nouvelles recherches dans les nécropoles grecques: Le signalement des tombes d'enfants* (Travaux de la Maison René-Ginouvès 12), ed. A.-M. Guimier-Sorbets and Y. Morizot, Paris, pp. 111–128.

Bouterie, A. M. 2004. "Hydrocephalus," in *Case Based Pediatrics for Medical Students and Residents,* ed. L. G. Yamamoto, A. S. Inaba, J. K. Okamoto, M. E. Patrinos, and V. K. Yamashiroya, Honolulu, pp. 577–580, http://www.hawaii.edu/medicine/pediatrics/pedtext/pedtext5.pdf.

Bradley, K. R. 1980. "Sexual Regulations in Wet-Nursing Contracts

from Roman Egypt," *Klio* 62, pp. 321–325.
Braun, K. 1970. "Der Dipylon-Brunnen B1: Die Funde," *AM* 85, pp. 129–269.
Breccia, E. 1912. *La necropoli di Sciatbi* (Catalogue général des antiquités égyptiennes [Musée d'Alexandrie] 63, 64), Cairo.
Brothwell, D. 1991. "Nils-Gustaf Gejvall 1911–1991," *International Journal of Osteoarchaeology* 1, p. 283.
Brown, S. 1991. *Late Carthaginian Child Sacrifice and Sacrificial Monuments in their Mediterranean Context* (JSOT/ASOR Monograph Series 3), Sheffield.
Brückner, A. 1909. *Der Friedhof am Eridanos bei der Hagia Triada zu Athen,* Berlin.
Brulé, P. 1992. "Infanticide et abandon d'enfants: Pratiques grecques et comparaisons anthropologiques," *Dialogues d'histoire ancienne* 18, pp. 53–90.
Bucovală, M. 1967. *Necropole elenistice la Tomis,* Constanţa.
Buikstra, J. E., and D. H. Ubelaker, eds. 1994. *Standards for Data Collection from Human Skeletal Remains: Proceedings of a Seminar at the Field Museum of Natural History* (Arkansas Archeological Survey Research Series 44), Fayetteville, Ark.
Burkert, W. 1985. *Greek Religion,* trans. J. Raffan, Cambridge, Mass.
Burnston, S. A. 1982. "Babies in the Well: An Underground Insight into Deviant Behavior in Eighteenth-Century Philadelphia," *Pennsylvania Magazine of History and Biography* 106, pp. 151–186.
———. 1997. "Babies in the Well: An Insight into Deviant Behavior in Eighteenth-Century Philadelphia," in *In Remembrance: Archaeology and Death,* ed. D. A. Poirier and N. F. Bellantoni, Westport, Conn., pp. 51–63.
Burt, W. H. 1960. *Bacula of North American Mammals* (Museum of Zoology, University of Michigan, Miscellaneous Publications 113), Ann Arbor.
Camp, J. McK., II. 1977. "The Water Supply of Ancient Athens from 3000 to 86 B.C." (diss. Princeton Univ.).
Capps, E. 1933. "Foreword," *Hesperia* 2, pp. 90–95.
Caracostea, G. 2003. "Systematic Review on the Incidence/Prevalence of Stillbirths," http://www.gfmer.ch/Endo/Course2003/Stillbirths.htm; accessed July 1, 2017.
Centlivres Challet, C.-E. 2016. "Tire-lait ou biberons romains? Fonctions, fonctionnalités et affectivité," *AC* 85, pp. 157–180.
Charbonneaux, J., R. Martin, and F. Villard. 1973. *Hellenistic Art, 330–50 B.C.* (The Arts of Mankind 18), trans. P. Green, New York.
Charitonides, S. I. 1958. "Ἀνασκαφὴ κλασσικῶν τάφων παρὰ τὴν πλατεῖαν Συντάγματος," *ArchEph* 1958, pp. 1–152.
———. 1979. "Ἀνασκαφὴ παρὰ τὸν Ἅγιον Δημήτριον τὸν Λουμπαρδιάρην ἐν Ἀθήναις," *ArchEph* 1979, pp. 161–187.
Charlier, P. 2003. "La mortalité infantile: Données paléopathologiques," in Gourevitch, Moirin, and Rouquet 2003, pp. 101–104.
Chenal-Velarde, I. 2006. "Food, Rituals? The Exploitation of Dogs from Eretria (Greece) during the Helladic and Hellenistic Periods," in *Dogs and People in Social, Working, Economic, or Symbolic Interaction. Proceedings of the 9th ICAZ Conference, Durham 2002,* ed. L. M. Snyder and E. A. Moore, Oxford, pp. 24–31.
Clement, A., S. Hillson, and M. Michalaki-Kollia. 2009. "The Ancient Cemeteries of Astypalaia, Greece," *Archaeology International* 12, pp. 17–21.
Cocks, A. H. 1921. "A Romano-British Homestead, in the Hambleden Valley, Bucks," *Archaeologia* 71, pp. 141–198.
Collis, J. 1977. "Owslebury (Hants) and the Problem of Burials on Rural Settlements," in *Burial in the Roman World* (Council for British Archaeology Research Report 22), ed. R. Reece, London, pp. 26–34.
Consp. = E. Ettlinger, B. Hedinger, B. Hoffmann, P. M. Kenrick, G. Pucci, K. Roth-Rubi, G. Schneider, S. von Schnurbein, C. M. Wells, and S. Zabehlicky-Scheffenegger, eds. *Conspectus formarum terrae sigillatae italico modo confectae* (Materialien zur römisch-germanischen Keramik 10), Bonn 1990.
Corinth XII = G. R. Davidson, *The Minor Objects* (*Corinth* XII), Princeton 1952.
Corvisier, J.-N., and W. Suder. 2000. *La population de l'Antiquité classique,* Paris.
Couve, L., and E. Bourguet. 1893. "Inscriptions inédites du mur polygonal de Delphes," *BCH* 17, pp. 343–409.
Cunliffe, B. 1975. *Excavations at Portchester Castle* I: *Roman* (Reports of the Research Committee of the Society of Antiquaries of London 32), London.
Dasen, V. 1993. *Dwarfs in Ancient Egypt and Greece,* Oxford.
———. 2013. "Becoming Human: From the Embryo to the Newborn Child," in Evans Grubbs and Parkin 2013, pp. 17–39.
Day, L. P. 1984. "Dog Burials in the Greek World," *AJA* 88, pp. 21–32.
Dedet, B., H. Duday, and A.-M. Tillier. 1991. "Inhumations de foetus, nouveau-nés, et nourrissons dans les habitats protohistoriques du Languedoc: L'exemple de Gailhan (Gard)," *Gallia* 48, pp. 59–108.
Dickemann, M. 1975. "Demographic Consequences of Infanticide in Man," *Annual Review of Ecology and Systematics* 6, pp. 107–137.
———. 1979. "Female Infanticide, Reproductive Strategies, and Social Stratification: A Preliminary Model," in *Evolutionary Biology and Human Social Behavior: An Anthropological Perspective,* ed. N. A. Chagnon and W. Irons, North Scituate, Mass., pp. 321–367.
Didelot, O. 1997. "Réchauds d'époque hellénistique: La diffusion des signatures," in *Le moulage en terre cuite dans l'Antiquité: Création et production dérivée, fabrication et diffusion. Actes du XVIIIe Colloque du Centre de Recherches Archéologiques–Lille III (7–8 déc. 1995),* ed. A. Muller, Villeneuve, pp. 376–395.
Donohue, A. A. 1988. *Xoana and the Origins of Greek Sculpture* (American Classical Studies 15), Atlanta.
Ducrey, P., and S. G. Schmid. 1997. "Les activités de l'École suisse

d'archéologie en Grèce 1996," *AntK* 40, pp. 103–108.

Duday, H., F. Laubenheimer, and A.-M. Tillier. 1995. *Sallèles d'Aude: Nouveau-nés et nourrissons gallo-romains* (Annales littéraires de l'Université de Besançon 563, Centre de recherches d'histoire ancienne 144, série amphores 3), Paris.

Dupras, T. L., H. P. Schwarcz, and S. I. Fairgrieve. 2001. "Infant Feeding and Weaning Practices in Roman Egypt," *American Journal of Physical Anthropology* 115, pp. 204–212.

Durand, R. 2003. "La mortalité infantile en Gaule romaine," in Gourevitch, Moirin, and Rouquet 2003, pp. 97–99.

Dye, T. J., D. Lucy, and A. M. Pollard. 1995. "The Occurrence and Implications of Post-mortem 'Pink Teeth' in Forensic and Archaeological Cases," *International Journal of Osteoarchaeology* 5, pp. 339–348.

Economist, "Gendercide" = "Gendercide: The Worldwide War on Baby Girls," *Economist*, March 6th, 2010, pp. 11, 72–75.

Edwards, C. M. 1984. "Aphrodite on a Ladder," *Hesperia* 53, pp. 59–72.

Edwards, G. R. 1957. "Panathenaics of Hellenistic and Roman Times," *Hesperia* 26, pp. 320–349.

Edwards, M. L. 1996. "The Cultural Context of Deformity in the Ancient Greek World: 'Let There Be a Law That No Deformed Child Shall Be Reared,'" *Ancient History Bulletin* 10, pp. 79–92.

Eleftheratou, S. 1996–1997. "Δύο τελετουργικές πυρές από την ανασκαφή για το 'Μετρό' στο 'οικόπεδο Μακρυγιάννη,'" *ArchDelt* 51–52, A′, pp. 99–118.

Empereur, J.-Y., and Y. Garlan. 1987. "Bulletin archéologique: Amphores et timbres amphoriques (1980–1986)," *RÉG* 100, pp. 58–109.

Engels, D. 1980. "The Problem of Female Infanticide in the Greco-Roman World," *CP* 75, pp. 112–120.

Eretria VIII = P. Ducrey, I. R. Metzger, and K. Reber, *Le quartier de la Maison aux mosaïques* (*Eretria: Fouilles et recherches* VIII), Lausanne 1993.

Espinoza, E. O., and M.-J. Mann. 2000. *Identification Guide for Ivory and Ivory Substitutes*, 3rd ed., Richmond.

EtThas IV = A.-M. Bon and A. Bon, *Les timbres amphoriques de Thasos* (*Études thasiennes* IV), Paris 1957.

Evans Grubbs, J. 2013. "Infant Exposure and Infanticide," in Evans Grubbs and Parkin 2013, pp. 83–107.

Evans Grubbs, J., and T. Parkin, eds. 2013. *The Oxford Handbook of Childhood and Education in the Classical World*, Oxford.

Eyben, E. 1980–1981. "Family Planning in Graeco-Roman Antiquity," *Ancient Society* 11–12, pp. 5–82.

Faerman, M., G. Kahila Bar-Gal, D. Filon, C. L. Greenblatt, L. Stager, A. Oppenheim, and P. Smith. 1998. "Determining the Sex of Infanticide Victims from the Late Roman Era through Ancient DNA Analysis," *JAS* 25, pp. 861–865 (repr. in Stager, Schloen, and Master 2008, pp. 537–540).

Farnell, L. R. 1896. *The Cults of the Greek States*, 5 vols., Oxford.

Fazekas, I. G., and F. Kósa 1978. *Forensic Fetal Osteology*, Budapest.

Feresu, S. A., S. D. Harlow, K. Welch, and B. W. Gillespie. 2005. "Incidence of Stillbirth and Perinatal Mortality and Their Associated Factors among Women Delivering at Harare Maternity Hospital, Zimbabwe: A Cross-Sectional Retrospective Analysis," *BMC Pregnancy and Childbirth* 5:9, doi: 10.1186/1471-2393-5-9.

Ferguson, W. S. 1911. *Hellenistic Athens: An Historical Essay*, London.

Fildes, V. A. 1986. *Breasts, Bottles, and Babies: A History of Infant Feeding*, Edinburgh.

Finkielsztejn, G. 2001. *Chronologie détaillée et révisée des éponymes amphoriques rhodiens, de 270 à 108 av. J.-C. environ: Premier bilan* (*BAR-IS* 990), Oxford.

———. 2004. "Koan Amphorae Imported in the Southern Levant in the Hellenistic Period," in *The Hellenistic Polis of Kos: State, Economy, and Culture. Proceedings of an International Seminar Organized by the Department of Archaeology and Ancient History, Uppsala University, 11–13 May, 2000* (Boreas: Uppsala Studies in Ancient Mediterranean and Near Eastern Civilizations 28), ed. K. Höghammar, Uppsala, pp. 153–164.

Foster, G. V. 1984. "The Bones from the Altar West of the Painted Stoa," *Hesperia* 53, pp. 73–82.

Foster, S. O. 1984. "Immunizable and Respiratory Diseases and Child Mortality," in *Child Survival: Strategies for Research* (Suppl. to *Population and Development Review* 10), ed. W. H. Mosley and L. C. Chen, Cambridge, pp. 119–140.

Franchini, M., and D. Veneri. 2005. "Recent Advances in Hereditary Hemochromatosis," *Annals of Hematology* 84, pp. 347–352.

Frere, S. S. 1987. *Britannia: A History of Roman Britain,* 3rd ed., London.

Frier, B. 1982. "Roman Life Expectancy: Ulpian's Evidence," *HSCP* 86, pp. 213–251.

Galanakis, E. 1998. "Apgar Score and Soranus of Ephesus," *Lancet* 352, pp. 2012–2013.

Gallant, T. W. 1991. *Risk and Survival in Ancient Greece: Reconstructing the Rural Domestic Economy,* Stanford.

Galloway, A., ed. 1999. *Broken Bones: Anthropological Analysis of Blunt Force Trauma,* Springfield, Ill.

Garland, R. 1990. *The Greek Way of Life: From Conception to Old Age,* Ithaca.

———. 1995. *The Eye of the Beholder: Deformity and Disability in the Graeco-Roman World,* Ithaca.

Garnand, B. K. 2002. "From Infant Sacrifice to the ABC's: Ancient Phoenicians and Modern Identities," *Stanford Journal of Archaeology* 1, https://web.stanford.edu/dept/archaeology/journal/newdraft/garnand/; accessed January 18, 2018.

Garnsey, P., and R. Saller. 1987. *The Roman Empire: Economy, Society, and Culture,* London.

Gawlinski, L. 2014. *The Athenian Agora: Museum Guide,* Princeton.

Ghosh, D., P. Gupta, and S. Prabhakar. 1999. "Systemic Brucellosis with Chronic Meningitis: A Case Report," *Neurology India* 47, pp. 58–60.

Gill, D. W. J. 2008. "Inscribed Silver Plate from Tomb II at Vergina: Chronological Implications," *Hesperia* 77, pp. 335–358.

Golden, M. 1981. "Demography and the Exposure of Girls at Athens," *Phoenix* 35, pp. 316–331.

———. 1988. "Did the Ancients Care When Their Children Died?" *GaR* 35, pp. 152–163.

———. 1990. *Children and Childhood in Classical Athens,* Baltimore.

———. 1997. "Change or Continuity? Children and Childhood in Hellenistic Historiography," in *Inventing Ancient Culture: Historicism, Periodization, and the Ancient World,* ed. M. Golden and P. Toohey, London, pp. 176–191.

Gomme, A. W. 1933. *The Population of Athens in the Fifth and Fourth Centuries B.C.* (Glasgow University Publications 28), Oxford.

Goodburn, R., R. P. Wright, M. W. C. Hassall, and R. S. O. Tomlin. 1976. "Roman Britain in 1975," *Britannia* 7, pp. 290–392.

Goodman, A. H., and G. J. Armelagos. 1989. "Infant and Childhood Morbidity and Mortality Risks in Archaeological Populations," *World Archaeology* 21, pp. 225–243.

Gourevitch, D., and J. Chamay. 1992. "Femme nourrissant son enfant au biberon," *AntK* 35, pp. 78–81.

Gourevitch, D., A. Moirin, and N. Rouquet, eds. 2003. *Maternité et petite enfance dans l'Antiquité romaine. Catalogue de l'exposition, Bourges, Muséum d'histoire naturelle, 6 novembre 2003–28 mars 2004,* Bourges.

Goutas, N., S. Simopoulou, V. Petraki, and E. Agapitos. 1993. "Limb Reduction Defects—Autopsy Study," *Fetal and Pediatric Pathology* 13, pp. 29–35.

Gowland, R. L., and A. T. Chamberlain. 2002. "A Bayesian Approach to Ageing Perinatal Skeletal Material from Archaeological Sites: Implications for the Evidence for Infanticide in Roman Britain," *JAS* 29, pp. 677–685.

Grace, V. R. 1949. "Standard Pottery Containers of the Ancient Greek World," in *Commemorative Studies in Honor of Theodore Leslie Shear* (*Hesperia* Suppl. 8), Princeton, pp. 175–189.

———. 1971. "Samian Amphoras," *Hesperia* 40, pp. 52–95.

———. 1979. *Amphoras and the Ancient Wine Trade* (*AgoraPicBk* 6), rev. ed., Princeton.

———. 1985. "The Middle Stoa Dated by Amphora Stamps," *Hesperia* 54, pp. 1–54.

Grace, V. R., and M. Savvatianou-Petropoulakou. 1970. "Les timbres amphoriques grecs," in P. Bruneau et al., *L'îlot de la Maison des comédiens* (*Délos* XXVII), Paris, pp. 277–382.

Graepler, D. 1997. *Tonfiguren im Grab: Fundkontexte hellenistischer Terrakotten aus der Nekropole von Tarent,* Munich.

Graham, E. E. 1908. "Infant Mortality," *Journal of the American Medical Association* 51, pp. 1045–1050.

Greco, E., ed. 2011. *Topografia di Atene: Svilupo urbano e monumenti dalle origini al III secolo d.C.* 2: *Colline sud-occidentali, Valle dell'Ilisso,* Athens.

Green, E. C., A. Jurg, and A. Djedje. 1994. "The Snake in the Stomach: Child Diarrhea in Central Mozambique," *Medical Anthropology Quarterly* n.s. 8, pp. 4–24.

Greenewalt, C. H., Jr. 1978. *Ritual Dinners in Early Historic Sardis* (Classical Studies 17), Berkeley.

Greenguard, J. 1964. "The Battered-Child Syndrome," *American Journal of Nursing* 64, pp. 98–100.

Haas, J. D., H. Balcazar, and L. Caulfield. 1987. "Variation in Early Neonatal Mortality for Different Types of Fetal Growth Retardation," *American Journal of Physical Anthropology* 73, pp. 467–473.

Habicht, C. 1997. *Athens from Alexander to Antony,* trans. D. L. Schneider, Cambridge, Mass.

Hadzisteliou-Price, T. 1978. *Kourotrophos: Cults and Representations of the Greek Nursing Deities* (Studies of the Dutch Archaeological and Historical Society 8), Leiden.

Hamilton, R. 1984. "Sources for the Athenian Amphidromia," *GRBS* 25, pp. 243–251.

———. 2000. *Treasure Map: A Guide to the Delian Inventories,* Ann Arbor.

Hampe, R., and U. Jantzen. 1937. "Eisengeräte und Waffen," *OlBer* 1, pp. 49–64.

Hansen, M. H. 1985. *Demography and Democracy: The Number of Athenian Citizens in the Fourth Century B.C.,* Herning.

———. 1988. *Three Studies in Athenian Demography* (Historisk-filosofiske Meddelelser 56), Copenhagen.

Harris, W. V. 1982. "The Theoretical Possibility of Extensive Infanticide in the Graeco-Roman World," *CQ* 32, pp. 114–116.

Hassan, F. A. 1981. *Demographic Archaeology,* New York.

Hassan, N. A.-M., K. A. Brown, J. Eyers, T. A. Brown, and S. Mays. 2014. "Ancient DNA Study of the Remains of Putative Infanticide Victims from the Yewden Roman Villa Site at Hambleden, England," *JAS* 43, pp. 192–197.

Hausfater, G. 1984. "Infanticide: Comparative and Evolutionary Perspectives," *CurrAnthr* 25, pp. 500–502.

Hayes, J. W. 1985. "Sigillate orientali," in *Atlante delle forme ceramiche* II: *Ceramica fine romana nel bacino mediterraneo (tardo ellenismo e primo impero)* (*EAA* Suppl. 2), Rome, pp. 1–96.

Hillson, S. 2009. "The World's Largest Infant Cemetery and Its Potential for Studying Growth and Development," in *New Directions in the Skeletal Biology of Greece* (*Hesperia* Suppl. 43), ed. L. A. Schepartz, S. C. Fox, and C. Bourbou, Princeton, pp. 137–154.

Hirsch, J. H., F. C. Killien, and R. H. Troupin. 1976. "The Arthropathy of Hemochromatosis," *Radiology* 118, pp. 591–596.

Hobbs, C. J. 1989. "ABC of Child Abuse: Head Injuries," *British Medical Journal* 298, pp. 1169–1170.

Hooper, B. 1975. "The Human Bones," in Cunliffe 1975, pp. 375–377.

Hopkins, K. 1983. *Death and Renewal* (Sociological Studies in Roman History 2), Cambridge.

Houby-Nielsen, S. 2000. "Child Burials in Ancient Athens," in *Children and Material Culture,* ed. J. Sofaer Derevenski, London, pp. 151–166.

Houghton, A., and C. Lorber. 2002. *Seleucid Coins: A Comprehensive Catalogue* I: *Seleucus I through Antiochus III,* New York.

Hughes, D. D. 1991. *Human Sacrifice in Ancient Greece,* London.

Huttmann, A., H. Greiling, U. Tillmanns, and M. Riedel. 1989. "Inhaltsanalysen römischer Säuglingstrinkgefässe," *KölnJb* 22, pp. 365–372.

Huys, M. 1989. "Ἔκθεσις and Ἀπόθεσις: The Terminology of Infant Exposure in Greek Antiquity," *AntCl* 58, pp. 190–197.

Jäger, H. J., U.-M. Mehring, G. F. Götz, M. Neise, R. Erlemann, H. J. Kapp, and K. D. Mathias. 1997. "Radiological Features of the Visceral and Skeletal Involvement of Hemochromatosis," *European Radiology* 7, pp. 1199–1206.

Jankauskas, R., and M. Schultz. 1995. "Meningeal Reactions in a Late Medieval–Early Modern Child Population from Alytus, Lithuania," *Journal of Paleopathology,* 7, p. 106 (abstract).

Jefremow, N. 1995. *Die Amphorenstempel des hellenistischen Knidos* (Quellen und Forschungen zur antiken Welt 19), Munich.

Johnston, S. I. 1990. *Hekate Soteira: A Study of Hekate's Roles in the Chaldean Oracles and Related Literature* (American Classical Studies 21), Atlanta.

———. 1995. "Defining the Dreadful: Remarks on the Greek Child-Killing Demon," in *Ancient Magic and Ritual Power* (Religions in the Graeco-Roman World 129), ed. M. Meyer and P. Mirecki, Leiden, pp. 361–387.

Jöhrens, G. 1999. *Amphorenstempel im Nationalmuseum von Athen: Zu den von H. G. Lolling aufgenommenen "unedierten Henkelinschriften,"* Mainz.

Jordan, D. R., and S. I. Rotroff. 1999. "A Curse in a Chytridion: A Contribution to the Study of Athenian Pyres," *Hesperia* 68, pp. 147–154.

Jouanna, J. 1999. *Hippocrates,* trans. M. B. DeBevoise, Baltimore.

Kaltsas, N., E. Vlachogianni, and P. Bouyia. 2012. *The Antikythera Shipwreck: The Ship, the Treasures, the Mechanism,* Athens.

Katzenberg, M. A., D. A. Herring, and S. R. Saunders. 1996. "Weaning and Infant Mortality: Evaluating the Skeletal Evidence," *Yearbook of Physical Anthropology* 39, pp. 177–199.

Kemp, A. M., F. Dunstan, S. Harrison, S. Morris, M. Mann, K. Rolfe, S. Datta, D. P. Thomas, J. R. Sibert, and S. Maguire. 2008. "Patterns of Skeletal Fractures in Child Abuse: Systematic Review," *British Medical Journal* 337, pp. 1–8, doi: 10.1136/bmj.a1518.

Kerameikos = *Kerameikos: Ergebnisse der Ausgrabungen*
V.i = K. Kübler, *Die Nekropole des 10. bis 8. Jahrhunderts,* Berlin 1954.
IX = U. Knigge, *Der Südhügel,* Berlin 1976.
XIV = W. Kovacsovics, *Die Eckterrasse an der Gräberstrasse des Kerameikos,* Berlin 1990.
XVII = U. Knigge, *Der Bau Z,* Munich 2005.

Kevill-Davies, S. 1991. *Yesterday's Children: The Antiques and History of Childcare,* Woodbridge.

Kitamura, H., and B. S. Kraus. 1964. "Visceral Variations and Defects Associated with Cleft Lip and Palate in Human Fetuses: A Macroscopic Description," *Cleft Palate Journal* 16, pp. 99–115.

Knigge, U. 1966. "Eridanos–Nekropole II. Gräber hS 205–230," *AM* 81, pp. 112–134.

Knodel, J. E. 1988. *Demographic Behavior in the Past: A Study of Fourteen German Village Populations in the Eighteenth and Nineteenth Centuries,* Cambridge.

Knoepfler, D. 1993. "Les *kryptoi* du stratège Épicharès à Rhamnonte et le début de la guerre de Chrémonidès," *BCH* 117, pp. 327–341.

———. 1995. "Les relations des cités eubéennes avec Antigone Gonatas et la chronologie delphique au début de l'époque étolienne," *BCH* 119, pp. 137–159.

Koch, G. 1984. "Zum Grabrelief der Helena," *GettyMusJ* 12, pp. 59–72.

Kochar, D. K., B. L. Kumawat, N. Agarwal, Shubharakaran, S. Aseri, B. V. Sharma, and A. Rastogi. 2000. "Meningoencephalitis in Brucellosis," *Neurology India* 48, pp. 170–173.

Koehler, C. G., and P. M. W. Matheson. 2004. "Knidian Amphora Chronology, Pergamon to Corinth," in *Transport Amphorae and Trade in the Eastern Mediterranean. Acts of the International Colloquium at the Danish Institute at Athens, September 26–29, 2002* (Monographs of the Danish Institute at Athens 5), ed. J. Eiring and J. Lund, Aarhus, pp. 163–169.

Konigsberg, L. W., and S. R. Frankenberg. 1992. "Estimation of Age Structure in Anthropological Demography," *American Journal of Physical Anthropology* 89, pp. 235–256.

Konigsberg, L. W., and M. A. Liston. 2013. "Paleodemography and Perinatal Mortality from the Agora Well, Athens, Greece," *American Journal of Physical Anthropology* 150 (S56), p. 171 (abstract).

Koukouli-Chrysanthaki, C. 1983. "Ἀνασκαφικὲς ἔρευνες στὴν ἀρχαία Τράγιλο," in *Ancient Macedonia* III: *Papers Read at the Third International Symposium Held in Thessaloniki, September 21–25, 1977,* Thessaloniki, pp. 123–146.

Kozin, S. H. 2007. "Radial Clubhand," http://www.emedicine.com/article/1243998-overview; accessed May 12, 2008.

Kraus, T. 1960. *Hekate: Studien zu Wesen und Bild der Göttin in Kleinasien und Griechenland* (Heidelberger kunstgeschichtliche Abhandlungen 5), Heidelberg.

Kroll, J. H. 1982. "The Ancient Image of Athena Polias," in *Studies in Athenian Architecture, Sculpture, and Topography Presented to Homer A. Thompson* (*Hesperia* Suppl. 20), Princeton, pp. 65–76.

Krstić, V. 2004. "Hellenistic Pottery from Budva from the Greek Collection of the National Museum of Belgrade," in *ΣΤ΄ Επιστημονική συνάντηση για την ελληνιστική κεραμική: Προβλήματα χρονολόγησης κλειστά, σύνολα-εργαστήρια, Βόλος 17–23 Απριλίου 2000,* ed. M. Kazakou, Athens, pp. 585–592.

Kunze, M. 1992. *Die Antikensammlung im Pergamonmuseum und in Charlottenburg,* Mainz.

Kuo, S. 2004. "Congenital and Perinatal Infections," in *Case Based Pediatrics for Medical Students and Residents,* ed. L. G. Yamamoto, A. S. Inaba, J. K. Okamoto, M. E. Patrinos, and V. K. Yamashiroya, Honolulu, pp. 107–110, http://www.hawaii.edu/medicine/pediatrics/pedtext/pedtext5.pdf.

Lacey, W. K. 1968. *The Family in Classical Greece,* London.

Lacombe, D. 2004. "Genetic Osteoarticular Diseases under the Molecular Biology Spotlight," *Joint Bone Spine* 71, pp. 486–492.

Lalonde, G. V. 2006. "*IG* I[3] 1055 B and the Boundary of Melite and Kollytos," *Hesperia* 75, pp. 83–119.

Langenegger, E. 1996. "'Hominem priusquam genito dente cremari mos genitum non est' (Plinius): Zu den Neonatengräbern im römischen Gutshof von Neftenbach ZH," *ArchSchw* 19, pp. 156–158.

Langlotz, E. 1954. *Aphrodite in den Gärten* (*SBHeid* 2), Heidelberg.

Latte, K., ed. 1953. *Hesychii Alexandrini lexicon* 1, Copenhagen.

Lawall, M. L. 2002. "Early Excavations at Pergamon and the Chronology of Rhodian Amphora Stamps," *Hesperia* 71, pp. 295–324.

Lewis, M. E. 2004. "Endocranial Lesions in Non-adult Skeletons: Understanding Their Aetiology," *International Journal of Osteoarchaeology* 14, pp. 82–97.

———. 2007. *The Bioarchaeology of Children: Perspectives from Biological and Forensic Anthropology* (Cambridge Studies in Biological and Evolutionary Anthropology 50), Cambridge.

Lewis, M. E., and R. Gowland. 2007. "Brief and Precarious Lives: Infant Mortality in Contrasting Sites from Medieval and Post-Medieval England (A.D. 850–1859)," *American Journal of Physical Anthropology* 134, pp. 117–129.

Lippolis, E. 2009. "Le moderne peregrinazioni di Apollo e di Afrodite nell'agorà di Atene," *ASAtene* 87, pp. 235–273.

Liston, M. A. 2017. "Human Skeletal Remains," in J. K. Papadopoulos and E. L. Smithson, *The Early Iron Age: The Cemeteries* (*Agora* XXXVI), Princeton, pp. 503–560.

Liston, M. A., and J. K. Papadopoulos. 2004. "The 'Rich Athenian Lady' Was Pregnant: The Anthropology of a Geometric Tomb Reconsidered," *Hesperia* 73, 7–38.

Liston, M. A., and S. I. Rotroff. 2013a. "Babies in the Well: Archaeological Evidence for Newborn Disposal in Hellenistic Greece," in Evans Grubbs and Parkin 2013, pp. 62–82.

———. 2013b. "Des bébés dans un puits: Un témoignage de l'abandon des nouveau-nés en Grèce hellénistique," *Dossiers d'Archéologie* 356, pp. 74–79.

Little, L. M. 1999. "Babies in Well G5:3: Preliminary Results and Future Analysis," *AJA* 103, p. 284 (abstract).

Little, L. M., and J. K. Papadopoulos. 1998. "A Social Outcast in Early Iron Age Athens," *Hesperia* 67, pp. 375–404.

Livi-Bacci, M. 1991. *Population and Nutrition: An Essay on European Demographic History* (Cambridge Studies in Population, Economy, and Society in Past Time 14), trans. T. Croft-Murray, Cambridge.

Lovejoy, C. O., R. S. Meindl, T. R. Pryzbeck, and R. P. Mensforth. 1985. "Chronological Metamorphosis of the Auricular Surface of the Ilium: A New Method for the Determination of Adult Skeletal Age at Death," *American Journal of Physical Anthropology* 68, pp. 15–28.

Lüdorf, G. 2000. *Die Lekane: Typologie und Chronologie einer Leitform der attischen Gebrauchskeramik des 6.–1. Jahrhunderts v. Chr.* (Internationale Archäologie 61), Rahden.

Lummaa, V., T. Vuorisalo, R. G. Barr, and L. Lehtonen. 1998. "Why Cry? Adaptive Significance of Intensive Crying in Human Infants," *Evolution and Human Behaviour* 19, pp. 193–202.

Lyman, R. L. 1994. *Vertebrate Taphonomy,* Cambridge.

———. 2008. *Quantitative Paleozoology,* Cambridge.

Martorell, R., and T. González-Cossío. 1987. "Maternal Nutrition and Birth Weight," *Yearbook of Physical Anthropology* 30, pp. 195–220.

Masson, O. 1950. "À propos d'un rituel hittite pour la lustration d'une armée," *RHR* 137, pp. 5–25.

Mauzy, C. A. 2009. "A Pictorial History of the Agora Excavations," in *The Athenian Agora: New Perspectives on an Ancient Site,* ed. J. McK. Camp II and C. A. Mauzy, Mainz, pp. 87–112.

Mays, S. 1993. "Infanticide in Roman Britain," *Antiquity* 67, pp. 883–888.

———. 2003. "Comment on 'A Bayesian Approach to Ageing Perinatal Skeletal Material from Archaeological Sites: Implications for the Evidence for Infanticide in Roman Britain,' by R. L. Gowland and A. T. Chamberlain," *JAS* 30, pp. 1695–1700.

Mays, S., and J. Eyers. 2011. "Perinatal Infant Death at the Roman Villa Site at Hambleden, Buckinghamshire, England," *JAS* 38, pp. 1931–1938.

Mays, S., and M. Faerman. 2001. "Sex Identification in Some Putative Infanticide Victims from Roman Britain Using Ancient DNA," *JAS* 28, pp. 555–559.

Meindl, R. S., C. O. Lovejoy, R. P. Mensforth, and R. A. Walker. 1985. "A Revised Method of Age Determination Using the Os Pubis, with a Review and Tests of Accuracy of Other Current Methods of Pubic Symphyseal Ageing," *American Journal of Physical Anthropology* 68, pp. 29–45.

Metzger, H. 1965. *Recherches sur l'imagerie athénienne* (Publications de la Bibliothèque Salomon Reinach 2), Paris.

Meyer, C. L., and M. Oberman. 2001. *Mothers Who Kill Their Children: Understanding the Acts of Moms from Susan Smith to the "Prom Mom,"* New York.

Mikalson, J. D. 1998. *Religion in Hellenistic Athens* (Hellenistic Culture and Society 29), Berkeley.

Miller, S. G. 1974. "Menon's Cistern," *Hesperia* 43, pp. 194–245.

Mittler, D. M., and S. G. Sheridan. 1992. "Sex Determination in Subadults Using Auricular Surface Morphology: A Forensic Science Perspective," *Journal of Forensic Sciences* 37, pp. 1068–1075.

Moalem, S., E. D. Weinberg, and M. E. Percy. 2004. "Hemochromatosis and the Enigma of Misplaced Iron: Implications for Infectious Disease and Survival," *BioMetals* 17, pp. 135–139.

Molleson, T. 2003. "The Archaeology of Family Planning and the Role of Infanticide," *Archaeological Review from Cambridge* 16, pp. 117–127.

Monaco, M. C. 2001. "Contributi allo studio di alcuni santuari ateniesi I: Il *temenos* del *Demos* e delle *Charites,*" *ASAtene* 79, pp. 103–150.

Morris, I. 1992. *Death-Ritual and Social Structure in Classical Antiquity,* Cambridge.
Morris, S. P. 1985. "ΛΑΣΑΝΑ: A Contribution to the Ancient Greek Kitchen," *Hesperia* 54, pp. 393–409.
Munsell Soil Color Charts, rev. ed., Baltimore 1994.
Murail, P., B. Maureille, D. Peresinotto, and F. Geus. 2004. "An Infant Cemetery of the Classic Kerma Period (1750–1500 B.C., Island of Saï, Sudan)," *Antiquity* 78, pp. 267–277.
Mutolo, M. J., L. L. Jenny, A. R. Buszek, T. W. Fenton, and D. R. Foran. 2012. "Osteological and Molecular Identification of Brucellosis in Ancient Butrint, Albania," *American Journal of Physical Anthropology* 147, pp. 254–263.
Mylonas, G. E. 1948. "Homeric and Mycenaean Burial Customs," *AJA* 52, pp. 56–81.
Naidu, S., J. Moodley, M. Adhikari, R. Ramsaroop, N. Morar, and O. O. Dunmoye. 2001. "Clinico-pathological Study of Causes of Perinatal Mortality in a Developing Country," *Journal of Obstetrics and Gynaecology* 21, pp. 443–447.
Narchi, H. 2013. "Hypernatremia in Children," *Journal of Pediatric Biochemistry* 3, pp. 213–224.
Nasheit, N. A. 2003. "Perinatal and Neonatal Mortality and Morbidity in Iraq," *Journal of Maternal-Fetal and Neonatal Medicine* 13, pp. 64–67.
Nauck = A. Nauck, *Tragicorum graecorum fragmenta,* 2nd ed., Leipzig 1889.
Nicolaou, I. 1989. "Les bouillottes thérapeutiques de Paphos et leurs parallèles hors de Chypre," *BCH* 113, pp. 301–318.
Nilsson, M. P. 1941. *Geschichte der griechischen Religion* 1 (Handbuch der Altertumswissenschaft 5.2), Munich.
Ohly, D. 1965. "Kerameikos-Grabung: Tätigkeitsbericht 1956–1961," *AA* 80, cols. 277–376.
Oliver, J. S. 1993. "Carcass Processing by the Hadza: Bone Breakage from Butchery to Consumption," in *From Bones to Behavior: Ethnoarchaeological and Experimental Contributions to the Interpretation of Faunal Remains* (Center for Archaeological Investigations Occasional Paper 21), ed. J. Hudson, Carbondale, Ill., pp. 200–227.
Olynthus = Excavations at Olynthus, Baltimore
V = D. M. Robinson, *Mosaics, Vases, and Lamps of Olynthus Found in 1928 and 1931,* 1933.
XI = D. M. Robinson, *Necrolynthia: A Study in Greek Burial Customs and Anthropology,* 1942.
XIII = D. M. Robinson, *Vases Found in 1934 and 1938,* 1950.
Ortner, D. J. 2003. *Identification of Pathological Conditions in Human Skeletal Remains,* 2nd ed., San Diego.
Osanna, M. 1988–1989. "Il problema topografico del santuario di Afrodite Urania ad Atene," *ASAtene* 66–67, pp. 73–95.
Osborne, R. 1985. *Demos: The Discovery of Classical Attika,* Cambridge.
———. 1987. *Classical Landscape with Figures: The Ancient Greek City and Its Countryside,* London.
Owsley, D. W., and R. L. Jantz. 1985. "Long Bone Lengths and Gestational Age Distributions of Post-contact Period Arikara Indian Perinatal Infant Skeletons," *American Journal of Physical Anthropology* 68, pp. 321–328.
Pagenstecher, R. 1913. *Die Gefässe in Stein und Ton, Knochenschnitzereien* (Expedition Ernst von Sieglin, Die griechisch-ägyptische Sammlung Ernst von Sieglin II.3), Leipzig.
Pandermalis, D. 2004. *Alexander the Great: Treasures from an Epic Era of Hellenism,* New York.
Papadopoulos, J. K. 2000. "Skeletons in Wells: Towards an Archaeology of Social Exclusion in the Ancient Greek World," in *Madness, Disability, and Social Exclusion: The Archaeology and Anthropology of "Difference"* (One World Archaeology 40), ed. J. Hubert, London, pp. 96–118.
Papagrigorakis, M. J., C. Yapijakis, P. N. Synodinos, and E. Baziotopoulou-Valavani. 2006. "DNA Examination of Ancient Dental Pulp Indicates Typhoid Fever as a Probable Cause of the Plague of Athens," *International Journal of Infectious Diseases* 10, pp. 206–214.
Paradise, J. L., C. D. Bluestone, and H. Felder. 1969. "The Universality of Otitis Media in 50 Infants with Cleft Palate," *Pediatrics* 44, pp. 35–42.
Paradiso, A. 1988. "L'agrégation du nouveau-né au foyer familial: Les Amphidromies," *Dialogues d'histoire ancienne* 14, pp. 203–218.
Parfitt, A. M. 1998. "Osteomalacia and Related Disorders," in *Metabolic Bone Disease and Clinically Related Disorders,* ed. L. V. Avioli and S. M. Krane, 3rd ed., San Diego, pp. 327–386.
Parker, H. N. 1999. "Greek Embryological Calendars and a Fragment from the Lost Work of Damastes, *On the Care of Pregnant Women and of Infants,*" *CQ* 49, pp. 515–534.
Parker, R. 1983. *Miasma: Pollution and Purification in Early Greek Religion,* Oxford.
Parkin, T. G. 1992. *Demography and Roman Society,* Baltimore.
Parlama, L., and N. C. Stampolides. 2000. *Athens: The City beneath the City. Antiquities from the Metropolitan Railway Excavations,* Athens.
Patterson, C. 1985. "'Not Worth the Rearing': The Causes of Infant Exposure in Ancient Greece," *TAPA* 115, pp. 103–123.
PCG = R. Kassel and C. Austin, eds., *Poetae comici graeci,* 8 vols., Berlin 1983–.
Penn, W. S. 1967. "Possible Evidence from Springhead for the Great Plague of A.D. 166," *Archaeologia cantiana* 82, pp. 263–271.
Petsas, P. M. 1963. "Ἀνασκαφὴ ἀρχαίου νεκροταφείου Βεργίνης," *ArchDelt* 18, B′2, pp. 217–232.
———. 1966. *Ὁ τάφος τῶν Λευκαδίων* (Βιβλιοθήκη τῆς ἐν Ἀθήναις Ἀρχαιολογικῆς Ἑταιρείας 57), Athens.
Pingiatoglou, S. 1981. *Eileithyia,* Würzburg.
Pirenne-Delforge, V. 1994. *L'Aphrodite grecque: Contribution à l'étude de ses cultes et de sa personnalité dans le panthéon archaïque et classique* (*Kernos* Suppl. 4), Athens.
Plunkett, J. 2001. "Fatal Pediatric Head Injuries Caused by Short-Distance Falls," *American Journal of Forensic Medicine and Pathology* 22, pp. 1–12.
Pomeroy, S. B. 1983. "Infanticide in Hellenistic Greece," in *Images of Women in Antiquity,* ed. A. Cameron and A. Kuhrt, Detroit, pp. 207–222.

Pounder, R. L. 1983. "A Hellenistic Arsenal in Athens," *Hesperia* 52, pp. 233–256.

Prosser, I., Z. Lawson, A. Evans, S. Harrison, S. Morris, S. Maguire, and A. M. Kemp. 2012. "A Timetable for the Radiologic Features of Fracture Healing in Young Children," *American Journal of Roentgenology* 198, pp. 1014–1020, doi: 10.2214/AJR.11.6734.

Pullinger, J. 1978. "The Cambridge Shrine," *Current Archaeology* 61, pp. 57–60.

Rahmani, L. Y. 1984. "Hellenistic Brazier Fragments from Israel," *IEJ* 34, pp. 224–231.

Reese, D. S. 1989. "Faunal Remains from the Altar of Aphrodite Ourania, Athens," *Hesperia* 58, pp. 63–70.

Rega, E. 1997. "Age, Gender, and Biological Reality in the Early Bronze Age Cemetery at Mokrin," in *Invisible People and Processes: Writing Gender and Childhood into European Archaeology,* ed. J. Moore and E. Scott, London, pp. 229–247.

Remouchamps, A. E. 1926. *Griechische Dolch- und Schwertformen: Ein Beitrag zur Chronologie der europäischen Bronzezeit,* Leiden.

Resnick, D. 1995. *Diagnosis of Bone and Joint Disorders,* 3rd ed., 6 vols., Philadelphia.

Resnick, P. J. 1970. "Murder of the Newborn: A Psychiatric Review of Neonaticide," *American Journal of Psychiatry* 126, pp. 1414–1420.

Richards, G. D., and S. C. Anton. 1991. "Craniofacial Configuration and Postcranial Development of a Hydrocephalic Child (ca. 2500 B.C.–500 A.D.): With a Review of Cases and Comment on Diagnostic Criteria," *American Journal of Physical Anthropology* 85, pp. 185–200.

Richter, G. M. A. 1966. *The Furniture of the Greeks, Etruscans, and Romans,* London.

Rihl, M., and H. Kellner. 2004. "Die Arthropathie der hereditären Hämochromatose," *Zeitschrift für Rheumatologie* 63, pp. 22–29.

Riley, J. A. 1979. "The Coarse Pottery from Berenice," in *Excavations at Sidi Khrebish, Benghazi (Berenice)* II (*LibAnt* Suppl. 5.2), ed. J. A. Lloyd, Tripoli, pp. 91–467.

Roberts, C. A., and J. E. Buikstra. 2003. *The Bioarchaeology of Tuberculosis: A Global View on a Reemerging Disease,* Gainesville, Fla.

Rogers, J., and T. Waldron. 1995. *A Field Guide to Joint Disease in Archaeology,* New York.

Rohde, E. 1925. *Psyche: The Cult of Souls and Belief in Immortality among the Greeks,* 8th ed., trans. W. B. Hillis, New York.

Rosenzweig, R. 2004. *Worshipping Aphrodite: Art and Cult in Classical Athens,* Ann Arbor.

Rosivach, V. J. 1993. "The Distribution of Population in Attica," *GRBS* 34, pp. 391–407.

Rostovtzeff, M. 1941. *The Social and Economic History of the Hellenistic World,* Oxford.

Rotroff, S. I. 1983. "Three Cistern Systems on the Kolonos Agoraios," *Hesperia* 52, pp. 257–297.

———. 1988. "The Long-Petal Bowl from the Pithos Settling Basin," *Hesperia* 57, pp. 87–93.

———. 1999. "The Artifacts from Well G5:3 and Some Conclusions Concerning the Deposit," *AJA* 103, pp. 284–285 (abstract).

———. 2001. Rev. of G. de Luca and W. Radt, *Sondagen im Fundament des Grossen Altars* (Pergamenische Forschungen 12), *AJA* 105, 129–130.

———. 2011a. "Ceramic Measures in Hellenistic Athens," in *Ζ΄ Επιστημονική συνάντηση για την ελληνιστική κεραμική, Αίγιο, 4–9 Απριλίου 2005,* Athens, pp. 699–704.

———. 2011b. "The Date of the Long-Petal Bowl: A Review of the Contextual Evidence," in *Ζ΄ Επιστημονική συνάντηση για την ελληνιστική κεραμική, Αίγιο, 4–9 Απριλίου 2005,* Athens, pp. 635–644.

———. 2011c. "Mended in Antiquity: Repairs to Ceramics at the Athenian Agora," in *Pottery in the Archaeological Record: Greece and Beyond. Acts of the International Colloquium Held at the Danish and Canadian Institutes in Athens, June 20–22, 2008,* ed. M. L. Lawall and J. Lund, Aarhus, pp. 117–134.

———. 2013. *Industrial Religion: The Saucer Pyres of the Athenian Agora* (*Hesperia* Suppl. 47), Princeton.

———. 2014. "The Pottery from the Agora Bone Well," in *Η΄ Επιστημονική συνάντηση για την ελληνιστική κεραμική, Ιωάννινα, 5–9 Μαΐου 2009,* Athens, pp. 517–527.
Rouquet, N. 2003. "Les biberons, les tire-lait ou les tribulations d'une tubulure peu commune . . ." in Gourevitch, Moirin, and Rouquet 2003, pp. 171–177.
Russell, J. C. 1958. *Late Ancient and Medieval Population* (*TAPS* 48.3), Philadelphia.
Sabetai, V. 2000. "Παιδικές τάφες Ακραιφίας," in *Επετηρίς της Εταιρείας Βοιωτικών Μελετών. Γ΄ Διεθνές Συνέδριο Βοιωτικών Μελετών, Θήβα, 4–8 Σεπτεμβρίου 1996,* pp. 494–535, Athens.
Salamine de Chypre III = Y. Calvet, *Les timbres amphoriques (1965–1970)* (*Salamine de Chypre* III), Paris 1972.
Sallares, R. 1991. *The Ecology of the Ancient Greek World,* Ithaca.
Sallares, R., and S. Gomzi. 2001. "Biomolecular Archaeology of Malaria," *Ancient Biomolecules* 3, pp. 195–213.
Sallares, R., S. Gomzi, A. Bouwman, C. Anderung, and T. Brown. 2003. "Identification of a Malaria Epidemic in Antiquity Using Ancient DNA," in *Archaeological Sciences 1999. Proceedings of the Archaeological Sciences Conference, University of Bristol, 1999* (*BAR-IS* 1111), ed. K. A. Robson Brown, Oxford, pp. 120–125.
Schaeffer, C. F.-A. 1962. *Ugaritica* IV: *Découvertes des XVIII*e *et XIX*e *campagnes, 1951–1955* (Mission de Ras Shamra 15; Bibliothèque archéologique et historique 74), Paris.
Scheidel, W. 2001. "Roman Age Structure: Evidence and Models," *JRS* 91, pp. 1–26.
Scheuer, J. L., J. H. Musgrave, and S. P. Evans. 1980. "The Estimation of Late Fetal and Perinatal Age from Limb Bone Length by Linear and Logarithmic Regression," *Annals of Human Biology* 7, pp. 257–265.
Scheuer, L., and S. Black. 2000. *Developmental Juvenile Osteology,* San Diego.
———. 2004. *The Juvenile Skeleton,* London.
Schlörb-Vierneisel, B. 1966. "Eridanos-Nekropole I: Gräber und Opferstellen hS 1–204," *AM* 81, pp. 4–111.
Schmid, S. G. 2000. "A Group of Early Hellenistic Pottery from a Well in Eretria," in *Ε΄ Επιστημονική συνάντηση για την ελληνιστική κεραμική, Χανιά, Απρίλιος 1997,* Athens, pp. 361–372.
Schmidt, M. 1983–1984. "Hephaistos lebt: Untersuchungen zur Frage der Behandlung behinderter Kinder in der Antike," *Hephaistos* 5–6, pp. 133–161.
Schmitt, M., ed. 1858. *Hesychii Alexandrini lexicon* 1, Jena.
Schoch, K. 2009. *Die doppelte Aphrodite: Alt und Neu bei griechischen Kultbildern,* Göttingen.
Schutkowski, H. 1987. "Sex Determination of Fetal and Neonate Skeletons by Means of Discriminant Analysis," *International Journal of Anthropology* 2, pp. 347–352.
———. 1993. "Sex Determination of Infant and Juvenile Skeletons: I. Morphognostic Features," *American Journal of Physical Anthropology* 90, pp. 199–205.
Schwartz, J. H. 1993. *What the Bones Tell Us,* New York.
Schwidetzky, I. 1965. "Sonderbestattungen und ihre paläodemographische Bedeutung," *Homo* 16, pp. 230–247.
Scott, E. 1991. "Animal and Infant Burials in Romano-British Villas: A Revitalization Movement," in *Sacred and Profane. Proceedings of a Conference on Archaeology, Ritual, and Religion, Oxford, 1989* (Oxford University Committee for Archaeology Monograph 32), ed. P. Garwood, D. Jennings, R. Skeates, and J. Toms, Oxford, pp. 115–121.
———. 1999. *The Archaeology of Infancy and Infant Death* (*BAR-IS* 819), Oxford.
———. 2001. "Killing the Female? Archaeological Narratives of Infanticide," in *Gender and the Archaeology of Death* (Gender and Archaeology 2), ed. B. Arnold and N. L. Wicker, Walnut Creek, pp. 3–21.
Scott, S., S. R. Duncan, and C. J. Duncan. 1995. "Infant Mortality and Famine: A Study in Historical Epidemiology in Northern England," *Journal of Epidemiology and Community Health* 49, pp. 245–252.
Shay, T. 1985. "Differentiated Treatment of Deviancy at Death as Revealed in Anthropological and Archaeological Material," *JAnthArch* 4, pp. 221–241.
Shear, T. L. 1933. "The Campaign of 1932," *Hesperia* 2, pp. 451–474.
———. 1938. "The Campaign of 1937," *Hesperia* 7, pp. 311–362.
———. 1939. "The Campaign of 1938," *Hesperia* 8, pp. 201–246.
Shear, T. L., Jr. 1969. "The Athenian Agora: Excavations of 1968," *Hesperia* 38, pp. 382–417.
———. 1973a. "The Athenian Agora: Excavations of 1971," *Hesperia* 42, pp. 121–179.
———. 1973b. "The Athenian Agora: Excavations of 1972," *Hesperia* 42, pp. 359–407.
———. 1984. "The Athenian Agora: Excavations of 1980–1982," *Hesperia* 53, pp. 1–57.
Sherwood, R. J., R. S. Meindl, H. B. Robinson, and R. L. May. 2000. "Fetal Age: Methods of Estimation and Effects of Pathology," *American Journal of Physical Anthropology* 113, pp. 305–315.
Silver, I. A. 1969. "The Aging of Domestic Animals," in *Science in Archaeology: A Survey of Progress and Research,* ed. D. R. Brothwell and E. Higgs, rev. ed., London, pp. 283–302.
Sim, S. Y., S. H. Yoon, and S. Y. Kim. 2012. "Quantitative Analysis of Developmental Process of Cranial Suture in Korean Infants," *Journal of the Korean Neurosurgery Society* 51, pp. 31–36.
Simmons, G. B., C. Smucker, S. Bernstein, and E. Jensen. 1982. "Post-neonatal Mortality in Rural India: Implications of an Economic Model," *Demography* 19, pp. 371–389.
Smith, P., and G. Kahila. 1992. "Identification of Infanticide in Archaeological Sites: A Case Study from the Late Roman–Early Byzantine Periods at Ashkelon, Israel," *JAS* 19, pp. 667–675.
Smithson, E. L. 1974. "A Geometric Cemetery on the Areopagus: 1897, 1932, 1947," *Hesperia* 43, pp. 325–390.
Sneed, D. 2018. "Nourishing Infants: The Function of Ancient Greek Feeding Bottles," *Archaeological*

Institute of America, 119th Annual Meeting Abstracts 41, Boston, pp. 270–271 (abstract).

Snyder, L. M. 1999. "The Animal Bones from Well G5:3: Domestic Debris, Industrial Debris, and Possible Evidence for the Sacrifice of Domestic Dogs in Late Hellenistic Athens," *AJA* 103, p. 284 (abstract).

Soren, D. 2003. "Can Archaeologists Excavate Evidence of Malaria?" *World Archaeology* 35, pp. 193–209.

Soren, D., and N. Soren, eds. 1999. *A Roman Villa and a Late Roman Infant Cemetery: Excavation at Poggio Gramignano, Lugnano in Teverina* (Bibliotheca archaeologica 23), Rome.

Sourlas, D. 2017. "In Search of Eileithyia and Aphrodite Pandemos: Two New Classical Reliefs from Athens," in *Kulte und Heiligtümer in Griechenland: Neue Funde und Forschungen,* ed. H. Frielinghaus and J. Stroszeck, Möhnesee, pp. 163–191.

Stager, L. E. 1982. "Carthage: A View from the Tophet," in *Phönizier im Westen: Die Beiträge des Internationalen Symposiums über "Die phönizische Expansion im westlichen Mittelmeerraum" in Köln vom 24. bis 27. April 1979,* ed. H. G. Niemeyer, Mainz, pp. 155–166.

———. 1991a. "Eroticism and Infanticide at Ashkelon," *Biblical Archaeology Review* 17(4), pp. 35–53 (repr. in L. E. Stager, *Ashkelon Discovered: From Canaanites and Philistines to Romans and Moslems,* Washington, D.C., 1991, pp. 38–57).

———. 1991b. "Why Were Hundreds of Dogs Buried at Ashkelon?" *Biblical Archaeology Review* 17(3), pp. 27–42 (repr. in L. E. Stager, *Ashkelon Discovered: From Canaanites and Philistines to Romans and Moslems,* Washington, D.C., 1991, pp. 20–36).

Stager, L. E., J. D. Schloen, and D. M. Master. 2008. *Ashkelon* I: *Introduction and Overview (1985–2006),* Winona Lake.

Stager, L. E., J. D. Schloen, D. M. Master, M. D. Press, and A. Aja. 2008. "Stratigraphic Overview," in Stager, Schloen, and Master 2008, pp. 213–323.

Steel, T. 1975. *The Life and Death of St. Kilda,* London.

Stevens, G. P. 1950. "A Tile Standard in the Agora of Ancient Athens," *Hesperia* 19, pp. 174–188.

Stewart, A. 2012. "Hellenistic Freestanding Sculpture from the Athenian Agora, Part 1: Aphrodite," *Hesperia* 81, pp. 267–342.

———. 2017. "Hellenistic Freestanding Sculpture from the Athenian Agora, Part 3: Agathe Tyche, Aphrodite, Artemis, Athena, Eileithyia," *Hesperia* 86, pp. 83–127.

Storey, R. 1986. "Perinatal Mortality at Pre-Columbian Teotihuacan," *American Journal of Physical Anthropology* 69, pp. 541–548.

Tanzi, M. G., and M. P. Gabay. 2002. "Association between Honey Consumption and Infant Botulism," *Pharmacotherapy* 22, pp. 1479–1483.

Tarn, W. W. 1930. *Hellenistic Civilization,* 2nd ed., London.

Temkin, O., trans. 1956. *Soranus' Gynecology* (Publications of the Institute of the History of Medicine, 2nd ser., Texts and Documents 3), Baltimore.

The, T. L., and C. O. Trouth. 1976. "Sexual Dimorphism in the Basilar Part of the Occipital Bone of the Dog (*Canis familiaris*)," *Acta Anatomica* 95, pp. 565–571.

Themelis, P. G. 1999. "Ἀνασκαφὴ Μεσσήνης," *Prakt* 154, pp. 69–111.

———. 2000. "Ἀνασκαφὴ Μεσσήνης," *Prakt* 155, pp. 75–105.

Thompson, D. B. 1954. "Three Centuries of Hellenistic Terracottas: I, B and C," *Hesperia* 23, pp. 72–107.

———. 1963. *Troy: The Terracotta Figurines of the Hellenistic Period* (*Troy* Suppl. 3), Princeton.

———. 1971. *An Ancient Shopping Center: The Athenian Agora* (*AgoraPicBk* 12), Princeton.

Thompson, H. A. 1934. "Two Centuries of Hellenistic Pottery," *Hesperia* 3, pp. 311–480.

———. 1951. "Excavations in the Athenian Agora: 1950," *Hesperia* 20, pp. 45–60.

Tillier, A.-M., B. Arensburg, H. Duday, and B. Vandermeersch. 2001. "An Early Case of Hydrocephalus: The Middle Paleolithic Qafzeh 12 Child

(Israel)," *American Journal of Physical Anthropology* 114, pp. 166–170.
Todd, T. W. 1920. "Age Changes in the Pubic Bone: I. The Male White Pubis," *American Journal of Physical Anthropology* 3, pp. 285–334.
Touratsoglou, I. 1986. "Το ξίφος της Βέροιας: Συμβολή στη μακεδονική οπλοποιία των ύστερων κλασικών χρόνων," in *Ancient Macedonia* IV: *Papers Read at the 4th International Symposium Held in Thessaloniki, September 21–25, 1983,* Thessaloniki, pp. 611–651.
Travlos, J. 1949. "The West Side of the Athenian Agora Restored," in *Commemorative Studies in Honor of Theodore Leslie Shear* (*Hesperia* Suppl. 8), Princeton, pp. 383–392.
———. 1960. *Πολεοδομικὴ ἐξέλιξις τῶν Ἀθηνῶν ἀπὸ τῶν προϊστορικῶν χρόνων μέχρι τῶν ἀρχῶν τοῦ 19ου αἰῶνος,* Athens.
———. 1971. *Pictorial Dictionary of Ancient Athens,* London.
Treasures of Ancient Macedonia = K. Ninou, ed., *Treasures of Ancient Macedonia,* Thessaloniki n.d.
Triantaphyllou, S., and M. Bessios. 2005. "A Mass Burial at Fourth Century B.C. Pydna, Macedonia, Greece: Evidence for Slavery?" *Antiquity, Project Gallery* 79 (305), http://antiquity.ac.uk/ProjGall/triantaphyllou305/; accessed January 9, 2017.
Trotter, M., and G. C. Gleser. 1952. "Estimation of Stature from Long Bones of American Whites and Negroes," *American Journal of Physical Anthropology* 10, pp. 463–514.
Trouth, C. O., S. Winter, K. C. Gupta, R. M. Millis, and J. A. Holloway. 1977. "Analysis of the Sexual Dimorphism in the Basioccipital Portion of the Dog's Skull," *Acta Anatomica* 98, pp. 469–473.
Tsakirgis, B. 2005. "Living and Working around the Athenian Agora: A Preliminary Case Study of Three Houses," in *Ancient Greek Houses and Households: Chronological, Regional, and Social Diversity,* ed. B. A. Ault and L. C. Nevett, Philadelphia, pp. 67–82.
———. 2009. "Living near the Agora: Houses and Households in Central Athens," in *The Athenian Agora: New Perspectives on an Ancient Site,* ed. J. McK. Camp II and C. A. Mauzy, Mainz, pp. 47–54.
Ubelaker, D. H. 1989. *Human Skeletal Remains: Excavation, Analysis, Interpretation,* 2nd ed., Washington, D.C.
Ucko, P. J. 1969. "Ethnography and Archaeological Interpretation of Funerary Remains," *World Archaeology* 1, pp. 262–280.
Uhlenbrock, J. P. 2004. "Dorothy Burr Thompson, 1900–2001," *AJA* 108, pp. 631–633.
Vanderas, A. P. 1987. "Incidence of Cleft Lip, Cleft Palate, and Cleft Lip and Palate among Races: A Review," *Cleft Palate Journal* 24, pp. 216–225.
Van Hook, L. 1920. "The Exposure of Infants at Athens," *TAPA* 51, pp. 134–145.
Vatin, C. 1970. *Recherches sur le mariage et la condition de la femme mariée à l'époque hellénistique* (*BÉFAR* 216), Paris.
Vermeule, C. 1968. "The Basel Dog: A Vindication," *AJA* 72, pp. 95–101.
Vermeule, E. 1979. *Aspects of Death in Early Greek Art and Poetry* (Sather Classical Lectures 46), Berkeley.
Viljoen, G. van N. 1959. "Plato and Aristotle on the Exposure of Infants at Athens," *Acta Classica* 2, pp. 58–69.
Virolleaud, C. 1956. "Les nouvelles tablettes alphabétiques de Ras-Shamra (19e campagne, 1955)," *CRAI* 100, pp. 60–67.
Vokotopoulou, I. 1986. *Βίτσα: Τα νεκροταφεία μιας μολοσσικής κώμης* (Publications of *ArchDelt* 33), Athens.
Walbank, M. B. 2013. "Greek Inscriptions from the Athenian Agora: Fragments of a Financial Nature," *Hesperia* 82, pp. 301–339.
Waldron, T. 2000. "Hidden or Overlooked? Where Are the Disadvantaged in the Skeletal Record?" in *Madness, Disability, and Social Exclusion: The Archaeology and Anthropology of "Difference"* (One World Archaeology 40), ed. J. Hubert, London, pp. 29–45.
Walker, P. L., D. C. Cook, and P. M. Lambert. 1997. "Skeletal Evidence for Child Abuse: A Physical Anthropological Perspective," *Journal of Forensic Sciences* 42, pp. 196–207.
Wapnish, P., and B. Hesse. 1993. "Pampered Pooches or Plain Pariahs? The Ashkelon Dog Burials," *Biblical Archaeologist* 56(2), pp. 55–80 (repr. as "The Ashkelon Dog Burials: Data and Interpretations" in Stager, Schloen, and Master 2008, pp. 541–564).
Watts, D. J. 1989. "Infant Burials and Romano-British Christianity," *ArchJ* 146, pp. 372–383.
Weaver, D. S. 1980. "Sex Differences in the Ilia of a Known Sex and Age Sample of Fetal and Infant Skeletons," *American Journal of Physical Anthropology* 52, pp. 191–195.
Weber, M. 2006. "Die Kultbilder der Aphrodite Urania der zweiten Hälfte des 5. Jhs. v. Chr. in Athen/Attika und das Bürgerrechtsgesetz von 451/0 v. Chr.," *AM* 121, pp. 165–223.
Weinfeld, M. 1972. "The Worship of Molech and of the Queen of Heaven and Its Background," *UgaritF* 4, pp. 133–154.
West, S. 1998. "Whose Baby? A Note on P. Oxy 744," *ZPE* 121, pp. 167–172.
Wheeler, S. M., L. Williams, P. Beauchesne, and T. L. Dupras. 2013. "Shattered Lives and Broken Childhoods: Evidence of Physical Child Abuse in Ancient Egypt," *International Journal of Paleopathology* 3, pp. 71–82.
Wheeler, S. M., L. Williams, P. Beauchesne, and J. E. Molto. 2007. "Fractured Childhood: A Case of Probable Child Abuse from Ancient Egypt," *SAS Bulletin: Newsletter of the Society for Archaeological Sciences* 30(4), pp. 6–9.
Whitbread, I. K. 1995. *Greek Transport Amphorae: A Petrological and Archaeological Study* (Fitch Laboratory Occasional Paper 4), Athens.
Whitehead, D. 1986. *The Demes of Attica: 508/7–ca. 250 B.C.: A Political and Social Study,* Princeton.
Whittemore, R. D., and E. A. Beverly. 1996. "Mandinka Mothers and Nurslings: Power and

Reproduction," *Medical Anthropology Quarterly,* n.s. 10, pp. 45–62.

Wicker, N. L. 1998. "Selective Female Infanticide as Partial Explanation for the Dearth of Women in Viking Age Scandinavia," in *Violence and Society in the Early Medieval West,* ed. G. Halsall, Woodbridge, pp. 205–221.

Williamson, L. 1978. "Infanticide: An Anthropological Analysis," in *Infanticide and the Value of Life,* ed. M. Kohl, Buffalo, pp. 61–75.

Wilson, L. A., N. MacLeod, and L. T. Humphrey. 2008. "Morphometric Criteria for Sexing Juvenile Human Skeletons Using the Ilium," *Journal of Forensic Sciences* 53, pp. 269–278.

Woods, R. 1993. "On the Historical Relationship between Infant and Adult Mortality," *Population Studies* 47, pp. 195–219.

Workum, P., R. J. Purvis, and G. W. Thomas. 1971. "A Case of Thoracic Outlet Syndrome Occurring in Infancy," *Pediatrics* 48, pp. 462–463.

World Health Organization. 2006. *Neonatal and Perinatal Mortality: Country, Regional, and Global Estimates,* Geneva.

Wrede, H. 1985. *Die antike Herme* (Trierer Beiträge zur Altertumskunde 1), Mainz.

Young, E. J. 1995. "An Overview of Human Brucellosis," *Clinical Infectious Diseases* 21, pp. 283–289.

Young, R. S. 1939. *Late Geometric Graves and a Seventh Century Well in the Agora* (*Hesperia* Suppl. 2), Princeton.

———. 1951a. "An Industrial District of Ancient Athens," *Hesperia* 20, pp. 135–288.

———. 1951b. "Sepulturae intra urbem," *Hesperia* 20, pp. 67–134.

Zaganiaris, N. J. 1975. "Sacrifices de chiens dans l'Antiquité classique," *Platon* 27, pp. 322–329.

Zorn, J. R. 1994. "Estimating the Population Size of Ancient Settlements: Methods, Problems, Solutions, and a Case Study," *BASOR* 295, pp. 31–48.

GENERAL INDEX

INDEX OF OBJECTS

INDEX OF DEPOSITS